2011
YEAR BOOK OF
SURGERY®

The 2011 Year Book Series

Year Book of Anesthesiology and Pain Management™: Drs Chestnut, Abram, Black, Gravlee, Lien, Mathru, and Roizen

Year Book of Cardiology®: Drs Gersh, Cheitlin, Elliott, Gold, Graham, and Thourani

Year Book of Critical Care Medicine®: Drs Dellinger, Parrillo, Balk, Dorman, Dries, and Zanotti-Cavazzoni

Year Book of Dermatology and Dermatologic Surgery™: Dr Del Rosso

Year Book of Diagnostic Radiology®: Drs Osborn, Abbara, Elster, Manaster, Oestreich, Offiah, Rosado de Christenson, Stephens, and Walker

Year Book of Emergency Medicine®: Drs Hamilton, Bruno, Handly, Mullin, Quintana, and Ramoska

Year Book of Endocrinology®: Drs Schott, Apovian, Clarke, Eugster, Ludlam, Meikle, Ovalle, Schinner, Schteingart, and Toth

Year Book of Gastroenterology™: Drs Talley, DeVault, Harnois, Murray, Pearson, Philcox, Picco, and Smith

Year Book of Hand and Upper Limb Surgery®: Drs Yao and Steinmann

Year Book of Medicine®: Drs Barker, Garrick, Gersh, Khardori, LeRoith, Seo, Talley, and Thigpen

Year Book of Neonatal and Perinatal Medicine®: Drs Fanaroff, Benitz, Donn, Neu, Papile, Polin, and van Marter

Year Book of Neurology and Neurosurgery®: Drs Klimo and Rabinstein

Year Book of Obstetrics, Gynecology, and Women's Health®: Drs Dungan and Shulman

Year Book of Oncology®: Drs Arceci, Bauer, Chiorean, Gordon, Lawton, Murphy, Thigpen, and Tsao

Year Book of Ophthalmology®: Drs Rapuano, Cohen, Flanders, Hammersmith, Milman, Myers, Nelson, Penne, Pyfer, Sergott, Shields, and Vander

Year Book of Orthopedics®: Drs Morrey, Beauchamp, Huddleston, Swiontkowski, and Trigg

Year Book of Otolaryngology-Head and Neck Surgery®: Drs Sindwani, Balough, Franco, Gapany, and Mitchell

Year Book of Pathology and Laboratory Medicine®: Drs Raab, Parwani, Bejarano, and Bissell

Year Book of Pediatrics®: Dr Stockman

Year Book of Plastic and Aesthetic Surgery™: Drs Miller, Gosain, Gurtner, Gutowski, Ruberg, Salisbury, and Smith

Year Book of Psychiatry and Applied Mental Health®: Drs Talbott, Ballenger, Buckley, Frances, Krupnick, and Mack

Year Book of Pulmonary Disease®: Drs Barker, Jones, Maurer, Raza, Tanoue, and Willsie

Year Book of Sports Medicine®: Drs Shephard, Cantu, Feldman, Jankowski, Khan, Lebrun, Nieman, Pierrynowski, and Rowland

Year Book of Surgery®: Drs Copeland, Behrns, Daly, Eberlein, Fahey, Huber, Klodell, Mozingo, and Pruett

Year Book of Urology®: Drs Andriole and Coplen

Year Book of Vascular Surgery®: Drs Moneta, Gillespie, Starnes, and Watkins

2011

The Year Book of SURGERY®

Editor-in-Chief
Edward M. Copeland III, MD
Distinguished Professor of Surgery, Department of Surgery, University of Florida, Gainesville, Florida

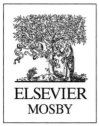

ELSEVIER
MOSBY

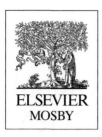

ELSEVIER
MOSBY

Vice President, Continuity: Kimberly Murphy
Editor: Jessica McCool
Production Supervisor, Electronic Year Books: Donna M. Skelton
Electronic Article Manager: Emily Ogle
Illustrations and Permissions Coordinator: Dawn Vohsen

2011 EDITION

Composition by TNQ Books and Journals Pvt Ltd, India

Editorial Office:
Elsevier
1600 John F. Kennedy Blvd.
Suite 1800
Philadelphia, PA 19103-2899

International Standard Serial Number: 0090-3671
International Standard Book Number: 978-0-323-08427-7

Printed and bound by CPI Group (UK) Ltd, Croydon, CR0 4YY

Transferred to Digital Print 2011

Table of Contents

Journals Represented

Journals represented in this YEAR BOOK are listed below.

American Journal of Gastroenterology
American Journal of Infection Control
American Journal of Pathology
American Journal of Surgery
American Journal of Transplantation
American Surgeon
Anaesthesia and Intensive Care
Anesthesia & Analgesia
Annals of Plastic Surgery
Annals of Surgery
Annals of Surgical Oncology
Annals of Thoracic Surgery
Annals of Vascular Surgery
Archives of Surgery
British Journal of Surgery
Burns
Cancer
Chest
Critical Care Medicine
Dermatologic Surgery
Diabetes Care
Digestive Diseases and Sciences
Diseases of the Colon and Rectum
European Journal of Endocrinology
European Journal of Vascular and Endovascular Surgery
European Urology
Foot & Ankle International
Gastroenterology
Gastrointestinal Endoscopy
Gut
Injury
Intensive Care Medicine
Journal of Bone and Joint Surgery
Journal of Burn Care & Research
Journal of Clinical Endocrinology & Metabolism
Journal of Clinical Investigation
Journal of Clinical Oncology
Journal of Heart and Lung Transplantation
Journal of Hepatology
Journal of Immunology
Journal of Parenteral and Enteral Nutrition
Journal of Pediatric Gastroenterology and Nutrition
Journal of Pediatric Orthopaedics
Journal of Shoulder and Elbow Surgery
Journal of Surgical Research
Journal of the American College of Surgeons
Journal of the American Geriatrics Society

Journal of the American Medical Association
Journal of the American Society of Nephrology
Journal of Thoracic and Cardiovascular Surgery
Journal of Trauma
Journal of Vascular and Interventional Radiology
Journal of Vascular Surgery
Lancet
Laryngoscope
Liver Transplantation
Metabolism
Nephrology Dialysis Transplantation
New England Journal of Medicine
Orthopedics
Pediatric Research
Plastic and Reconstructive Surgery
Proceedings of the National Academy of Sciences of the United States of America
Scandinavian Journal of Gastroenterology
Surgery
Transplantation
World Journal of Surgery
Wound Repair and Regeneration

STANDARD ABBREVIATIONS

The following terms are abbreviated in this edition: acquired immunodeficiency syndrome (AIDS), cardiopulmonary resuscitation (CPR), central nervous system (CNS), cerebrospinal fluid (CSF), computed tomography (CT), deoxyribonucleic acid (DNA), electrocardiography (ECG), health maintenance organization (HMO), human immunodeficiency virus (HIV), intensive care unit (ICU), intramuscular (IM), intravenous (IV), magnetic resonance (MR) imaging (MRI), ribonucleic acid (RNA), and ultrasound (US).

NOTE

The YEAR BOOK OF SURGERY is a literature survey service providing abstracts of articles published in the professional literature. Every effort is made to assure the accuracy of the information presented in these pages. Neither the editors nor the publisher of the YEAR BOOK OF SURGERY can be responsible for errors in the original materials. The editors' comments are their own opinions. Mention of specific products within this publication does not constitute endorsement.

To facilitate the use of the YEAR BOOK OF SURGERY as a reference tool, all illustrations and tables included in this publication are now identified as they appear in the original article. This change is meant to help the reader recognize that any illustration or table appearing in the YEAR BOOK OF SURGERY may be only one of many in the original article. For this reason, figure and table numbers appear to be out of sequence within the YEAR BOOK OF SURGERY.

1 General Considerations

Association Between Implementation of a Medical Team Training Program and Surgical Mortality

Neily J, Mills PD, Young-Xu Y, et al (Dartmouth Med School, Hanover, NH; et al)

JAMA 304:1693-1700, 2010

Context.—There is insufficient information about the effectiveness of medical team training on surgical outcomes. The Veterans Health Administration (VHA) implemented a formalized medical team training program for operating room personnel on a national level.

Objective.—To determine whether an association existed between the VHA Medical Team Training program and surgical outcomes.

Design, Setting, and Participants.—A retrospective health services study with a contemporaneous control group was conducted. Outcome data were obtained from the VHA Surgical Quality Improvement Program (VASQIP) and from structured interviews in fiscal years 2006 to 2008. The analysis included 182 409 sampled procedures from 108 VHA facilities that provided care to veterans. The VHA's nationwide training program required briefings and debriefings in the operating room and included checklists as an integral part of this process. The training included 2 months of preparation, a 1-day conference, and 1 year of quarterly coaching interviews.

Main Outcome Measure.—The rate of change in the mortality rate 1 year after facilities enrolled in the training program compared with the year before and with nontraining sites.

Results.—The 74 facilities in the training program experienced an 18% reduction in annual mortality (rate ratio [RR], 0.82; 95% confidence interval [CI], 0.76-0.91; $P = .01$) compared with a 7% decrease among the 34 facilities that had not yet undergone training (RR, 0.93; 95% CI, 0.80-1.06; $P = .59$). The risk-adjusted mortality rates at baseline were 17 per 1000 procedures per year for the trained facilities and 15 per 1000 procedures per year for the nontrained facilities. At the end of the study, the rates were 14 per 1000 procedures per year for both groups. Propensity matching of the trained and nontrained groups demonstrated that the decline in the risk-adjusted surgical mortality rate was about 50% greater in the training group (RR, 1.49; 95% CI, 1.10-2.07; $P = .01$) than in the nontraining group. A dose-response relationship for additional quarters of the training program was also demonstrated: for every quarter of the training program, a reduction of 0.5 deaths per 1000 procedures occurred (95% CI, 0.2-1.0; $P = .001$).

Conclusion.—Participation in the VHA Medical Team Training program was associated with lower surgical mortality.

▶ The surgical community, through the American College of Surgeons, has acknowledged that the National Surgical Quality Improvement Project (NSQIP) has produced the best outcome measures currently available in this country. In fact, it is to the advantage of every hospital to participate in the NSQIP, for the data have been ratified by the surgical community and accepted by those institutions that have participated. This program is not one forced upon us by a government agency. The promise of the new health care bill is to force quality by setting up measures that will dictate reimbursement. Better surgeons control the quality data than an agency of the federal government. The Veterans Affairs (VA) system is a government agency, but the program was initiated and embraced by surgeons working within the VA system.

This report is another example of the Veterans Health Administration's ability to identify and implement quality improvement. Appropriate characteristics of teamwork among health care professionals who participate in the operative experience of a patient have been identified and implemented within 108 VA hospitals. Mortality is an unarguable end point. The VA Surgical Quality Improvement Program (VASQIP) sampled 182 409 surgical procedures. This volume provides a large enough sample from diverse sources to prove the teamwork mechanisms instituted by the program lowered mortality. The longitudinal follow-up identified a further lowering of mortality as the teamwork programs matured.

The training program included didactic sessions, retreats, and observed implementation. The question is, will non-VA hospitals embrace this program? NSQIP has not been embraced by most community and academic hospitals, 1 reason being the expense incurred by the hospitals. The VASQIP will require time away from work to be trained.

Health care employees will be required to spend time that is not income productive. Simply stated, a reduction of mortality is worth every penny.

E. M. Copeland III, MD

Communication Practices on 4 Harvard Surgical Services: A Surgical Safety Collaborative
ElBardissi AW, Regenbogen SE, Greenberg CC, et al (Brigham and Women's Hosp, Boston, MA; Massachusetts General Hosp, Boston; et al)
Ann Surg 250:861-865, 2009

Background.—Communication breakdowns between surgical residents and attending physicians in the pre- and postoperative setting are common contributors to patient injury. These communication transactions might offer an opportunity for safety improvement, but it remains unknown how often resident-attending communication fails, what the current level of attending involvement is, and how often attending input changes the plan for patient care. We conducted a prospective study at 4 Harvard teaching hospitals to address these issues.

Methods.—Three prospective data collection strategies were employed: (1) we randomly selected surgical services and queried residents for the occurrence of predefined critical patient events and the characteristics of attending communications that ensued, (2) on weekends, randomly selected patients were interviewed and their charts reviewed to identify the frequency of attending visitation and how such visits affected processes of care, and (3) on weekends, senior residents on randomly selected surgical services were queried regarding the occurrence of attending-resident discussion of patients in their care.

Results.—Of 80 critical patient events identified, 26 (33%) were not communicated to attending surgeons. Residents reported that, when contacted, all attending physicians were receptive to communication, whether they were the primary surgeon or providing cross-coverage. Although residents felt that attending contact was unnecessary for safe patient care in 61 (76%) of these events, discussions with attending physicians changed management in 33% (18/54) of cases in which they occurred. Attending surgeons were found to visit their patients on randomly selected weekend days 42% (n = 37) of the time, while 21% (n = 19) had not visited for 2 or greater days. When attending physicians visited patients, however, resident management was modified 46% (n = 36) of the time. Though residents frequently discussed patient management with attending physicians on randomly selected weekends, they failed to do so 16% (n = 58) of the time, which appeared to be related to service-specific variation ($\chi^2 = 269$, $P < 0.0001$).

Conclusions.—In the context of both critical patient events and routine patient care, residents often fail to obtain attending surgeons' input for management decisions. These failures seem to derive more from residents' perception of necessity than from attending physicians' receptiveness or interest in being contacted. Once involved, attending physicians frequently modify resident's management decisions. It seems, therefore, that there is significant potential for communication failure and information loss among our 4 institutions.

▶ My initial reaction upon reading this article was "Holy mackerel! If these frightening data emanate from Harvard hospitals, thought to be the best in the world, what about the resident behavior in all the other hospitals?" I congratulate the chairs of the Harvard surgical services on their willingness to share these data with us and to share the corrective actions taken.

Except for some public hospitals, almost every patient in a US hospital has an assigned attending surgeon, and a bill for services is submitted. The surgical bill for an operation is global, and daily fees for services are, therefore, uncommon.

Consequently, I assume that some attending surgeons do not feel the need to see patients daily, especially if the residents are as qualified as those residents in the Harvard system. It was obviously the opinion of the residents that they are qualified to provide some critical care services without the input of the attending surgeons (Table 1 in the original article). Nevertheless, all attending surgeons were eager for the communication to take place and, when contacted, often changed the medical management prescribed by the residents to include an emergent operation.

I am forced to wonder whether this behavior is the product of the new training paradigm caused by the 80-hour workweek. The new paradigm was supposed to result in more patient management by the attending surgeon. Similarly, the night float residents, who knew very little about the patients whom they were called to evaluate, would be forced to communicate with a more senior surgeon. Possibly the new paradigm has had the opposite effect!

E. M. Copeland III, MD

Working With a Fixed Operating Room Team on Consecutive Similar Cases and the Effect on Case Duration and Turnover Time
Stepaniak PS, Vrijland WW, de Quelerij M, et al (Erasmus Univ Rotterdam, the Netherlands; St Franciscus Hosp, Rotterdam, the Netherlands)
Arch Surg 145:1165-1170, 2010

Hypothesis.—If variation in procedure times could be controlled or better predicted, the cost of surgeries could be reduced through improved scheduling of surgical resources. This study on the impact of similar consecutive cases on the turnover, surgical, and procedure times tests the perception that repeating the same manual tasks reduces the duration of these tasks. We hypothesize that when a fixed team works on similar consecutive cases the result will be shorter turnover and procedure duration as well as less variation as compared with the situation without a fixed team.

Design.—Case-control study.

Setting.—St Franciscus Hospital, a large general teaching hospital in Rotterdam, the Netherlands.

Patients.—Two procedures, inguinal hernia repair and laparoscopic cholecystectomy, were selected and divided across a control group and a study group. Patients were randomly assigned to the study or control group.

Main Outcome Measures.—Preparation time, surgical time, procedure time, and turnover time.

Results.—For inguinal hernia repair, we found a significantly lower preparation time and 10 minutes less procedure time in the study group, as compared with the control group. Variation in the study group was lower, as compared with the control group. For laparoscopic cholecystectomy, preparation time was significantly lower in the study group, as compared with the control group. For both procedures, there was a significant decrease in turnover time.

Conclusions.—Scheduling similar consecutive cases and performing with a fixed team results in lower turnover times and preparation times. The procedure time of the inguinal hernia repair decreased significantly and has practical scheduling implications. For more complex surgery, like laparoscopic cholecystectomy, there is no effect on procedure time.

▶ Having the same operating team for surgical procedures would seem obvious, but remarkably, in the 2 institutions where I have worked, this plan took a long time to implement (although implementation was eventually obtained with results more dramatic than those in this study). The barrier to implementation was the nursing philosophy that every nurse should be familiar with the needs of each surgeon, or at least each operating service. This philosophy was to make the operating room nurses more flexible. The outcome was that no nurse was familiar with any of the needs of any service. (This may be a bit strong, but you get my point.) Specialty services were the first to get dedicated nurses, for example, orthopedics, otolaryngology, and neurosurgery. The last service for implementation was general surgery, the thought being that we were all the same with the same needs. This thought process is immediately untrue for me since I operate left-handed! The time wasted in getting the proper instruments is enormous, not to mention the frustration for the surgeon and the fact that the proper but absent equipment is needed often at critical time points during the operation.

The constant scrub nurse can survey the instrument table to be sure that the proper instruments are available before the case begins. For the last 15 years of my career, I had the same nursing team in the operating room with me. An often overlooked benefit of the same team is proper positioning and preparation of the patient prior to the incision. The nurses are constant compared with the residents since the residents rotate on a 6-week or 3-month basis. I was always present during the critical portions of every operation but did trust the residents to participate without me during the noncritical portions of the case. However, when I wasn't in the room, I told the residents to do exactly what my nurses told them to do. And the nurses knew to call me if there was any deviation in procedure.

Nursing constants are even more important in the new training paradigm in which residents may come and go during a case as they attempt to comply with the rigors of the 80-hour work week.

This study was of 2 rather simple procedures. I would predict that the more complex operations, such as low anterior colon resections and difficult upper abdominal procedures, would show a much greater disparity, and complications resulting from this disparity would evolve.

E. M. Copeland III, MD

Can Aviation-Based Team Training Elicit Sustainable Behavioral Change?

Sax HC, Browne P, Mayewski RJ, et al (The Warren Alpert Med School of Brown Univ, Providence, Rhode Island; Univ of Rochester Med Ctr, NY; Indelta Learning Systems, LLC, Pittsford, NY)
Arch Surg 144:1133-1137, 2009

Objective.—To quantify effects of aviation-based crew resource management training on patient safety–related behaviors and perceived personal empowerment.

Design.—Prospective study of checklist use, error self-reporting, and a 10-point safety empowerment survey after participation in a crew resource management training intervention.

Setting.—Seven hundred twenty-two–bed university hospital; 247-bed affiliated community hospital.

Participants.—There were 857 participants, the majority of whom were nurses (50%), followed by ancillary personnel (28%) and physicians (22%).

Main Outcome Measures.—Preoperative checklist use over time; number and type of entries on a Web-based incident reporting system; and measurement of degree of empowerment (1-5 scale) on a 10-point survey of safety attitudes and actions given prior to, immediately after, and a minimum of 2 months after training.

Results.—Since 2003, 10 courses trained 857 participants in multiple disciplines. Preoperative checklist use rose (75% in 2003, 86% in 2004, 94% in 2005, 98% in 2006, and 100% in 2007). Self-initiated reports increased from 709 per quarter in 2002 to 1481 per quarter in 2008. The percentage of reports related to environment as opposed to actual events increased from 15.9% prior to training to 20.3% subsequently ($P < .01$). Perceived self-empowerment, creating a culture of safety, rose by an average of 0.5 point in all 10 realms immediately posttraining (mean [SD] rating, 3.0 [0.07] vs 3.5 [0.05]; $P < .05$). This was maintained after a minimum of 2 months. There was a trend toward a hierarchical effect with participants less comfortable confronting incompetence in a physician (mean [SD] rating, 3.1 [0.8]) than in nurses or technicians (mean [SD] rating, 3.4 [0.7] for both) ($P > .05$).

Conclusions.—Crew resource management programs can influence personal behaviors and empowerment. Effects may take years to be ingrained into the culture.

▶ Over the last several years there has been a lot of interest in comparing methods of increasing airline safety with patient safety. In fact, we invited members of aviation to give a presentation on the methods of improving airline safety for the Board of Regents. Rather than the pilot being a dictator with no interaction with the crew (I am overemphasizing here), the crew was trained to take more ownership of flight safety. As I listened to the presentation, I could agree with the concept, but I still wanted the pilot of the plane on which I was traveling to clearly be in charge but receptive to constructive criticism.

The adaptation of the airline safety techniques to patient safety techniques, especially in the operating room, has been rewarding as is demonstrated in this article. Usage of preoperative check lists improved to 100% within a short period of time. A feeling of empowerment of the personnel associated with the operative event also increased significantly as did self-reporting of adverse events. These latter 2 outcomes are to be commended, yet they could diminish the responsibility of the primary surgeon and have the responsibility of the operating surgeon so diffused that the surgeon no longer takes ownership of the patient, other than the technical component.

In my opinion, the patient pays the fee for the judgment and technical expertise of the surgeon. Therefore, the surgeon should be ultimately in charge just as the pilot of the plane should be ultimately in charge, especially in a crisis situation.

How an institution handles the self-reporting of adverse events and personnel empowerment are the key ingredients for the system to work. A committee to evaluate these events is recommended. There certainly are surgeons whose skills are lacking and whose behavior is inappropriate at times. But to act on isolated events could be detrimental to the confidence of the surgeon. If enough criticisms accumulate about the same surgeon, then there is a major problem with the surgeon and it must be dealt with appropriately.

E. M. Copeland III, MD

A closer look at surgical quality measures across different surgical specialties
Watkins JM, Qadan M, Battista C, et al (Taylor Regional Hosp, Campbellsville, KY; Univ of Louisville School of Medicine, KY)
Am J Surg 200:90-96, 2010

Background.—Most studies of surgical quality improvement have been performed in large and/or teaching hospitals; the efficacy of safety and quality efforts in smaller hospitals have not been reported.

Methods.—Four smaller hospitals joined a collaborative to study process measures through an expanded surgical time-out and some outcomes. The data were collected in real time.

Results.—Well-performing hospitals (all 4) improved further but variably. Gynecologic and orthopedic surgeons performed more consistently in most measures than did general surgeons.

Conclusions.—These small hospitals readily accepted a time-out—based real-time data collection and with their surgical staff improved in most parameters.

▶ This study originates from the University of Louisville School of Medicine, where Dr Hiram Polk has taken a great interest in quality assessment and control, especially since his retirement as Chairman of Surgery of the Department of Surgery. I mention this fact only because I have been impressed with the work on quality issues from this group. Here they compare quality measures among different specialties of orthopedic, gynecologic, and general surgery within smaller community hospitals (approximately 150 beds). These data were then compared with compliance with these standard quality measures among physicians in urban hospitals. Compliance was similar among specialties and hospitals.

I was at first surprised that deep vein thrombosis (DVT) prophylaxis preoperatively was used seldom by orthopedic surgeons. I guess I am behind the information curve, and DVT prophylaxis is not currently recommended preoperatively for patients undergoing joint replacements. Yet in these patients, DVT prophylaxis was used liberally in the immediate postoperative period. It is within these patients who are undergoing hip fracture reduction and stabilization that DVT prophylaxis was originally shown to be advantageous. I remain old school and use low-dose heparin preoperatively and compression stockings intraoperatively in patients who do not have a contraindication. I have had no complications from this treatment and have had no clinically evident pulmonary emboli. I did have the latter before accepting this treatment philosophy. I may fly in the face of currently indicated evidence-based medicine, but why change something that has worked for years and is relatively inexpensive?

Nevertheless, among specialties and regardless of hospital size, there was very little variation among quality measures that were evaluated in this study.

E. M. Copeland III, MD

An Evaluation of Information Transfer Through the Continuum of Surgical Care: A Feasibility Study
Nagpal K, Vats A, Ahmed K, et al (Imperial College, London, UK)
Ann Surg 252:402-407, 2010

Objective.—To evaluate information transfer and communication (ITC) across the surgical care pathway with the use of Information Transfer and Communication Assessment Tool for Surgery (ITCAS).

Background.—Communication failures are the leading cause of surgical errors and adverse events. It is vital to assess the ITC across the entire surgical continuum of care to understand the process, to study teams, and to prioritize the phases for intervention.

Methods.—Twenty patients undergoing major gastrointestinal procedures were followed through their entire surgical care, and ITC process was assessed using ITCAS. ITCAS consisted of 4 checklists for 4 phases of the surgical care.

Results.—ITC failures are distributed across the entire surgical continuum of care. Preprocedural teamwork and postoperative handover phases have the maximum number of ITC failures (61.7% and 52.4%, respectively). Moreover, it was found that information degrades as it crosses from one phase to another. Of patients, 75% had clinical incidents or adverse events because of ITC failures.

Conclusions.—The study demonstrated that ITC failures are ubiquitous across surgical care pathway and there is an imminent need to modify current ITC practices. Standardization of ITC through use of checklists, protocols, or information technology is essential to reduce these communication failures.

▶ This study was done in London and within a teaching hospital. The working hours restrictions have been in place in England now for many years. So the results of this study can represent an end point of this training process, which requires multiple hand-offs. The data include communication errors from both physicians and nurses. Essential information was defined as errors that could or did result in a major complication. The most disturbing issues for me were that 55% of essential information was not transmitted from the operating room to the recovery room and 44% of the essential information was not transmitted from the recovery room to the floor. If my math is accurate, only 25% of the essential information, as defined by this questionnaire, actually made it from the operating room to the floor. As an isolated result, this information transfer is troublesome. Whether this failure is limited to this hospital or only to teaching hospitals awaits comparative data from other institutions.

Residency programs in this country now have limited work hours, not as limited as in the United Kingdom, but more limited work hours are in upcoming recommendations from our residency governing organizations. The major complaint of our current system is diminished communication among health care providers. This study quantifies the communication errors in 1 hospital. I wonder if a reduction in resident working hours creates an atmosphere of shift work that breeds a lack of communication among all health care providers. I hope that I am wrong, but it is better to quantify the communication errors before having to quantify the resultant complications.

E. M. Copeland III, MD

Arguments for and Against a Career in Surgery: A Qualitative Analysis
Businger A, Villiger P, Sommer C (St Claraspital Basel, Switzerland; Kantonsspital Graubunden, Chur, Switzerland)
Ann Surg 252:390-396, 2010

Objective.—To evaluate arguments given by board-certified surgeons in Switzerland for and against a career in surgery.

Background Data.—Currently, the surgical profession in most Western countries is experiencing a labor shortage because of a declining interest in a surgical career among new graduates, a changed public opinion of medicine and its representatives, and as a consequence of the increasing influence of health economists and politicians on the professional independence of surgeons. Reports that focus primarily on the reasons that board-certified surgeons remain within the surgical profession are rare.

Methods.—Surgeons were asked to answer 2 questions concerning arguments for and against a career in surgery. Of 749 surgeons the arguments of 334 (44.6%) were analyzed using Mayring's content analysis. The surgeons were also asked whether they would choose medicine as a career path again.

TABLE 2.—Examples of Surgeons' Arguments for and Against a Career in Surgery

Category of Arguments	Arguments for a Career in Surgery	Arguments Against a Career in Surgery
Personal experience in daily professional life	"In this highly complex profession, one's will to bear up is trained daily"	"Work conditions which are not improved despite the limited 50 h per week"
	"High satisfaction by intellectual challenge"	"Lacking incentives for young surgeons (Senseless work-hour limitation, inadequate case load)"
	"Satisfaction through immediately visible results"	"Outdated role models, lacking female role models in an increasing
	"Complete demand of the job"	feminization of surgery are seen daily"
Work-related conditions	"Unique opportunity to combine intellectual and technical skills"	"Dismantling of the profession by administration and politics"
	"Surgery doesn't belong to humanities: it is necessary to acquire both knowledge and competence"	"Influence of politics, family unfriendly professional ethics, and health economy turn surgery into an unattractive profession"
	"Technological development has contributed to a enormous heightening of regard for surgery"	
Doctor-patient interaction	"Patients' gratitude gives power."	"Increasing unrealistic patients' expectations and achievement guarantee make a patient-doctor dialog difficult"
	"The contact with patients is not restricted to conversation"	"Nowadays, patients are more ready for malpractice litigation"
Work-life balance	"The work-hour limitations permit spending more time with friends and family"	"Surgery does not allow to ideally combine job and family due to lacking role models as before"
	"Social live is newly defined due to work-hour requirements"	"The job has an enormous influence on the personal disposability"
		"There's a neglect of women's needs in surgery"
Further professional perspectives	"Social life is now compatible with a professional career (work-hour limitations)"	"Feminization of surgery"
	"Job security because surgeons will always be needed"	"Few possibilities to go into a practice outside governmental institutions"
	"Academic possibilities of development"	"Decreasing case load due to extension of interventional techniques"
Specific training conditions	"The result of our work is immediately visible"	"The training takes a long time and is frequently not structured because of lacking networking of clinics and is therefore inefficient (blanket subsidies)"
	"One's own capability and experience has a direct influence on outcome"	"Lacking culture of training- and education; it is stopped on the level—see one, do one, teach one—(Halstedian paradigm)"
	"Extremely problem-focused job"	"The today's sub-specialization and the falling case load does not allow a timely training"
	"Everyday training of decision-making and resilience"	
Professional interactions	"The exchange with colleagues and in an interdisciplinary team is stimulating"	"Hierarchy and resulting power struggle"
	"Teamwork is daily new defined (Work in the operation room and on the ward)"	"Dependence on goodwill of seniors"
		"Slipping work ethic of next generation of surgeons"
		"A culture of shame and blame without a culture of communication"

(*Continued*)

TABLE 2. *(continued)*

Category of Arguments	Arguments for a Career in Surgery	Arguments Against a Career in Surgery
Environment of the profession	"The employment law causes lifestyle to conform to surgery"	"Excessive regimentation has caused the loss of a creative approach in surgery" "The actual health policy underestimates the manual practice and restricts surgeons' livelihood (TARMED)" "Increasing interference of external players (politics, administration, law) made surgery unattractive"
Prestige/social appreciation	"The Swiss health care system holds the surgeon dear"	"Increasing social-political downgrading of the medical profession with the highest impact on surgeons" "Demontage of the surgical myth" "Changed role of surgeon, even to the point of service provider" "Increasing interventional techniques in medicine and thereby loss of value of surgery"
Income	"Assured income by ongoing demand of surgical services"	"Continuous loss of fee and concurrent increase in work" "Practice work is difficult because of increasing financial restrictions" "Low income despite long training, constant availability, high social demands, and a shifting domain"

Results.—The 334 participating surgeons provided 790 statements for and 981 statements against a career in surgery. Fifty-nine surgeons (17.7%) would not choose medicine as a career again. Mayring's content analysis of the statements yielded 10 categories with arguments both for and against a career in surgery. "Personal Experience in Daily Professional Life" (18.7%) was the top-ranked category in favor of a career in surgery, and "Specific Training Conditions" (20%) was the top-ranked category against the choice of such a career. Ordinal logistic regression showed that the category "Personal Experience in Daily Professional Life" (OR, 2.39; 95% CI, 1.13—5.07) was independently associated with again studying medicine, and the category "Work-life Balance" (OR, 0.37; 95% CI, 0.20—0.70) was associated with not studying medicine again.

Conclusion.—This qualitative study revealed unfavorable working conditions and regulations as surgeons' main complaints. It is concluded that new organizational frameworks and professional perspectives are required to retain qualified and motivated surgeons in the surgical profession (Table 2).

▶ I will use my space for this commentary with the publication of Table 2, "Examples of Surgeons' Arguments for and Against a Career in Surgery." I cannot summarize the arguments any better than those summarized in this table. Although this study originates from Switzerland, it could just as easily have come from the United States or many other countries. One of my joys of the office of the President of the American College of Surgeons in 2007 was the opportunity to interact with surgeons around the world and in their home countries. Table 2 is a reflection of the status of surgical training, bias, and perspective in North America, South America, Europe, Asia, and Australia.

E. M. Copeland III, MD

Collateral damage: The effect of patient complications on the surgeon's psyche
Patel AM, Ingalls NK, Mansour MA, et al (Grand Rapids Med Education Partners/Michigan State Univ General Surgery Residency Program)
Surgery 148:824-830, 2010

Background.—The effect of patient complications on physicians is not well understood. Our objective was to determine the impact of a surgeon's complication(s) on his/her emotional state and job performance.

Methods.—An anonymous survey was distributed to Midwest Surgical Society members and attending surgeons within the Grand Rapids, Michigan, community.

Results.—There were 123 respondents (30.5% response rate). For the majority of participants, the first complication that had a significant emotional impact on them occurred during residency (51.2%). Most respondents reported this did not impair their professional functioning (77.2%). If a major complication was first experienced after residency, this had a greater likelihood of causing impairment ($P < .05$). Surgeons primarily dealt with the emotional impact by discussing it with a surgical partner (87.8%). Alcohol or other substance use increased in 6.5% of those surveyed. Most respondents (58.5%) felt it was difficult to handle the emotional effects of complications throughout their careers and this did not improve with experience.

Conclusion.—The majority of surgeons agreed that it was difficult to handle the emotional effects of complications throughout their careers. Efforts should be made to increase awareness of unrecognized emotional effects of patient complications and improve access to support systems for surgeons.

▶ How we are affected emotionally by a significant complication is something that many of us do not actively think about until asked to do so. Certainly I fit into that category. Surgeons who do elective surgery are taught to prepare the patient and themselves (know the anatomy of the operative site and get appropriate rest the night before are 2 examples) for the operative event. Errors can be divided into 3 categories: unavoidable, omission, and commission. If we eliminate the errors of omission and commission, almost by definition, the complications can be classified as unavoidable. Unavoidable complications should not tax the surgeons' emotional state. The other 2 classifications should be emotionally unsettling since by definition an appropriate preoperative evaluation was not done or an intraoperative event occurred that could have been avoided.

If surgeons morph into individuals who are not emotionally disturbed by patient complications that could have been avoided, then the profession is in trouble. One of the internal monitors of a surgeon's behavior is the fear of doing harm and of the emotional consequences that follow. We should not be paralyzed by an avoidable complication but should evaluate the circumstances that led to the complication in order to avoid it in the future. Being distraught over a complication that occurred in the past could negatively impact your ability to provide appropriate surgical care to patients in the present.

I will give an example. Once I was doing a somewhat difficult abdominal operation with the chief resident and as the first case in the morning. A report of the morning hemoglobin being 6 gm% was transmitted to us in the operating room. The chief resident almost froze. I asked him if he had seen the patient before coming to the operating room. He had, and the patient was stable, had no active bleeding, and had no complaints. Since he had seen the patient and no emergency existed (the patient was calibrating from prior blood loss), I told him to relax and get on with the operation at hand. Since he had acted appropriately by evaluating the patient before coming to the operating room, he did not need to be anxious about a problem that could safely be handled at the end of the current operation. Now, had he not seen the patient that morning, the situation would have been entirely different and stressful for both of us.

E. M. Copeland III, MD

Do Student Perceptions of Surgeons Change during Medical School? A Longitudinal Analysis during a 4-Year Curriculum
Naylor RA, Reisch JS, Valentine RJ (UT Southwestern Med Ctr, Dallas, TX)
J Am Coll Surg 210:527-532, 2010

Background.—Student recruiting is a top priority for surgical educators. Efforts have focused on improving the junior clerkship, but earlier interventions might prove to be more effective. This study was performed to determine students' perceptions of surgeons across all 4 years, with special emphasis on the effect of the 3rd-year clerkship.

Study Design.—During 2004 to 2007, medical students at all levels were surveyed with 21 statements about surgeons' behavior, lifestyle issues, and potential as role models. Subjects responded anonymously using a 5-point Likert scale (1 = strongly agree). Surveys were administered annually to medical student year 1 (MS1), MS2, and MS4, and before and after the clerkship to MS3. Data were analyzed using chi-square contingency table analyses.

Results.—Three-thousand and sixty surveys were analyzed (MS1, n = 833; MS2, n = 670; MS3, n = 1,193; and MS4, n = 364). Responses among MS1 and MS2 confirm that students enter medical school with negative impressions of surgeons. The surgical clerkship had a positive impact, but this effect was lost by senior year. Changes in perceptions were statistically significant for 20 of 21 statements. This is underscored by the fact that the proportion of students applying to general surgery from our medical school remains essentially unchanged (2004, 5.3%; 2005, 7.4%; 2006, 10%; 2007, 7.4%; and 2008, 6%).

Conclusions.—These data suggest that the junior surgery clerkship has a favorable but transient impact on the negative perceptions that medical students have about surgeons. Perceptions return to negative values within 1 year of the clerkship. Recruiting efforts should be focused on earlier interaction with students rather than concentrating on a 2- to 3-month rotation in the junior year.

▶ The static number of medical students applying for general surgical residencies has been evaluated at least on an annual basis for several years; the results have been the same; the recommendations have been the same; and there has been no increase in the number of applicants. Possibly medical schools should be evaluated individually, and those schools that have a relatively high number of medical students applying for general surgical residencies should be studied to see if there are any similarities in the surgical experience for students from these schools. These data exist; maybe I will do it. I expect that the experience varies among classes in any individual school, so meaningful data may be hard to define.

The impending shortage of general surgeons in this country, combined with the increase in the elderly population, has been described as the perfect storm. No amount of evaluating medical students' career desires is going to change the preference for lifestyle-friendly specialties, especially with the percent of women in medical school classes at 52% and rising. No criticism of gender implied. In fact, I have 5 physicians for my various maladies and they are all women (remembering that I am in the unique position, as are you, of being able to choose the best physicians available). Nevertheless, ophthalmology, radiology, group family practice, radiation therapy, and other specialties that allow for controlled lifestyle will continue to attract women and are now attracting men for the same reasons.

What to do about it? Make general surgery a lifestyle-friendly profession. This is occurring on its own. General surgery is being broken down into its components such as breast surgery, which requires very little on-call time and is easily organized to meet the private demands of the surgeon.

Who then will be left to provide acute care? The specialty of trauma and acute-care surgery has already evolved and is rapidly attracting women into it, at least at the University of Florida. Why? The specialty is now well organized, and the work time is almost finitely defined. You are either on call or you are not, and there is a partner that sees all patients in the office or hospital for a set period of time. Because most acute-care patients do not select their surgeon, the patients appear at the hospital and are relegated to the surgeon on call. The patients readily accept this physician schedule. So the potentially demanding surgical specialty has been organized in a lifestyle-friendly manner.

The bottom line is to keep teaching students the surgical disciplines, and the rest will sort itself out.

E. M. Copeland III, MD

Resident fatigue: is there a patient safety issue?
Mitchell CD, Mooty CR, Dunn EL, et al (Methodist Dallas Med, TX)
Am J Surg 198:811-816, 2009

Background.—In 2003, the 80-hour resident workweek was implemented in response to concerns that fatigued residents led to substandard patient care. Existing evidence links fatigue with impaired human performance; however, this has not consistently translated into similar impairment in the clinical arena. There is now discussion of additional work hour restrictions. Sentinel events are major medical mistakes tracked by the Joint Commission (JC). Root cause analysis of these events can determine if resident fatigue plays a role in medical errors.

Methods.—A retrospective review of sentinel events in our health system from January 2004 to July 2008 was performed. A root cause analysis for each event was performed. The JC national databank of sentinel events from 1995 to 2007 was also reviewed. In addition, a literature search was performed.

Results.—At our institution, 110 sentinel events were identified. Root cause analysis showed no evidence of resident fatigue involvement. The JC's national databank includes 4,817 sentinel events. No documented evidence of resident fatigue was found.

Conclusions.—Our data did not provide any evidence to support the contention that resident fatigue leads to increased medical errors. Clinical data supporting a direct relationship between resident fatigue and compromised patient safety must be demonstrated before further work hour restrictions are made. More research must be done. The JC should consider monitoring sentinel events for resident fatigue.

▶ There needs to be a compromise between resident working hours, resident education, and patient safety. Numerous articles on the 3 issues have been studied with varying results. I think the consensus agrees with the authors here, at least in the patient safety area. The authors are trying to prevent further reductions in work hours and have primarily focused on sentinel events after the 80-work hours restrictions were implemented. Comparisons between the eras before and after the 80-work hours implementation have also not uniformly demonstrated an improvement in patient safety. The problem has been with the night-float system in which a resident on call at night knows very little about the patients for whom the resident is responsible. Nevertheless, the 80-hour workweek has been in place long enough for most residency programs to adapt to it, and, at least, our residents and faculty members now feel more comfortable with the changes required to comply with the 80-hour rule.

To further limit work hours makes no sense, and studies like this one, which are being done prospectively, that is, before any other restrictions are put in place, are very important to prevent any further restrictions. Yes, several European countries have further restricted resident work hours, but I am unaware of anyone who is satisfied with it. These countries have handled the issue in several ways. One is to hire the residents to work after hours to take care of their own patients. A second is to ignore the rule. A third is to embrace it because no residents or faculty members operate much until they reach senior status. And last but not least, a fourth is to ignore the residents because the faculty members are forced to provide all patient care anyway.

These solutions are not applicable to resident training in this country.

E. M. Copeland III, MD

Moral angst for surgical residents: a qualitative study
Knifed E, Goyal A, Bernstein M (Univ of Toronto, Ontario, Canada)
Am J Surg 199:571-576, 2010

Background.—The ethical dilemmas that residents experience throughout their training have not been explored qualitatively from surgical residents' perspectives.

Methods.—Grounded theory methodology was used. All University of Toronto surgical, otolaryngology, and obstetrics and gynecology residents were invited to participate. Twenty-eight face-to-face interviews were conducted. Interviews were transcribed and analyzed by 3 reviewers.

Results.—Five encompassing themes emerged: (1) residents prefer operating with another resident while the staff watches; (2) residents felt that patients were rarely well informed about their role; (3) residents develop good relationships with patients; (4) residents felt ethically obliged to disclose intraoperative errors; and (5) residents experience ethical distress in certain teaching circumstances.

Conclusions.—Residents encounter ethical dilemmas leading to moral angst during their surgical training and need to feel safe to discuss these openly. Staff and residents should work together to establish optimal communication and teaching situations.

▶ This study originates from the Canadian system but is probably reflective of at least some training programs in the United States. When those of us who are older trained, operating with a more senior resident, usually on the public (ward) service, was standard. A faculty member was called if needed. Medicare and Medicaid changed this training paradigm because to be reimbursed, the responsible attending surgeon had to be present for the critical portion of the operation, a requirement that already had been instituted for patients with commercial insurance.

I began my career in 1972 at the University of Texas Medical School at Houston and worried that the decrease in independent operations (all operations were required to be under direct supervision by the responsible attending surgeon) would produce a surgical resident who was insufficiently trained. In fact, I soon discovered that the residents finishing in this new system were better trained both technically and judgmentally. At the University of Florida, my current institution, this method of training persists today and my observations remain the same. Interestingly, the dictated 80-hour workweek has decreased the contact of residents with the surgical faculty members both in the operating room and on teaching rounds and has thus created somewhat of an oxymoron.

The current Veterans Administration (VA) system requires documentation of the participation of the responsible surgeon and does allow for some operations to be done with the responsible surgeon watching within the operating room. Surgical quality issues and outcomes have already been documented by hospitals in VA system, and there seems to be no adverse effect of the responsible surgeon only observing on certain procedures.

In the Canadian medical system of national health insurance, I expect all patients could be considered private or all could be considered ward. I expect that there is a combination of these 2 categories, and the anxieties identified by the residents from Toronto could emanate from a potential confusion of the roles. Is this a picture of things to come in our new health care reform?

E. M. Copeland III, MD

Temporal Trends in Rates of Patient Harm Resulting from Medical Care
Landrigan CP, Parry GJ, Bones CB, et al (Brigham and Women's Hosp and Harvard Med School, Boston, MA; Children's Hosp Boston and Harvard Med School, MA; Inst for Healthcare Improvement, Cambridge, MA; et al)
N Engl J Med 363:2124-2134, 2010

Background.—In the 10 years since publication of the Institute of Medicine's report *To Err Is Human,* extensive efforts have been undertaken to improve patient safety. The success of these efforts remains unclear.

Methods.—We conducted a retrospective study of a stratified random sample of 10 hospitals in North Carolina. A total of 100 admissions per quarter from January 2002 through December 2007 were reviewed in random order by teams of nurse reviewers both within the hospitals (internal reviewers) and outside the hospitals (external reviewers) with the use of the Institute for Healthcare Improvement's Global Trigger Tool for Measuring Adverse Events. Suspected harms that were identified on initial review were evaluated by two independent physician reviewers. We evaluated changes in the rates of harm, using a random-effects Poisson regression model with adjustment for hospital-level clustering, demographic characteristics of patients, hospital service, and high-risk conditions.

Results.—Among 2341 admissions, internal reviewers identified 588 harms (25.1 harms per 100 admissions; 95% confidence interval [CI], 23.1 to 27.2). Multivariate analyses of harms identified by internal reviewers showed no significant changes in the overall rate of harms per 1000 patient-days (reduction factor, 0.99 per year; 95% CI, 0.94 to

1.04; P = 0.61) or the rate of preventable harms. There was a reduction in preventable harms identified by external reviewers that did not reach statistical significance (reduction factor, 0.92; 95% CI, 0.85 to 1.00; P = 0.06), with no significant change in the overall rate of harms (reduction factor, 0.98; 95% CI, 0.93 to 1.04; P = 0.47).

Conclusions.—In a study of 10 North Carolina hospitals, we found that harms remain common, with little evidence of widespread improvement. Further efforts are needed to translate effective safety interventions into routine practice and to monitor health care safety over time. (Funded by the Rx Foundation.)

▶ The Institute of Medicine (IOM) is probably the most prestigious medical organization in the United States. Membership is limited and acceptance as a member is arduous. The publication *To Err Is Human* has set in motion many attempts to improve patient safety. A number of the members of the IOM are a bit distant from the active practice of medicine, the term *active* meaning the daily attempts at medical intervention to improve the care of a single patient. And for this reason, some critics would consider the report to be a bit ivory tower. In any system involving human beings or machines, errors and breakdowns that result in harm are inevitable. The question is as follows: What is the baseline below which these errors and breakdowns cannot or should not fall?

This study demonstrated that harm has remained rather common and has not significantly improved since the publication of the report by the IOM. Was a 50% reduction in medical errors within 10 years a goal that was set a bit high by the members of the IOM? The goal may not have been too high, but it was unobtainable. Does this mean that the baseline below which errors and breakdowns should not fall has been established by this study? No, trade-offs have occurred that have decreased errors on one front but have increased them on another. An example is the limitations in work hours that have improved the working environment for residents and students and reduced errors of commission because of lack of sleep, but several studies have demonstrated that communication errors of omission have increased from the lack of appropriate longitudinal patient care, ie, handoffs.

All harms to patients were identified by this report, and the report is most appropriate to determine what global impact the publication of the IOM has had. However, there has been significant improvement in targeted areas such as reduction in nosocomial infections and in surgical complications of surgical procedures selected for study.

North Carolina is the poster child for the reduction of medical errors because a concentrated focus on reduction of errors has been done by this state. Therefore, the data from this report possibly indicate the best that has been accomplished in the United States to reduce medical errors across the global spectrum of possible errors.

The target of reducing medical errors by 50% was naive. I hope that this report does not create more regulations that will have an upside that is counteracted by a downside. I know that subset analysis is frowned upon, but I would recommend having this study broken down into subsets of harm to identify where progress has been made.

E. M. Copeland III, MD

Effect of the 50-Hour Workweek Limitation on Training of Surgical Residents in Switzerland
Businger A, Guller U, Oertli D (Univ Hosp Basel, Switzerland; Univ Hosp Bern, Switzerland)
Arch Surg 145:558-563, 2010

Hypothesis.—The 50-hour workweek limitation for surgical residents in Switzerland has a major effect on surgical training, resident quality of life, and patient care.

Design.—Survey study.

Setting.—Residencies in Switzerland.

Participants.—Surgical residents and surgical consultants.

Main Outcome Measures.—An anonymous survey was conducted in Switzerland. Of 93 surgical departments contacted, 52 (55.9%) responded; of their 281 surgical residents and 337 surgical consultants, 405 (65.5%) returned a completed survey.

Results.—Residents and consultants indicated a negative effect of the 50-hour workweek limitation on surgical training (62.8% and 77.2%, respectively) and on quality of patient care (43.0% and 70.1%, respectively) ($P < .001$ for both). Most residents and consultants reported that operative time (76.9% and 73.4%, respectively) and overall operating room experience (73.8% and 84.8%, respectively) were negatively affected by the work hour limitation. Only 8.1% of residents and 4.9% of consultants perceived the work hour limitation as beneficial to surgical training. Conversely, 58.4% of residents and 81.5% of consultants considered that residents' quality of life had improved ($P < .001$).

Conclusions.—Most surgical residents and surgical consultants perceive the work hour limitation as having a negative effect on surgical training and on the quality of patient care. Despite somewhat improved resident quality of life, the work hour limitation for surgical residencies in Switzerland appears to be a failure.

▶ This study is easy to discuss. If the results of the 80-hour workweek in this country have not improved patient care and possibly have had a negative impact, then the introduction of a 50-hour workweek should be even less desirable. Voila! The more interesting outcome from this study was the lack of an increased satisfaction with the surgical profession in a large percentage of the resident respondents. Likewise, the assumption was made that the residents would be better read and better prepared for the operations in which they participated. Wrong! The residents were, however, more adept at social interaction as viewed by both male and female residents and the attending staff members. Yet here were a significant number of residents and staff members who felt that patient care had suffered.

What do these entire results mean: happier residents more satisfied with surgery as a profession; better educated residents because of an increase in time to be devoted to study; surgeons who feel more confident with their surgical skills? The answer is no to all of these questions. One would conclude, at least from the patients' perspective, that the 50-hour workweek experiment is a dismal failure. Why then do some of the governmental and not-for-profit regulatory agencies in this country pursue a reduction in work hours for residents from 80 to some smaller number? Beats me!

E. M. Copeland III, MD

The VA is critical to academic development
Robinson CN, Freischlag J, Brunicardi FC, et al (Baylor College of Medicine, Houston, TX; Johns Hopkins Univ School of Medicine, Baltimore, MD)
Am J Surg 200:628-631, 2010

Background.—A principal responsibility for surgical chairs is the development of academic programs. This has been challenging in light of the current economic downturn, declining reimbursement, and changes in funding. The aim of this study was to determine the importance that surgical chairs place on the US Department of Veterans Affairs (VA) regarding their ability to develop academic programs.

Methods.—A Web-based survey was constructed and the link sent to 122 university-based surgical department chairs in the United States in 2009 to evaluate previous and current VA affiliations as well as attitudes associated with academic program development.

Results.—A total of 58 of 122 surveys (47.5%) were completed. Seventy percent of surgical chairs received some of their training at VA facilities, and 65% have held VA appointments. Although only 62% of programs were affiliated with VA centers, 91% of chairs believed that VA affiliations were important for their training programs. Additionally, 91% felt that the VA was a good place for faculty development. Finally, 78% indicated that the opportunity to obtain VA research funding is important for academic faculty development.

Conclusion.—Academic program development is an important part of a chair's responsibilities. The overwhelming majority of surgical chairs view a VA affiliation as an important resource in building academic surgical programs.

▶ I chose this article not because of hard science but because I agree with the results. I wanted an opportunity to share my experience with our affiliation with the Malcom Randall VA in Gainesville, Florida. The only contact I had in my career before coming to the University of Florida in 1982 was a chief resident rotation at the Philadelphia VA, which had just become affiliated with the Hospital of the University of Pennsylvania. Everything was great except the nurses were accustomed to removing orders from the chart only once a day. We made rounds twice a day, which produced a conflict that was shortly resolved in our favor.

The chief executive officer of the Gainesville VA was Malcom Randall, who had a lot of experience dealing with medical school chairs at the University of Florida. We discussed that everyone hired to be on the surgical staff at the Department of Veterans Affairs (VA) and at Shands Hospital, our teaching private hospital, would be equal; in fact, all surgical faculty members were less than 8/8 (1 full-time equivalent) at the VA. This included such notable faculty members as Kirby Bland, now Chairman of Surgery at The University of Alabama at Birmingham, and Wiley Souba, the current dean at Dartmouth Medical School. Their time at the VA was 5/8 in order for them to qualify for VA research funding. Since 5/8 represents 25 hours of a 40-hour day, a person working 60 to 80 hours a week had no problem meeting the minimum time requirement at the VA and usually exceeded it. The fact that the VA is across the street and connected by a tunnel to the Medical School was an obvious help.

Our faculty members treated the VA fairly, and the VA reciprocated. At the time, VA salaries were not equivalent to those of the same rank at the Medial School, so the salaries were appropriately subsidized. VA funding through the Merit Review System was available, and if obtained, the VA provided a laboratory equivalent to the funding. How much better can it get!!

I expect that my experience with our VA might have been somewhat unique. Full-time salaries in the VA system are now more equivalent to full-time medical school salaries. And most of our VA faculty members are full time (8/8), which means that they are often nearing retirement and like the regimentation of the VA or their interests are primarily research and funding is available via the VA system.

The current system prevents the VA from being taken advantage of, but I felt a closer kindred with the part-time VA faculty members who also had offices and operated at Shands Hospital.

Like many older academic surgeons, I enjoy applauding the past. Yet the relationship that we had with the Malcom Randall VA hospital was a benefit to all, as proven by the successful surgeons, both in academic and private practice, who both worked there or had a substantial experience at our VA during their surgical training.

E. M. Copeland III, MD

A Novel Method for Reproducibly Measuring the Effects of Interventions to Improve Emotional Climate, Indices of Team Skills and Communication, and Threat to Patient Outcome in a High-Volume Thoracic Surgery Center

Nurok M, Lipsitz S, Satwicz P, et al (Brigham and Women's Hosp, Boston, MA; Newton Wellesley Hosp, MA; et al)
Arch Surg 145:489-495, 2010

Objective.—To create and test a reproducible method for measuring emotional climate, surgical team skills, and threats to patient outcome by conducting an observational study to assess the impact of a surgical team skills and communication improvement intervention on these measurements.

Design.—Observational study.

Setting.—Operating rooms in a high-volume thoracic surgery center from September 5, 2007, through June 30, 2008.

Participants.—Thoracic surgery operating room teams.

Interventions.—Two 90-minute team skills training sessions focused on findings from a standardized safety culture survey administered to all participants and highlighting positive and problematic aspects of team skills, communication, and leadership. The sessions created an interactive forum to educate team members on the importance of communication and to role-play optimal interactive and communication strategies.

Main Outcome Measures.—Calculated indices of emotional climate, team skills, and threat to patient outcome.

Results.—The calculated communication and team skills score improved from the preintervention to postintervention periods, but the improvement extinguished during the 3 months after the intervention ($P < .001$). The calculated threat-to-outcome score improved following the team training intervention and remained statistically improved 3 months later ($P < .001$).

Conclusions.—Using a new method for measuring emotional climate, teamwork, and threats to patient outcome, we were able to determine that a teamwork training intervention can improve a calculated score of team skills and communication and decrease a calculated score of threats to patient outcome. However, the effect is only durable for threats to patient outcome.

▶ The most disappointing result from this study was the lack of longevity of the team skills demonstrated throughout the active period of observation of the study parameters. In fact, this deterioration in team interaction may be the most important result. The operating theater is a dynamic entity. Different nurses report to work at different times, residents change services both in surgery and anesthesia, a different surgical affect exists for difficult versus easy surgical procedures, etc. The intervention to improve skills and teamwork lasted for a defined period of time. A simple conclusion from this study would be the need to repeat the intervention sessions at the time of decay of the positive outcomes. The observers standing in the operating rooms were a significant variable. Possibly observers could participate at intervals not previously known to the study participants, especially if the same study participants were to be reeducated and the study repeated.

I go into this detail because I am impressed with the time and effort of the authors put into developing a reproducible study vehicle. There is a critique at the end of the printed article and a list of limitations enumerated by the authors. Nevertheless, the durability of the positive outcomes of the study cannot be criticized. And this outcome can be used as a benchmark for the future to improve the methodology of studying the interactive human environment of the operating room with the aim of producing a durable positive outcome.

E. M. Copeland III, MD

2 Trauma

Computed Tomography Alone Versus Computed Tomography and Magnetic Resonance Imaging in the Identification of Occult Injuries to the Cervical Spine: A Meta-Analysis

Schoenfeld AJ, Bono CM, McGuire KJ, et al (Brigham and Women's Hosp, Boston, MA; Harvard Med School, Boston, MA)

J Trauma 68:109-114, 2010

Background.—Ruling out injuries of the cervical spine in obtunded blunt trauma patients is controversial. Although computed tomography (CT) readily demonstrates fractures and malalignment, it provides limited direct evaluation of ligamentous integrity, leading some to advocate a magnetic resonance imaging (MRI) in obtunded patients. Thus, the question remains: does adding an MRI provide useful information that alters treatment when a CT scan reveals no evidence of injury?

Methods.—Published studies from 2000 to 2008 involving patients undergoing MRI for the purposes of further cervical spine evaluation after a "negative" CT scan were identified via a literature search of online databases. Data from eligible studies were pooled and original scale meta-analyses were performed to calculate overall sensitivity, specificity, positive and negative predictive values, likelihood ratios, and relative risk. The Q-statistic p value was used to evaluate heterogeneity.

Results.—Eleven studies met the inclusion criteria, yielding data on 1,550 patients with a negative CT scan after blunt trauma subsequently evaluated with a MRI. The MRI detected abnormalities in 182 patients (12%). Ninety traumatic injuries were identified, including ligamentous injuries (86/182), fractures, and dislocations (4/182). In 96 cases (6% of the cohort), the MRI identified an injury that altered management. Eighty-four patients (5%) required continued collar immobilization and 12 (1%) required surgical stabilization. The Q-statistic p value for heterogeneity was 0.99, indicating the absence of heterogeneity among the individual study populations.

Conclusions.—Reliance on CT imaging alone to "clear the cervical spine" after blunt trauma can lead to missed injuries. This study supports a role for the addition of MRI in evaluating patients who are obtunded, or unexaminable, despite a negative CT scan.

▶ The optimal imaging protocol for cervical spine and soft tissue clearance in the patient with obtunded blunt trauma remains controversial. Although CT scanning is highly sensitive in identifying bone abnormalities, the data presented in this selection demonstrate that CT scanning is not capable of detecting all clinically significant injuries. This meta-analysis supports a continued role for the addition of MRI in the evaluation of patients who cannot be cleared with a clinical physical examination, despite a normal CT scan result. There are several limitations to this meta-analysis. One of these is that 6 of the 11 studies included were retrospective. There is also not a specific definition of what constitutes a clinically significant CT or MRI finding. Instead, all studies included in this meta-analysis relied on radiologists' or surgeons' interpretations of CT and magnetic resonance images. Similarly, decisions in all studies regarding which cervical injuries required prolonged immobilization or surgery were made by the treating spine surgeons. An objective protocol that directed treatment based on specific criteria could not be identified in any of the studies. Such variation in practice is a major reason to do an investigation such as this. Currently, there are few specific data that correlate many of the identifiable MRI soft tissue findings with a clinical assessment of instability in a patient who cannot be fully examined.

D. W. Mozingo, MD

Bicyclists Injured by Automobiles: Relationship of Age to Injury Type and Severity—A National Trauma Databank Analysis

Lustenberger T, Inaba K, Talving P, et al (Univ of Southern California, Los Angeles, CA)
J Trauma 69:1120-1125, 2010

Background.—Bicycle riding is a popular recreational activity and a common mode of transportation. Impact with a motor vehicle, however, has the potential to result in significant injury to the rider. The magnitude of this problem, the incidence and types of injuries, and the effect of age on these variables are poorly defined in the literature.

Methods.—This was a National Trauma Databank study during a 5-year period. Injury Severity Score (ISS), specific injuries sustained by riders, and outcomes were analyzed according to age groups ($\leq$14 years, 15–35 years, 36–55 years, 56–65 years, and >65 years).

Results.—During the study period, there were 12,429 admissions as a result of bicycle-related injuries involving motor vehicles (0.7% of all trauma admissions). There were 4,095 patients (32.9%) $\leq$14 years, 3,806 (30.7%) 15 to 35 years, 3,413 (27.5%) 36 to 55 years, 688 (5.5%) 56 to 65 years, and 427 (3.4%) >65 years. The incidence of severe or critical trauma (ISS $\geq$16) in the five age strata was 20.3%, 19.2%, 26.4%, 33.4%, and 38.2%, respectively ($p < 0.001$). The most commonly encountered injuries consisted of extremity fractures (34.9%). Patients $\leq$14 years old were significantly more likely to suffer fractures to the lower extremity and less likely to sustain fractures to the upper extremity. The overall incidence of head injury was 28.3% and increased in a stepwise fashion with increasing age, ranging from 26.5% in the age stratum 15 to 35 years to 38.6% in the age stratum >65 years, $p < 0.001$. The overall

TABLE 5.—Bicyclists Injured by Automobiles: Outcome According to Age Group

	Age Group	Percent	n	Odds Ratio (95% CI)*	P*	Adjusted Odds Ratio (95% CI)*,†	Adjusted p*,†
Need for	≤14	4.8	196 of 4,095	1.0	—	1.0	—
rehabilitation	15−35	6.0	227 of 3,806	1.26 (1.04−1.54)	0.02	1.34 (1.04−1.73)	0.023
	36−55	10.5	357 of 3,413	2.32 (1.94−2.78)	<0.001	2.42 (1.93−3.05)	<0.001
	56−65	18.2	125 of 688	4.42 (3.47−5.62)	<0.001	4.72 (3.43−6.49)	<0.001
	>65	23.0	98 of 427	5.93 (4.54−7.74)	<0.001	6.86 (4.82−9.77)	<0.001
Mortality	≤14	2.4	99 of 4,073	1.0	—	1.0	—
	15−35	2.5	96 of 3,784	1.05 (0.79−1.39)	0.762	1.54 (1.00−2.37)	0.051
	36−55	4.9	165 of 3,397	2.05 (1.59−2.64)	<0.001	3.03 (2.00−4.59)	<0.001
	56−65	6.6	45 of 683	2.83 (1.97−4.07)	<0.001	5.28 (2.97−9.37)	<0.001
	>65	12.2	52 of 426	5.58 (3.93−7.94)	<0.001	10.04 (5.51−18.32)	<0.001

Percentage of patients with missing data (not available for multiple logistic regression): need for rehabilitation: 11.3%; mortality: 11.4%.
SBP, systolic blood pressure; GCS, Glasgow coma scale.
*Age group ≤14 yr used as reference for comparison.
†Multiple logistic regression adjusting for ISS, gender, SBP <90 mm Hg, GCS score ≤8, head injuries, spinal fractures, spinal cord injuries, extremity fractures, pelvic fractures, thoracic injuries.

mortality was 3.7% and ranged from 2.4% in the age stratum ≤14 years, to 12.2% in the stratum >65 years. After adjusting for differences in age groups, there was a stepwise increase in the risk of death for bicyclists >65 years old who were 10-fold more likely to die than those ≤14 years old (adj. $p < 0.001$).

Conclusion.—Bicycle-related injuries involving motor vehicles are associated with a high incidence of head injuries and extremity fractures. Age plays a critical role in the severity and anatomic distribution of injuries sustained, with a stepwise increase in mortality with increasing age. Further evaluation of specific preventative measures, especially for elderly bicyclists is warranted (Table 5).

▶ In the United States, about 540 000 injured bicyclists are treated in emergency rooms every year.

In 2007, 700 bicyclists died in the United States, with the vast majority involving crashes with motor vehicles. Consequently, bicycle-related injuries along with their long-term sequelae are associated with costs exceeding $8 billion annually. Age-related differences in anatomic and physiologic characteristics predispose patients to different injury patterns and outcomes, even with identical mechanisms of injury. Previous studies on bicycle-related injuries have been restricted to selected age groups or have focused primarily on head injuries. This study was selected because it examines a nationwide epidemiologic data set on bicycle-related injuries. In addition, the authors sought to evaluate the associations between age, injuries, and outcome for bicycle riders involved in crashes with motor vehicles. The authors of this study demonstrated that in bicycle-related injuries involving automobiles, age plays a critical role in the anatomic distribution and severity of injuries. Older bicyclists are more likely to sustain injury after being hit by a car, in particular head injury, and are more likely to die as a result. The need for rehabilitation also increased significantly with age, further increasing costs. Further evaluation of preventative measures, especially for elderly bicyclists, is warranted.

D. W. Mozingo, MD

Intraabdominal Vascular Injury: Are We Getting Any Better?
Paul JS, Webb TP, Aprahamian C, et al (Med College of Wisconsin, Milwaukee; Clement J Zablocki Veterans Affairs Hosp, Milwaukee, WI)
J Trauma 69:1393-1397, 2010

Background.—Intraabdominal vascular injury (IAVI) as a result of penetrating and blunt trauma carries a high mortality rate. This study was performed to compare current mortality rates with a previously reported historic control.

Methods.—The experience at our institution from 1970 to 1981 was previously reported with an overall mortality rate of 32% in 112 patients with penetrating IAVI. In a retrospective analysis, this historic cohort was compared with 248 patients with penetrating and blunt IAVI during a 138-month interval ending in June 2007.

Results.—Overall mortality rate was 28.6%. The most commonly injured arteries were the iliac artery, aorta, and superior mesenteric artery. The most commonly injured veins were the inferior vena cava, iliac vein, and portal vein. Injury to the aorta, IVC, and portal vein had the highest mortality rates of 67.8%, 42.1%, and 66.6%, respectively. One hundred forty-four patients with one vessel injured had a mortality rate of 18.7%, whereas those with more than one vessel injured had a mortality rate of 48.7% ($p < 0.001$). A total of 46% of 117 patients in shock died compared with 9.6% of 104 patients not in shock ($p < 0.001$). Patients with a base deficit of less than -15 had a mortality rate of 72%, whereas those with a base deficit of 0 to -15 ($p < 0.001$) had a mortality rate of 18.9%. There was no difference in the overall mortality rate for penetrating trauma compared with the previous study.

Conclusions.—Although over 20 years have passed, no significant changes have occurred in the mortality associated with IAVI. Patients presenting in shock with IAVI continue to have a high mortality rate.

▶ Intra-abdominal vascular injuries can be devastating injuries and a major cause of mortality in the patient population with trauma. These patients may have massive blood loss before hospital arrival, have injuries that are difficult to expose and repair operatively, and develop early and profound coagulopathy making hemostasis and resuscitation much more difficult. The mortality rate of intra-abdominal vascular injuries is reported to be between 32% and 54%. Shock, coagulopathy, the number of vessels injured, and acidosis have all been associated with increased mortality. In this selection, the authors discern that little has changed in the outcome of these patients over the past 30 years. Several limitations to this study exist. This is a single-institution study with a well-developed prehospital program. The data are retrospective, and several of the patients had missing data. There were enough data documented to develop reasonable conclusions about mortality. Morbidity data were not evaluated in this study, and important conclusions might have been made regarding complications. Also, because of the retrospective nature, the authors were unable to evaluate several aspects of care that have become of interest in the recent literature. The infusion of hypertonic solutions during transport, hypotensive strategies during early resuscitation, and use of massive transfusion protocols with higher fresh frozen plasma to packed red blood cell ratios all may be considered as potential strategies to apply in this patient population.

D. W. Mozingo, MD

Access to Trauma Systems in Canada
Hameed SM, for the Research Committee of the Trauma Association of Canada
(Res Committee of the Trauma Association of Canada, Calgary, Alberta)
J Trauma 69:1350-1361, 2010

Background.—Trauma is a leading cause of morbidity, potential years of life lost and health care expenditure in Canada and around the world. Trauma systems have been established across North America to provide comprehensive injury care and to lead injury control efforts. We sought to describe the current status of trauma systems in Canada and Canadians' access to acute, multidisciplinary trauma care.

Methods.—A national survey was used to identify the locations and capabilities of adult trauma centers across Canada and to identify the catchment populations they serve. Geographic information science methods were used to map the locations of Level I and Level II trauma centers and to define 1-hour road travel times around each trauma center. Data from the 2006 Canadian Census were used to estimate populations within and outside 1-hour access to definitive trauma care.

Results.—In Canada, 32 Level I and Level II trauma centers provide definitive trauma care and coordinate the efforts of their surrounding trauma systems. Most Canadians (77.5%) reside within 1-hour road travel catchments of Level I or Level II centers. However, marked geographic disparities in access persist. Of the 22.5% of Canadians who live more than an hour away from a Level I or Level II trauma centers, all are in rural and remote regions.

Discussion.—Access to high quality acute trauma care is well established across parts of Canada but a clear urban/rural divide persists. Regional efforts to improve short- and long-term outcomes after severe trauma should focus on the optimization of access to pre-hospital care and acute trauma care in rural communities using locally relevant strategies or novel care delivery options (Fig 1).

▶ Trauma systems have been implemented across Canada for many years. Fig 1 is included in this selection and demonstrates the extent of the Canadian trauma system. However, significant variations in trauma system structure and access

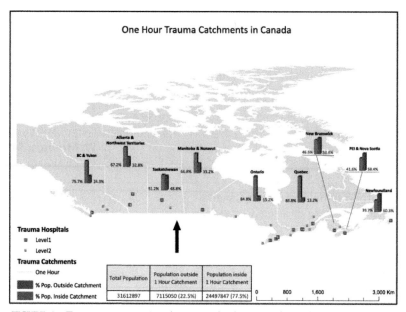

FIGURE 1.—Trauma systems in Canada. Geographic locations of Canada's Level 1 and Level 2 trauma centers and surrounding 1 hour catchments. Overall, 20% of the Canadian population, including 100% of the residents of the 3 territories, lives beyond 1 hour by road from definitive trauma care. (Reprinted from Hameed SM, for the Research Committee of the Trauma Association of Canada. Access to trauma systems in Canada. *J Trauma*. 2010;69:1350-1361, with permission from Lippincott Williams & Wilkins.)

are still present, and disparities in access persist in rural and remote communities. Depending on the local context and needs, access to critical trauma services can be improved by reducing emergency medical service response times by expanding the use of helicopter and fixed wing transport. Also, increasing the role and integration of level III and level IV trauma centers within regional trauma systems may provide better access in remote areas. In addition, the use of telemedicine and teleultrasound may potentially enlarge the geographical extent of trauma systems. More programs for injury prevention specific to remote areas could be developed. Further advances may result from intensified efforts to acquire and apply injury data to measure and standardize processes of trauma care within trauma systems and further develop national benchmarks for trauma care. It would also be interesting to explore regional differences in trauma outcome as a means of assessing and raising the standards of trauma care.

D. W. Mozingo, MD

Impact of Low-dose Vasopressin on Trauma Outcome: Prospective Randomized Study
Cohn SM, McCarthy J, Stewart RM, et al (Univ of Texas Health Science Ctr, San Antonio)
World J Surg 35:430-439, 2011

Background.—We previously found that regardless of the animal injury model used resuscitation strategies that minimize fluid administration requirements lead to better outcomes. We hypothesized that a resuscitation regimen that limited the total volume of fluid administered would reduce morbidity and mortality rates in critically ill trauma patients.

Methods.—We performed a double-blind randomized trial to assess the safety and efficacy of adding vasopressin to resuscitative fluid. Subjects were hypotensive adults who had sustained acute traumatic injury. Subjects were given fluid alone (control group) or fluid plus vasopressin (experimental group), first as a bolus (4 IU) and then as an intravenous infusion of 200 ml/h (vasopressin 2.4 IU/h) for 5 h.

Results.—We randomly assigned 78 patients to the experimental group ($n = 38$) or the control group ($n = 40$). The groups were similar in age, sex, preexisting medical illnesses, and mechanism and severity of injury. Serum vasopressin concentrations were higher in the experimental group than in the control group at admission, after infusion of vasopressin ($p = 0.01$), and 12 h later. The experimental group required a significantly lower total volume of resuscitation fluid over 5 days than did the control group ($p = 0.04$). The mortality rate at 5 days was 13% in the experimental group and 25% in the control group ($p = 0.19$). The rates of adverse events, organ dysfunction, and 30-day mortality were similar.

Conclusions.—This is the first trial to investigate the impact of vasopressin administration in trauma patients. Infusion of low-dose vasopressin maintained elevated serum vasopressin levels and decreased fluid requirements after injury.

▶ Improving our understanding of the optimal resuscitation strategy for patients with hemorrhagic shock may help reduce morbidity and mortality rates among civilian and military trauma patients. Vasopressin is an endogenous hormone that is crucial for maintaining vascular tone, and although studies have demonstrated that vasopressin has a clinical benefit for the resuscitation of patients with hemorrhagic shock, the results of numerous clinical investigations support the utility of adjunctive low-dose vasopressin for other critically ill patients. It is noteworthy that vasopressin does not act as a pressor agent in normal healthy volunteers or in patients with cardiogenic shock but is effective at very low doses in improving the blood pressure of patients with vasodilatory shock. The primary objective in this study was to evaluate the safety and efficacy of a new low-dose vasopressin resuscitation regimen. The investigators hypothesized that a protocol that would minimize the total volume of resuscitation fluid would lead to lower morbidity and mortality rates among critically ill trauma patients. This is the first trial to investigate the impact of vasopressin administration in trauma patients. This double-blind randomized clinical trial demonstrated that the infusion of low-dose vasopressin could maintain elevated serum vasopressin concentrations and decreased fluid requirements after injury. The administration of vasopressin was associated with a possible early survival advantage. This important finding suggests the need for a larger sufficiently powered trial to determine the potential benefits of this hormone in treating critically ill trauma patients.

D. W. Mozingo, MD

Blunt Cerebrovascular Injury Screening With 32-Channel Multidetector Computed Tomography: More Slices Still Don't Cut It
DiCocco JM, Emmett KP, Fabian TC, et al (Univ of Tennessee Health Science Ctr, Memphis)
Ann Surg 253:444-450, 2011

Objective.—We sought to determine the diagnostic accuracy of computed tomographic angiography (CTA) using 32-channel multidetector computed tomography for blunt cerebrovascular injuries (BCVIs).

Background.—Unrecognized BCVI is a cause of stroke in young trauma patients. Digital subtraction angiography (DSA), the reference standard, is invasive, expensive, and time-consuming. Computed tomographic angiography has been rapidly adopted by many institutions because of its availability, less resource intensive, and noninvasive nature. However, conflicting results comparing CTA and DSA have been reported. Studies with 16-channel CTA report a wide range of sensitivities for BCVI diagnosis.

Methods.—From January 2007 through May 2009, patients with risk factors for BCVI underwent *both* CTA and DSA. All CTAs were performed using a 32-channel multidetector CT scanner. Using DSA as the reference standard, the diagnostic accuracy of CTA for determination of BCVI was calculated.

Results.—There were 684 patients who met the inclusion criteria. Ninety patients (13%) had 109 injuries identified; 52 carotid and 57 vertebral injuries were diagnosed. CTA failed to detect 53 confirmed BCVI, yielding a sensitivity of 51%.

Conclusion.—Given the devastation of stroke, and high mortality from missed injuries, this study demonstrates that even with more advanced technology (32 vs 16 channel), CTA is inadequate for BCVI screening. Digital subtraction angiography remains the gold standard for the diagnosis of BCVI (Table 4).

▶ Before widespread screening for blunt cerebrovascular injury, many patients developed stroke because of unrecognized injuries. This complication is particularly devastating because trauma occurs mostly in the young people. Now, with more aggressive screening, blunt cerebrovascular injury is identified in nearly 2% of blunt trauma patients. Screening for blunt cerebrovascular injury

TABLE 4.—Sensitivity of Computed Tomography Angiography

	No. of Vessels	No Injury (DSA−) (CTA−) TN	(CTA+) FP	Injury (DSA+) (CTA−) FN	(CTA+) TP	Sensitivity (%)
Overall	2736	2552	75	53	56	51
Carotid	1368	1286	30	26	26	50
Vertebral	1368	1266	45	27	30	53

TN indicates true negative; FP, false positive; FN, false negative; TP, true positive.

allows for early detection and prompt intervention. Untreated blunt cerebrovascular injury results in stroke rates of 30% to 50%. Early intervention probably improves the prevalence of stroke to less than 10%. Despite the apparent benefits of early screening, there continues to be debate regarding the optimal screening modality for blunt cerebrovascular injury. Digital subtraction angiography (DSA) has long been the reference standard for screening; however, it is invasive and requires a substantial investment of personnel and time. Many institutions have adopted CT angiography (CTA) to replace DSA for screening. Mainly, the rapid acceptance of CTA is because of several perceived advantages of being less invasive and available in many hospitals. It is much less resource intensive and can be performed during the initial trauma evaluation, resulting in a decreased time to diagnosis. The potential benefits of CTA are negated if it is inaccurate. In the past year, both the Eastern Association for the Surgery of Trauma and the Western Trauma Association have made recommendations regarding blunt cerebrovascular injury. Both organizations acknowledge the role of DSA as the reference standard but suggest that 16-channel CTA may be an acceptable screening modality. These recommendations are based on 6 reports using 16-channel CTA, which reported a wide range of sensitivity. In light of the results in this selection, additional studies may need to be conducted or institutions will need to carefully define their protocols for screening for patients with blunt cerebrovascular injuries.

D. W. Mozingo, MD

"Damage Control" in the Elderly: Futile Endeavor or Fruitful Enterprise?
Newell MA, Schlitzkus LL, Waibel BH, et al (The Brody School of Medicine at East Carolina Univ, Greenville, NC; Univ Health Systems of Eastern Carolina, Greenville, NC)
J Trauma 69:1049-1053, 2010

Background.—Damage control laparotomy (DCL) provides effective management in carefully selected, exsanguinating trauma patients. However, the effectiveness of this approach has not been examined in the elderly. The purpose of this study was to characterize elderly DCL patients.

Methods.—The National Trauma Registry of the American College of Surgeons was queried for patients admitted to our Level I trauma center between January 2003 and June 2008. Patients who underwent a DCL were included in the study. Elderly (55 years or older) and young (16–54 years) patients were compared for demographics, injury severity, intraoperative transfusion volume, complications, and mortality.

Results.—During the study period, 62 patients met inclusion criteria. Elderly and young cohorts were similar in gender (male, 78.6% vs. 75.0%, $p = 0.78$), Injury Severity Score (25.1 ± 2.1 vs. 23.8 ± 1.7, $p = 0.49$), packed red blood cell transfusion volume (3036 mL ± 2760 mL vs. 2654 mL ± 2194 mL, $p = 0.51$), and number of complications (3.21 ± 0.48 vs. 3.33 ± 0.38, $p = 0.96$). Mortality was greater in the elderly cohort (42.9% vs. 12.5%, $p = 0.02$). The mean time to death for the elderly was 9.8 days ± 10.2 days and 26 days ± 21.5 days in the young ($p = 0.485$).

Conclusions.—Despite the severity of injury, the outcome of elderly DCL patients is better than what might be predicted. They succumb to their injuries more frequently and earlier in the hospital course compared with the young, but the majority of these patients survive. DCL in the elderly is not a futile endeavor (Table 4).

▶ Elderly trauma patients typically have poorer outcomes than younger patients with similar injury severity. Lack of physiologic reserve provides one explanation for these poor results. Although the approach of using damage control laparotomy has led to improved outcomes in trauma patients in general, the effectiveness of this approach in the elderly has not been studied. Considering the severity of injury, the need for intensive support, and the potential for prolonged use of costly resources in the patient undergoing damage control laparotomy, if outcomes in the elderly were poor, withholding this potentially futile treatment would have to be contemplated. Indeed, as an overwhelming amount of health care expense is spent on the elderly in general and for end-of-life care in particular, such determinations would need to be considered. However, if outcomes of using the damage control approach were similar in the elderly to those in the young, this would favor continuing to provide this aggressive management approach. The purpose of this study was to compare outcomes in elderly and young trauma patients undergoing damage control laparotomy. The lethal combination of hypothermia, acidosis, and coagulopathy denotes the limits of the patient's ability to survive the physiologic consequences of injury. In this selection, the authors have clearly demonstrated that the use of

TABLE 4.—Comparison of Outcomes in Elderly and Young Patients

	Elderly	Young	*p*
Hospital days (survivors)	32.9 ± 19.0	31.9 ± 21.2	0.805*
Hospital days (nonsurvivors)	9.8 ± 10.2	26.0 ± 21.4	0.485*
ICU days (survivors)	20.9 ± 9.7	16.8 ± 14.5	0.137*
Ventilator days (survivors)	21.5 ± 15.3	17.0 ± 19.0	0.194*
Mortality	42.9%	12.5%	0.020[†]

Data presented as percentage or mean ± SD.
*Mann-Whitney *U* test.
[†]Fisher's exact test.

damage control laparotomy in the elderly patient population warrants consideration. Their results show that it would be of benefit to many patients. The long-term consequences of this aggressive care, although not detailed in this report, show a trend toward long-term disability and loss of function of activities of daily living. Much more work needs to be done to categorize the outcomes in this increasing segment of the population.

D. W. Mozingo, MD

The Association Between Cost and Quality in Trauma: Is Greater Spending Associated With Higher-Quality Care?
Glance LG, Dick AW, Osler TM, et al (Univ of Rochester Med Centre, NY; RAND, Pittsburgh, PA; Univ of Vermont Med College, Burlington; et al)
Ann Surg 252:217-222, 2010

Objective.—To examine the association between trauma center quality and costs.

Background.—Current efforts to reduce health care costs and improve health care quality require a better understanding of the relationship between cost and quality.

Methods.—Using data from the Healthcare Cost and Utilization Projects Nationwide Inpatient Sample, we performed a retrospective observational study of 67,124 trauma patients admitted to 73 trauma centers. Generalized linear models were used to explore the association between hospital cost and in-hospital mortality, controlling for hospital and patient factors as follows: injury diagnoses, age, gender, mechanism of injury, comorbidities, teaching status, hospital ownership, geographic region, and hospital wages.

Results.—Patients treated in hospitals with low risk-adjusted mortality rates had significantly lower costs than those treated in average-quality hospitals. The relative cost of patients treated in high-quality hospitals was 0.78 (95% confidence interval: 0.64, 0.95) compared with average-quality hospitals. The cost of treating patients in average- and high-mortality trauma centers was similar.

Conclusion.—In this study based on the Healthcare Cost and Utilization Project Nationwide Inpatient Sample, the care of injured patients is less expensive in hospitals with lower risk-adjusted mortality rates. Hospitals with low risk-adjusted mortality rates have adjusted mortality rates that are 34% lower while spending nearly 22% less compared with average-quality hospitals.

▶ The findings in this selection suggest that higher-quality care for injured patients is associated with lower cost.

Focusing efforts of health care reform on improving quality of care may lead to lower health care spending for trauma patients. However, the findings in this study, although enticing, should be interpreted with caution, given the observational nature of this study. The mechanism underlying the finding that better hospital trauma mortality outcomes can be associated with lower costs is not certain. The cost savings associated with higher-quality patient care could result from higher-quality hospitals having fewer complications compared with lower-quality hospitals. It is plausible that hospitals with fewer complications may spend less on the care of trauma patients. Further investigation is necessary to explore this explanation for the association between better outcomes and lower cost in trauma patients. Proof will require prospective interventions designed to improve the quality of care while quantifying the impact on cost.

D. W. Mozingo, MD

Insurance status is a potent predictor of outcomes in both blunt and penetrating trauma

Greene WR, Oyetunji TA, Bowers U, et al (Howard Univ College of Medicine, Washington, DC; et al)
Am J Surg 199:554-557, 2010

Background.—Patients with penetrating injuries are known to have worse outcomes than those with blunt trauma. We hypothesize that within each injury mechanism there should be no outcome difference between insured and uninsured patients.

Methods.—The National Trauma Data Bank version 7 was analyzed. Patients aged 65 years and older and burn patients were excluded. The insurance status was categorized as insured (private, government/ military, or Medicaid) and uninsured. Multivariate analysis adjusted for insurance status, mechanism of injury, age, race, sex, injury severity score, shock, head injury, extremity injury, teaching hospital status, and year.

Results.—A total of 1,203,243 patients were analyzed, with a mortality rate of 3.7%. The death rate was significantly higher in penetrating trauma patients versus blunt trauma patients (7.9% vs 3.0%; $P < .001$), and higher in the uninsured (5.3% vs 3.2%; $P < .001$). On multivariate analysis, uninsured patients had an increased odds of death than insured patients, in both penetrating and blunt trauma patients. Penetrating trauma patients with insurance still had a greater risk of death than blunt trauma patients without insurance.

Conclusions.—Insurance status is a potent predictor of outcome in both penetrating and blunt trauma (Fig 1).

▶ This selection documents the importance of insurance status to trauma-related mortality. Patients who have insurance are less likely to die, but the magnitude of this problem is overshadowed by the complexities of the contributing factors. Many studies show the ethnic disparity in health care and now have attributed this to the care of the trauma patient. Trauma care is one of the most protocolized and standardized systems of care with direction provided by the American College of Surgeons—sponsored advanced trauma life support

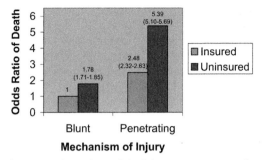

FIGURE 1.—Multivariate analysis of OR of death by insurance status and mechanism of injury. (Reprinted from The American Journal of Surgery, Greene WR, Oyetunji TA, Bowers U, et al. Insurance status is a potent predictor of outcomes in both blunt and penetrating trauma. *Am J Surg.* 2010;199:554-557. Copyright © 2010, with permission from Elsevier.)

education. Insurance status should have no effect on the trauma patient's access to the health care system. The confounding variables, which influence outcomes, may be multifactorial. The mechanism of injury regarding blunt or penetrating is well controlled in this study of more than one million patients from the National Trauma Database. However, they cannot control for the type of weapon used, the speed of the vehicle crash, and the prior health and socioeconomic status of the injured patient. Fig 1 depicts the discrepancy in outcomes. A prospective study needs to be done to address the additional patient-related factors that might contribute to the difference in outcomes between insured and uninsured patients.

D. W. Mozingo, MD

Arterial embolization for pelvic fractures after blunt trauma: are we all talk?

Costantini TW, Bosarge PL, Fortlage D, et al (Univ of California, San Diego)
Am J Surg 200:752-758, 2010

Background.—We hypothesized that arterial embolization for bleeding after pelvic fracture is used relatively infrequently. We sought to identify the true need for arterial embolization and define injury patterns associated with successful therapeutic angiographic embolization.

Methods.—A retrospective review identified patients admitted to our urban, Level 1 trauma center with pelvic fractures from 2001 to 2009. Patients requiring pelvic arterial angiogram and embolization of pelvic bleeding were reviewed for pelvic fracture pattern and pelvic injury mechanism.

Results.—There were 819 patients diagnosed with pelvic fractures, with only 31 patients (3.8%) undergoing diagnostic pelvic angiography. Of those, 18 patients (58.1%) had active bleeding requiring arterial embolization. Complex pelvic fracture patterns were common in patients undergoing angiogram. Patients undergoing pelvic angiography with an anteroposterior compression mechanism were more likely to have negative findings on angiogram.

Conclusions.—The actual need for angiography and therapeutic embolization is quite small in patients sustaining pelvic fracture. Although factors associated with the need for pelvic angiography frequently are debated, we may discuss angiography for pelvic fractures more often than it actually is performed.

▶ Traumatic pelvic fractures may result in serious hemorrhage that can be associated with significant morbidity and mortality. Patients with pelvic fractures that cause hemodynamic instability have a mortality exceeding 50% in some reports. Identification of patients at risk for severe bleeding due to their pelvic fracture and prompt mobilization of resources to treat those patients are of great importance. Bleeding from pelvic fractures can be generated from several sources including arterial and venous injury, as well as bleeding from fractured cancellous bone within the pelvis. Bleeding from fractured bone within the pelvis can be controlled with prompt stabilization of the fracture, which also can tamponade venous bleeding. Arterial injury caused by pelvic fracture may require therapeutic arterial embolization, which has been shown to be an important adjunct in the treatment of patients with pelvic hemorrhage. Thus, management of patients with pelvic fractures may require care from a multidisciplinary team of trauma surgeons, orthopedic surgeons, and interventional radiologists. In this selection, the authors found that the need for pelvic angiography was relatively rare in 819 patients admitted with pelvic fracture to a level 1 trauma center during the 9-year study period. Angiographic arterial embolization remained an important but infrequent treatment adjunct in severely injured patients with bleeding from pelvic fractures. Those patients sustaining complex pelvic fractures with associated hypotension and tachycardia not due to other obvious causes should be considered candidates for angiography.

D. W. Mozingo, MD

Field triage score (FTS) in battlefield casualties: validation of a novel triage technique in a combat environment
Eastridge BJ, Butler F, Wade CE, et al (United States Army Inst of Surgical Res, Fort Sam Houston, TX; et al)
Am J Surg 200:724-727, 2010

Background.—By the principles of Tactical Combat Casualty Care, battlefield casualties are preferentially triaged on the basis of pulse character and mental status. A weak or absent palpable pulse correlates with a systolic blood pressure (SBP) of ≤ 100 mm Hg. Furthermore, the motor component of the Glasgow Coma Scale (GCS-M) has been shown to correlate with outcomes. In a previous study, the authors developed a simple triage tool, the field triage score (FTS), on the basis of pulse character and GCS-M status, which provided a quick and effective means of predicting injury survival in the civilian trauma environment. The purpose of this analysis was to validate the predictive utility of the FTS in the battlefield trauma environment.

Methods.—The Joint Theater Trauma Registry was used to identify 4,988 battlefield casualties from Iraq and Afghanistan from January 2002 to September 2008 with requisite admission data elements of SBP, GCS-M status, and survival. SBP was stratified as ≤100 mm Hg, consistent with weak or absent pulse character, or >100 mm Hg, consistent with a normal pulse character. GCS-M status was stratified as either abnormal (<6) or normal (6). Casualties with presenting SBPs of 0 mm Hg were excluded from the analysis. As in the civilian trauma triage study, the FTS was derived by assigning a component value of 0 for weak or absent pulse or abnormal GCS-M status and a component value of 1 for either a normal pulse or normal GCS-M status. Adding the scores resulted in an aggregate FTS value of 0, 1, or 2.

Results.—For the overall population of 4,988 casualties, 87.5% (n = 4,366) had FTS of 2, with overall mortality of .1% (5 of 4,366). From the battlefield, 10.8% of patients (n = 540) presenting with FTS of 1 had a mortality rate that increased to 6.1% (33 of 540). In contrast, combat casualties presenting with FTS of 0 had a significantly higher mortality of 41.4% (34 of 82). The calculated lengths of stay were 6.1 (FTS 2), 9.2 (FTS 1), and 17.7 (FTS 0) days.

Conclusion.—This study has validated the utility of the FTS as a simple and practical triage instrument for use in the battlefield environment. Using the FTS, medics and medical providers will have a quick and effective measure to predict high-acuity combat casualties to triage evacuation and medical resources in austere military environments. This technique may have potential implications for domestic or foreign disaster or mass casualty situations in which supplies, medical resources, and facilities are limited (Figs 1 and 2).

▶ This selection evaluates a field triage score (FTS) in a database of combat casualties. A simple scoring system would be useful for triage in battlefield settings. The authors validated the FTS as a valid and efficacious trauma triage scoring system with the potential for profound implications in the prehospital

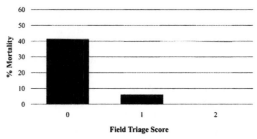

FIGURE 1.—Mortality associated with the combat FTS score. *P* < .05, all scores. (Reprinted from The American Journal of Surgery, Eastridge BJ, Butler F, Wade CE, et al. Field triage score (FTS) in battlefield casualties: validation of a novel triage technique in a combat environment. *Am J Surg.* 2010;200:724-727. Copyright © 2010, with permission from Elsevier Inc.)

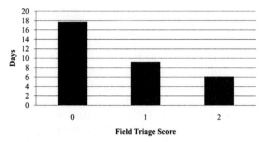

FIGURE 2.—Length of stay associated with the combat FTS. $P < .01$, all scores. (Reprinted from The American Journal of Surgery, Eastridge BJ, Butler F, Wade CE, et al. Field triage score (FTS) in battlefield casualties: validation of a novel triage technique in a combat environment. *Am J Surg.* 2010;200:724-727. Copyright © 2010, with permission from Elsevier Inc.)

triage of the combat casualty. Figs 1 and 2 are included and demonstrate the stratification with respect to length of stay and mortality rate. The application of the FTS in the combat environment could provide a simple and effective tool for classification of patients into categories for patient management in circumstances in which treatment prioritization requires the stratification of multiple simultaneous patients. In addition, this technique may have implications for domestic or foreign disaster or mass casualty situations in which supplies, medical resources, and facilities are limited. Prospective validation of this technique in the prehospital environment is needed.

D. W. Mozingo, MD

Abdominal trauma in primary blast injury
Owers C, Morgan JL, Garner JP (Rotherham NHS Foundation Trust, UK)
Br J Surg 98:168-179, 2011

Background.—Blast injury is uncommon, and remains poorly understood by most clinicians outside regions of active warfare. Primary blast injury (PBI) results from the interaction of the blast wave with the body, and typically affects gas-containing organs such as the ear, lungs and gastrointestinal tract. This review investigates the mechanisms and injuries sustained to the abdomen following blast exposure.

Methods.—MEDLINE was searched using the keywords 'primary blast injury', 'abdominal blast' and 'abdominal blast injury' to identify English language reports of abdominal PBI. Clinical reports providing sufficient data were used to calculate the incidence of abdominal PBI in hospitalized survivors of air blast, and in open- and enclosed-space detonations.

Results.—Sixty-one articles were identified that primarily reported clinical or experimental abdominal PBI. Nine clinical reports provided sufficient data to calculate an incidence of abdominal PBI; 31 ($3 \cdot 0$ per cent) of 1040 hospitalized survivors of air blast suffered abdominal PBI, the incidence ranging from $1 \cdot 3$ to 33 per cent. The incidence for open- and enclosed-space detonations was $5 \cdot 6$ and $6 \cdot 7$ per cent respectively. The

TABLE 1.—Zuckerman's Classification of Blast Injury[67]

Type of Blast Injury	Mechanism of Injury
Primary	Interaction of the blast wave with the body
Secondary	Energized fragments from the bomb itself or environmental debris accelerated by the blast wind
Tertiary	Physical displacement of the body by the blast wind, including tumbling and impact with stationary objects; crush from building collapse caused by blast wind
Quaternary	All other miscellaneous effects, including psychological effects of an explosion, burns and inhalational injury

Editor's Note: Please refer to original journal article for full references.

terminal ileum and caecum were the most commonly affected organs. Surgical management of abdominal PBI is similar to that of abdominal trauma of other causes.

Conclusion.—Abdominal PBI is uncommon but has the potential for significant mortality and morbidity, which may present many days after blast exposure. It is commoner after blast in enclosed spaces and under water (Table 1).

▶ The treatment of blast injuries in general, and those of the abdomen specifically, has traditionally been the expertise of military surgeons. Exceptions include instances of civilian terrorist bombings. Experience over the past 20 years has demonstrated that mass casualty bombing incidents have occurred across the world from London and Madrid to Bali and Oklahoma City involving weapons of mass destruction in civilian life. The frequency of explosive devices being used in acts of terrorism relates to the ready availability of precursor materials and commercial resources for making such devices. With the potential for creating a large number of injured individuals that may overwhelm the capacities of any civilian emergency system, an understanding of the pathophysiology of blast injuries is now required in civilian practice. This selection presents a clear and comprehensive overview of blast injuries with regard to mechanism, diagnosis, and treatment. Table 1 is included, as it reviews the classification of these injuries.

D. W. Mozingo, MD

Analysis of Compliance and Outcomes in a Trauma System With a 2-Hour Transfer Rule
Crandall ML, Esposito TJ, Reed RL, et al (Northwestern Univ, Chicago, IL; Loyola Univ Med Ctr, Maywood, IL)
Arch Surg 145:1171-1175, 2010

Hypothesis.—Minimizing time to definitive care in an effort to optimize outcomes is the goal of trauma systems. Toward this end, some systems have imposed standards on time to interfacility transfer. This study evaluates compliance and outcome in a system with a 2-hour transfer rule.

Design.—Retrospective review.

Setting.—State trauma registry data from 1999 to 2003.

Patients.—Trauma patients who underwent interfacility transfer and those who did not.

Main Outcome Measures.—Time to transfer; Injury Severity Score; mortality; and time to operating room at second facility. These variables were then stratified by time to transfer.

Results.—During the study period, there were 22 447 interfacility transfers. Overall transfer rate was 10.4%. Of the transfers, 4502 (20%) occurred within 2 hours. Median transfer time was 2 hours 21 minutes. Injury Severity Score, mortality, and number of patients with operation performed on same day of transfer were all higher for the group transferred within 2 hours in comparison with patients transferred on the same day of injury at greater than 2 hours.

Conclusions.—While the majority of transfers occur at greater than the mandated 2-hour interval, the most seriously injured patients are reaching definitive care within 2 hours. Markers of acuity for patients transferred at greater than 2 hours parallel those of the general trauma patient population. These data suggest that, in this system, provider-determined transfer time that exceeds 2 hours has no adverse effect on patient outcome. It appears to accomplish recognition and rapid transport of the most seriously ill. This may obviate the need for onerous system mandates that are not feasible or have poor compliance (Fig 2).

▶ This selection was included to demonstrate the analysis of a single state's trauma system compliance with a 2-hour transfer rule and influence on outcomes. Evidence suggests that there is poor compliance with a mandated 2-hour transfer window; however, the most severely injured patients are being recognized early and transferred within the 2-hour standard. It also may be that time to transfer has less influence on mortality than injury severity. Of greater note may be the nature of transfers from level II to level I centers that

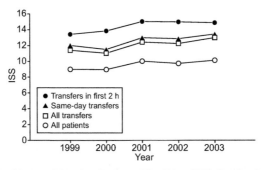

FIGURE 2.—Trend in mean Injury Severity Score (ISS) 1999 to 2003. (Reprinted from Crandall ML, Esposito TJ, Reed RL, et al. Analysis of compliance and outcomes in a trauma system with a 2-hour transfer rule. *Arch Surg.* 2010;145:1171-1175, with permission from American Medical Association.)

appear to be predicated on factors unrelated to injury severity and associated with a perceived reluctance to treat locally. Patients with traumatic brain injury and others with higher injury severity were likely to be transferred promptly. Fig 2 depicts the Injury Severity Score of transfers received over the different time intervals. Regulation of transfer indications, rather than the time to transfer, may be more relevant and beneficial to the system as a whole.

D. W. Mozingo, MD

"Never Be Wrong": The Morbidity of Negative and Delayed Laparotomies After Blunt Trauma
Crookes BA, Shackford SR, Gratton J, et al (Univ of Vermont College of Medicine, Burlington, VT; Scripps Mercy Health, San Diego, CA; et al)
J Trauma 69:1386-1392, 2010

Background.—The objective of this study was to investigate the 30-day morbidity of a negative laparotomy (NEGLAP) in blunt abdominal trauma. No previous work has exclusively examined blunt abdominal trauma patients, used a control group, or determined the complication burden incurred by a NEGLAP.

Methods.—In this retrospective cohort study of a prospectively maintained database, demographics, Injury Severity Score, Revised Trauma Score (TRISS), hospital length of stay, mortality, and findings at laparotomy (LAP) were analyzed. Patients were assigned to four groups as follows: NEGLAP (n = 28), positive LAP (n = 126), delay to LAP (DELAY, n = 18), and no LAP (NOLAP, n = 427). Complications during hospitalization and 30 days postdischarge were extracted from our complication database and adjusted for severity using a complication scoring system (Complication Impact Score [CIS]). The effect of LAP on the log transformed CIS was assessed using a linear regression model, controlling for age and TRISS.

Results.—Complications per patient ranged from 1.73 (DELAY) to 0.38 (NOLAP), and the average CIS per patient ranged from 7.29 (NEGLAP) to 1.8 (NOLAP). When controlled for TRISS and age, NEGLAP did not significantly increase the CIS ($p = 0.620$), whereas positive LAP ($p = 0.004$) and DELAY ($p = 0.034$) were associated with a significant increase in CIS.

Conclusions.—When controlled for TRISS and age, NEGLAP does not increase the complication burden compared with NOLAP. In blunt abdominal trauma patients, operations to establish diagnosis do not add significantly to complication burden (Table 4).

▶ In this selection, the authors present the first study to examine the morbidity of a negative or nontherapeutic trauma laparotomy using a validated concurrent tracking system to enumerate complications that occur during the 30-day perioperative period. It is the first such study to limit the analysis to patients with blunt trauma only, a group in which the decision to operate is often complex because of conflicting priorities in the management of associated injuries. It is

TABLE 4.—Linear Regression Model of the Effect of LAP Group on the Log of CIS

Log (Impact)	Coefficient	SE	95% Confidence Interval From	To	p
Age	0.010	0.003	0.003	0.016	0.003
TRISS	−1.174	0.186	−1.54	−0.808	0.000
NEGLAP	0.108	−0.218	−0.322	0.539	0.62
POSLAP	0.393	0.135	0.127	0.660	0.004
DELAY	0.609	0.285	0.047	1.171	0.034

SE, standard error.

the first study that used control groups of patients with similar Injury Severity Score (ISS) and age to compare morbidity and that used the severity of complications in estimating morbidity. They adequately assess the question of whether a control group is necessary since complications reflect not only the severity of patient illness but also the quality of the processes of care at a given trauma center. It is conceivable that the patients having a negative laparotomy might have the lowest complication rate than any of the trauma patients in previous reports. Without control groups, it is impossible to know the relative morbidity of a negative or nontherapeutic operation.

The authors found that their negative laparotomy group had a complication rate that was no different from patients in the observation group. Although these 2 groups were well matched for age, the ISS of the negative laparotomy group was statistically significantly higher than that of the no laparotomy group. Interestingly, the highest rate of complications per patient occurred in the delay group. They also noted that only 10 complications in the negative laparotomy group could be attributed to the surgery itself, and these were often of minor (90%) or moderate (10%) severity.

D. W. Mozingo, MD

Predictive Value of a Flat Inferior Vena Cava on Initial Computed Tomography for Hemodynamic Deterioration in Patients With Blunt Torso Trauma

Matsumoto S, Sekine K, Yamazaki M, et al (Saiseikai Yokohamashi Tobu Hosp, Tsurumi-ku, Kanagawa, Japan; et al)
J Trauma 69:1398-1402, 2010

Background.—We aimed to investigate the value of the diameter of the inferior vena cava (IVC) on initial computed tomography (CT) to predict hemodynamic deterioration in patients with blunt torso trauma.

Methods.—We reviewed the initial CT scans, taken after admission to emergency room (ER), of 114 patients with blunt torso trauma who were consecutively admitted during a 24-month period. We measured the maximal anteroposterior and transverse diameters of the IVC at the level of the renal vein. Flat vena cava (FVC) was defined as a maximal transverse to anteroposterior ratio of less than 4:1. According to the hemodynamic status, the patients were categorized into three groups. Patients with hemodynamic deterioration after the CT scans were defined as group D (n = 37). The other patients who remained hemodynamically stable after the CT scans were divided into two groups: patients who were hemodynamically stable on ER arrival were defined as group S (n = 60) and those who were in shock on ER arrival and responded to the fluid resuscitation were defined as group R (n = 17).

Results.—The anteroposterior diameter of the IVC in group D was significantly smaller than those in groups R and S (7.6 mm ± 4.4 mm, 15.8 mm ± 5.5 mm, and 15.3 mm ± 4.2 mm, respectively; $p < 0.05$). Of the 93 patients without FVC, 16 (17%) were in group D, 14 (15%) required blood transfusion, and 8 (9%) required intervention. However, of the 21 patients with FVC, all patients were in group D, 20 (95%) required blood transfusion, and 17 (80%) required intervention. The patients with FVC had higher mortality (52%) than the other patients (2%).

Conclusion.—In cases of blunt torso trauma, patients with FVC on initial CT may exhibit hemodynamic deterioration, necessitating early blood transfusion and therapeutic intervention.

▶ In the initial evaluation of patients with blunt trauma, transfusion of crystalloid solutions or blood products is conducted in those with hypotension. Early emergency surgery is required in nonresponders to transfusion loading. On the other hand, further examination is needed to determine whether nonsurgical treatment should be selected in patients with stable hemodynamics and those showing a rapid increase in blood pressure from a hypotensive state after transfusion loading. In these patients, the blood pressure may again become unstable in some patients, requiring further therapeutic intervention. The results of this study showed that independent factors for hemodynamic deterioration include the flat ratio of the inferior vena cava (IVC) and blood pressure on admission and that hemodynamic deterioration could be predicted by evaluating the IVC using CT in the initial treatment of trauma. In this study, the flat vena cava (FVC) sign is the most important factor for predicting therapeutic interventions or hemodynamic deterioration. However, there was a higher incidence in this study than previous reports: 84% of the patients who required interventional treatment had a FVC. This could have been because of a difference in the indication of therapeutic intervention. This interesting finding readily visible on CT scans should alert the trauma team for the potential deterioration of the patient and need for rapid intervention.

D. W. Mozingo, MD

Biomarkers to Predict Wound Healing: The Future of Complex War Wound Management

Hahm G, Glaser JJ, Elster EA (Natl Naval Med Ctr, Bethesda, MD; Naval Med Res Ctr, Silver Spring, MD; Uniformed Services Univ of Health Sciences, Bethesda, MD)

Plast Reconstr Surg 127:21S-26S, 2011

Background.—Currently, no biological assay exists to objectively assess wounds to aid in timing of wound closure and guide therapy. In this article, the authors review military investigations in biomarkers as a method of objectively determining acute traumatic wound physiology and their applicability in predicting healing of complex soft-tissue wounds.

Methods.—The civilian literature related to biomarkers and wound physiology related to chronic and acute wounds was reviewed as a basis for current research into acute traumatic soft-tissue wounds.

Results.—Analysis of serum and wound effluent from traumatic extremity soft-tissue combat wounds revealed changes in specific proinflammatory matrix metalloproteinases associated with impaired wound healing. Forsberg et al. analyzed serum and wound effluent for chemokines and cytokines. An increase in serum procalcitonin levels correlated with wound dehiscence. Lastly, serum, wound effluent, and wound bed tissue biopsy specimens were analyzed by Hawksworth et al. Consistent with previous studies, elevation in proinflammatory cytokines was associated with wound dehiscence.

Conclusions.—Changes in levels of proteases, protease inhibitors, and inflammatory markers have been correlated with wound healing. These findings further support the idea that inflammatory dysregulation and a persistent inflammatory state leads to failure of wound healing in the acute setting. These findings highlight potential targets for the development of a biological assay to individualize management of complex soft-tissue wounds, based on patient physiology and response, that would be applicable to not only military trauma but also civilian trauma. Ultimately, this would result in earlier wound closure, reduction in the number of operating room trips, and reduced health care costs.

▶ Timing of wound closure has been based historically on the subjective assessment of the surgeon. The wound appearance and the overall condition of the patient have been used as determinants in timing of wound closure. In this selection, the authors consider the use of biomarkers to help guide wound closure in particularly complex wounds, such as those incurred on the battlefield. The usual practice may lend to great variability, especially in the war wounded, in the number of operations patients undergo before definitive wound closure. The ability to objectively measure matrix metalloproteinases and their proportional relationship to tissue inhibitors of metalloproteinases correlates to healing of chronic wounds with a decrease in proinflammatory matrix metalloproteinases. Having the ability to objectively assess the suitability of a wound for closure and assess response to therapy based on analysis of tissue, serum, and wound effluent may change wound care management to a more objective assessment of stage of healing. A rapid, reliable, and cost-effective assay needs to be developed before widespread use of this approach is realized in the management of complex soft-tissue wounds. This selection reviews the accomplishments thus far on such an approach.

D. W. Mozingo, MD

Optimal Deployment of Trauma Personnel in the 80-Hour Work Week Era Based on Peak Times of Trauma Patient Arrival
Yaghoubian A, De Virgilio C, Destro L, et al (Harbor-UCLA Med Ctr, Torrance)
Am Surg 76:1039-1042, 2010

In the 80-hour work week era, optimal distribution of the residency workforce is critical. Little data exist as to whether current hours of hospital staffing parallel trends in trauma activity. The purpose of this study was to determine peak periods of trauma volume, severity, need for operative intervention, and mortality and determine if there are differences in mortality based on time period of arrival. We performed a retrospective analysis of the 17,167 patients admitted to our academic Level I trauma center between 2000 and 2007. Each admission was plotted against time of arrival and trends noted. A significant increase in activity occurred between 1700 and 0100 hours. Compared with other shifts, this shift had a disproportionately higher number of patients with penetrating injuries, need for operative intervention, Injury Severity Score (ISS) greater than 15, and death ($P < 0.0001$). After adjusting for ISS and penetrating trauma, arrival time was not predictive of mortality (OR 0.97, CI 0.87–1.08, $P = 0.6$). In conclusion, a peak in trauma activity occurs during an evening shift between 1700 and 0100 hours. In an era of optimizing resident training within the constraints of an 80-hour work week, strong consideration should be made for deploying personnel to match these findings.

▶ Now that the 80-hour workweek is here to stay and may possibly be even shorter in the future, concern has been raised about the effect of shorter duty hours on resident education as well as patient outcome. Using the resident workforce in ways to optimize educational goals and achieve outstanding patient care remains a challenge for many residency programs. Trauma care is different from many other patient care activities at academic institutions since it does not, for the most part, function on an established schedule. The workload of the trauma/acute general surgery service is dependent on the volume of patients in the emergency department and related to the variations in patient arrival times throughout the course of a day. In this selection, the investigators evaluated a single institution's daily trauma activity to determine if any trends could be identified that could optimize how the resident workforce was allocated. In evaluating peak times of activity, they identified that 44% of daily trauma arrivals, 48% of operative traumas, and 44% of severely injured patient admissions occurred during the shift from 1700 to 0100 hours. This evening shift was significantly busier than both the day and night shifts. Increases in both blunt and penetrating trauma admissions seem to contribute to this increase in activity. Whereas 56% of daily penetrating injuries present during these evening hours, the biggest influence on trauma activity is the increase in blunt trauma admissions. They also found that there was no difference in overall mortality between the time intervals studied. They did not evaluate the contribution of an emergency general surgery practice in this evaluation, nor any activities of an emergency inpatient consultation service if that is a component of their current practice. As more programs move toward acute care surgery, paradigms to total practice need to be evaluated.

D. W. Mozingo, MD

Functional Status after Injury: A Longitudinal Study of Geriatric Trauma
Kelley-Quon L, Min L, Morley E, et al (David Geffen School of Medicine at UCLA)
Am Surg 76:1055-1058, 2010

We evaluated self-rated functional status measured longitudinally in the year after injury in a geriatric trauma population. The longitudinal (L) group included 37 of 60 eligible trauma patients aged 65 years or older admitted December 2006 to November 2007 for greater than 24 hours who completed a Short Functional Status questionnaire (SFS) at 3, 6, and 12 months after injury. The SFS yields scores of 0 to 5 (5 = independent in all five activities of daily living [ADLs]) and has been validated among community-dwelling elders. The control (C) group included 63 trauma patients aged 65 years or older admitted December 2007 to July 2009 for greater than 24 hours who reported their preinjury functional status using the SFS at hospital admission. We used characteristics and scores of the C group to impute preinjury ADL scores for the L group. The groups were similar in baseline characteristics (age, ethnicity, Injury Severity Score, Charlson Comorbidity Index, and living arrangement; $P > 0.05$). For the C group, the preinjury ADL score was 4.6 (SD = 0.9). For the L group, ADL scores declined at all intervals reaching statistical significance at 12 months. We conclude that in the year after traumatic injury, geriatric patients lost the equivalent of approximately one ADL, increasing their risk of further functional decline, loss of independence, and death (Table 2).

▶ In this selection, the authors have prospectively described the long-term trajectory of functional capacity among geriatric patients who sustain trauma. This study was undertaken to describe the functional recovery of a small cohort of injured adults in their first year after injury. The investigators measured recovery after traumatic injury using self-reported ability to perform activities of daily living (ADLs) as an indicator of functional status. ADLs were assessed at 3 intervals in the year after injury to explore trends in recovery. They found

TABLE 2.—Functional Decline after Injury

	Months After Injury		
	3 Months (n = 12)	6 Months (n = 17)	12 Months (n = 35)
Calculated L group baseline ADL score	4.2	4.2	4.3
L group ADL score	3.7	3.8	3.3
Total number of ADLs lost	0.5	0.4	1
P	<0.14	<0.11	<0.0001

L, longitudinal; ADLs, activities of daily living.

that this population routinely loses 1 ADL because of their injury as depicted in Table 2. Past studies have shown that a loss of 1 ADL leads to future dependence, increased likelihood of admission to a skilled nursing facility, and increased mortality. Also, in the very elderly population (older than 85 years), once an ADL is lost, it is rarely regained. Clinical consequences may include increased risk of future decline, loss of independence, and mortality. The authors propose that the care of geriatric trauma patients should move beyond prevention of death and speak for multidisciplinary care targeted at prevention of permanent functional impairment.

D. W. Mozingo, MD

3 Burns

Systematic Care Management: A Comprehensive Approach to Catastrophic Injury Management Applied to a Catastrophic Burn Injury Population—Clinical, Utilization, Economic, and Outcome Data in Support of the Model
Kucan J, Bryant E, Dimick A, et al (Paradigm Management Services, Concord, CA; et al)
J Burn Care Res 31:692-700, 2010

The new standard for successful burn care encompasses both patient survival and the burn patient's long-term quality of life. To provide optimal long-term recovery from catastrophic injuries, including catastrophic burns, an outcome-based model using a new technology called systematic care management (SCM) has been developed. SCM provides a highly organized system of management throughout the spectrum of care that provides access to outcome data, consistent oversight, broader access to expert providers, appropriate allocation of resources, and greater understanding of total costs. Data from a population of 209 workers' compensation catastrophic burn cases with a mean TBSA of 27.9% who were managed under the SCM model of care were analyzed. The data include treatment type, cost, return to work, and outcomes achieved. Mean duration of management to achieve all guaranteed outcomes was 20 months. Of the 209 injured workers, 152 (72.7%) achieved sufficient recovery to be released to return to work, of which 97 (46.8%) were both released and competitively employed. Assessment of 10 domains of functional independence indicated that 47.2% of injured workers required total assistance at initiation of SCM. However, at termination of SCM, 84% of those injured workers were fully independent in the 10 functional activities. When compared with other burn research outcome data, the results support the value of the SCM model of care (Table 9).

▶ The goal of burn care is the optimal restoration, rehabilitation, and reintegration of the patient into society, including a return to gainful employment. This report describes the clinical experience of a national catastrophic care management organization in coordinating the care of a large group of burned workers using an established proprietary technology of care management that they call systematic care management. This methodology was developed, applied, and refined over nearly 20 years by a health systems management company specializing in complex clinical conditions such as spinal cord and traumatic brain injury, multiple trauma, and major burns. It was developed as an alternative to current managed care approaches for managing the most complex medical

TABLE 9.—Full SCM Sample vs Control (Industry Match)—Excluding Vocational
Rehabilitation

Return to Work Status	SCM, n (%)	Control (Industry Match Sample), n (%)	Persons χ^2	P (1 Tailed)	CL (95% 1 Tailed)
Released, competitively employed without restrictions	56 (30)	7 (15)	2.1296	.07224	(0.0019, 1)
Released, competitively employed with restrictions	41 (22)	0 (0)	—	—	—
Release employed total	97 (52)	7 (15)	13.9265	.00001	(0.1947, 1)
Released, not competitively employed	55 (29)	7 (15)	1.9565	.08094	(0.0028, 1)
Release not employed total	55 (29)	7 (15)	6.746	.004698	(0.0953, 1)
Overall released to RTW total	152 (81)	14 (30)	27.8484	.000001	(0.2871, 1)
Not released, but competitively employed	1 (1)	0 (0)	—	—	—
Not released, not competitively employed	35 (19)	32 (19)	—	—	—
Overall sample size (N)	188 (100)	46	—	—	—

SCM, systematic care management; RTW, return to work.

challenges such as catastrophic burns. The model provides a comprehensive projection of anticipated care pathways and the clinical results expected for each individual patient. By adopting the philosophy that "the best care is often the most economical," it encourages access to the best treatment centers and programs. Case management consistently provides for proactive intervention into patient problems. Their outcomes are clearly superior to the industry standard. Survival from the burn injury is no longer the standard by which successful burn care should be measured. The individual's quality of life after survival and ongoing improvement in quality of life demand a comprehensive program throughout the entire continuum of care.

D. W. Mozingo, MD

Treatment of heterotopic ossification of the elbow following burn injury: Recommendations for surgical excision and perioperative prophylaxis using radiation therapy
Maender C, Sahajpal D, Wright TW, et al (Univ of Florida, Gainesville)
J Shoulder Elbow Surg 19:1269-1275, 2010

Background.—Heterotopic ossification (HO) is reported to occur in 0.1-3.3% of elbows after a severe burn, and can significantly limit elbow motion and upper extremity function.

Methods.—The study included 9 patients (11 elbows) treated by the senior author (TW). The surgical technique consisted of making multiple small surgical approaches to remove heterotopic ossification (without raising cutaneous flaps) and concomitantly releasing the elbow capsule and skin contracture. Perioperative radiation therapy was performed to decrease heterotopic ossification recurrence. Outcome measures included postoperative elbow range of motion and Mayo Elbow Performance Score.

Results.—The average amount of body surface area burned was 54% (range, 10-86%) and mean time from injury to elbow surgery was 416 days (range, 175-860). All elbows had some degree of direct involvement with the thermal injury. Preoperative arc of motion averaged 39° in flexion/extension and 78° in supination/pronation. Four elbows had complete ankylosis in the flexion/extension plane and 1 had only 5° of motion. At last follow-up, arc of motion in flexion/extension averaged 116° and 139° in supination/pronation, an improvement of 77° and 61°, respectively. One recurrence of HO required re-excision.

Conclusion.—We recommend this multiple-approach surgical technique for treatment of heterotopic ossification and elbow contracture after burn injury, along with perioperative radiation therapy to decrease recurrence. Our surgical approach and treatment resulted in significant gains in elbow motion and upper extremity function with few complications (Fig 1).

▶ Heterotopic ossification (HO) after burn injuries is a rare but well-known complication. The elbow is the most common joint to be affected, and HO

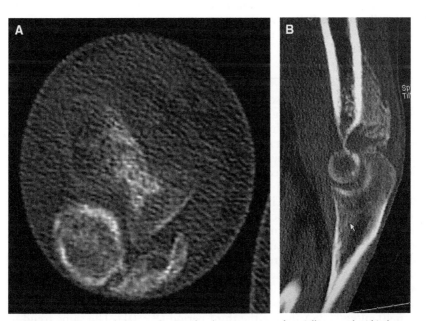

FIGURE 1.—(A) Sagittal CT scan showing the ulnar nerve circumferentially encased within heterotopic bone. (B) Coronal CT scan of same patient showing posterior heterotopic ossification. (Reprinted from Maender C, Sahajpal D, Wright TW, et al. Treatment of heterotopic ossification of the elbow following burn injury: recommendations for surgical excision and perioperative prophylaxis using radiation therapy. *J Shoulder Elbow Surg.* 2010;19:1269-1275, with permission from Journal of Shoulder and Elbow Surgery Board of Trustees.)

has been reported to occur in 0.1% to 3.3% of patients after severe burn. This can significantly affect elbow motion and upper extremity function. Fig 1 depicts the typical location of the HO and entrapment of the ulnar nerve. Outcome of surgical release of contracted elbows and excision of HO because of burns has rarely been reported. The previous studies that have been published have short average follow-up times and relatively high complication rates, including hematomas, wound problems, and HO recurrence. In addition, no studies have reported on functional scores in this population after surgical treatment. Preventing the recurrence of HO is important in this high-risk population, but it is controversial. Options include no prophylaxis, anti-inflammatory medications, and radiation therapy. This is the first reported series using radiation therapy for prophylaxis of HO recurrence about the elbow in burn patients. Also elbow function scores are reported and underscore the significant disability incurred from this complication. In this series, 10 of 11 elbows received perioperative radiation therapy. There was 1 recurrence of HO in a patient who received XRT. The shortcomings of the report, similar to most other series in the literature, are the retrospective nature of the review and lack of long-term follow-up in all the patients.

D. W. Mozingo, MD

The Impact of Opioid Administration on Resuscitation Volumes in Thermally Injured Patients

Wibbenmeyer L, Sevier A, Liao J, et al (The Univ of Iowa Carver College of Medicine, Iowa City)
J Burn Care Res 31:48-56, 2010

Administration of resuscitation volumes far beyond the estimates established by burn-body weight resuscitation formulas has been well documented. The reasons behind this increase are not clear. We sought to determine if our resuscitation volumes had increased and, if so, what factors were related to their increase. A retrospective chart review identified 154 patients admitted with burns greater than 20% of their BSA during the years of 1975−1976 (period 1), 1990−1991 (period 2), and 2006−2007 (period 3). Charts were reviewed for total fluids (crystalloid, colloid, and blood products) and opioids given before admission, during the first 8 hours of treatment, the next 16 hours of treatment, and the following 24 hours of treatment. Opioids were converted to opioid equivalents (OE). Multiple regression analysis was performed to determine the effects of variables of interest and control for confounders. Significance was assumed at the $P < .05$ level. Resuscitation fluid volumes increased significantly among adults from 3.97 ml/kg/%BSA during the first period to 6.40 ml/kg/%BSA during the third period ($P < .01$). The same trend in children <30 kg was not seen ($P = .72$). Fluid administered during the first 24 hours was significantly associated with age, BSA, intubation, latter two study periods, and opioid administration. Fluid administration was consistently associated with opioid administration at all measured time points. At 24 hours postburn, patients who received 2 to 4 OE/kg required an average of additional 3,650 ± 1,704 ml of fluid, those receiving 4 to 6 OE/kg had required an average of 25,154 ± 4,386 ml, and those who received >6 OE kg had required an average of 32,969 ± 3,982 ml. In this single center retrospective study, we have shown a statistically significant increase in resuscitation fluids (from 1975 to 2007) and an association of resuscitation volumes with opioids. Opioids have been shown to increase resuscitation volumes in critically ill patients through both central and peripheral effects on the cardiovascular system. Because increased fluid resuscitation has been associated with adverse consequences in other studies, further research on alternative pain control strategies in thermally injured patients is warranted.

▶ Burn patients have been resuscitated successfully by using formulas based on body weight and burn size for many years. A number of previous reports have documented that resuscitation fluid volumes have greatly surpassed those predicted by body weight and extent of burn. This trend has been associated with increased morbidity and mortality and termed fluid creep by some authors. An increased incidence of abdominal and extremity compartment syndromes, hospital-acquired infections, multiorgan failure, and death have all been associated with increased resuscitation volumes.

The reasons for this trend, although not completely known, are likely multifactorial, including patient-related factors and provider-related factors, such as excessive fluid administration before arrival at the burn center and inconsistent protocol application. The authors of this selection sought to determine the role of changing opioid use in their practice in the increase in resuscitation volume required for reversal of burn shock.

They reported an increase in resuscitation fluids in patients with burns greater than 20% of the body surface area. This trend was evident in the early 1990s, but by the mid 2000s, resuscitation fluid volumes had increased by more than 1.5% of estimated needs. Although increased needs were related to several well-reported variables, they were correlated to administered opioids at all measured time points. This important finding needs to be repeated in a large multicenter trial using a variety of outcome variables. It also suggests the need to consider other nonopioid methods of pain control as adjunctive treatment during resuscitation.

D. W. Mozingo, MD

Early Acute Kidney Injury Predicts Progressive Renal Dysfunction and Higher Mortality in Severely Burned Adults
Mosier MJ, Pham TN, Klein MB, et al (Univ of Washington Burn Ctr at Harborview Med Ctr, Seattle; et al)
J Burn Care Res 31:83-92, 2010

The incidence and prognosis of acute kidney injury (AKI) developing during acute resuscitation have not been well characterized in burn patients. The recently developed Risk, Injury, Failure, Loss, and End-stage (RIFLE) classification provides a stringent stratification of AKI severity and can allow for the study of AKI after burn injury. We hypothesized that AKI frequently develops early during resuscitation and is associated with poor outcomes in severely burned patients. We conducted a retrospective review of patients enrolled in the prospective observational multicenter study "Inflammation and the Host Response to Injury." A RIFLE score was calculated for all patients at 24 hours and throughout hospitalization. Univariate and multivariate analyses were performed to distinguish the impact of early AKI on progressive renal dysfunction, need for renal replacement therapy, and hospital mortality. A total of 221 adult burn patients were included, with a mean TBSA burn of 42%. Crystalloid resuscitation averaged 5.2 ml/kg/%TBSA, with urine output of 1.0 ± 0.6 ml/kg/hr at 24 hours. Sixty-two patients met criteria for AKI at 24 hours: 23 patients (10%) classified as risk, 32 patients (15%) as injury, and 7 (3%) as failure. After adjusting for age, TBSA, inhalation injury, and nonrenal Acute Physiology and Chronic Health Evaluation II ≥ 20, early AKI was associated with an adjusted odds ratio 2.9 for death (95% CI $1.1-7.5$, $P = .03$). In this cohort of severely burned patients, 28% of patients developed AKI during acute resuscitation. AKI was not always transient, with 29% developing progressive renal deterioration by RIFLE criteria. Early AKI was associated with early multiple organ dysfunction and higher mortality risk. Better understanding of how early AKI develops and which patients are at risk for progressive renal dysfunction may lead to improved outcomes.

▶ Acute renal failure with oliguria is uncommon during burn shock resuscitation. Transient oliguria and acute creatinine level elevations are seen commonly during burn resuscitation and are of uncertain prognostic significance. The incidence of acute renal dysfunction in burn units has varied widely from 15% to 40%, and few publications have evaluated the significance of transient renal dysfunction associated with burn resuscitation. The authors of this selection use the Risk, Injury, Failure, Loss, and End-stage (RIFLE) kidney classification system that was developed to characterize the severity of renal dysfunction in critically ill patients. The RIFLE classification system defines 3 grades of increasing severity of acute kidney injury, including risk, injury, and failure, based on changes in either serum creatinine or urine output and 2 outcome categories (loss and end-stage kidney disease). Using the data set of patient outcome variables collected under the Inflammation and Host Response to Injury Study, a collaborative program supported by the National Institute of General Medical Sciences with the primary intent to better define the proteomic and genomic responses to trauma and burn injuries, the authors sought to determine the significance of early and late acute kidney injury on outcome following burn injury. Fig 1 in the original article depicts the outcome of patients developing acute kidney injury during the early hospital course. They demonstrated that acute kidney injury after a burn occurs commonly, with a quarter of patients developing early acute kidney injury and nearly half developing acute kidney injury during the hospital stay. Early acute kidney injury was often progressive and associated with larger total body surface area burns.

D. W. Mozingo, MD

Colloid Administration Normalizes Resuscitation Ratio and Ameliorates "Fluid Creep"
Lawrence A, Faraklas I, Watkins H, et al (Univ of Utah College of Medicine, Salt Lake City)
J Burn Care Res 31:40-47, 2010

Although colloid was a component of the original Parkland formula, it has been omitted from standard Parkland resuscitation for over 30 years. However, some burn centers use colloid as "rescue" therapy for patients who exhibit progressively increasing crystalloid requirements, a phenomenon termed "fluid creep." We reviewed our experience with this procedure. With Institutional Review Board approval, we reviewed all adult patients with ≥20%TBSA burns admitted from January 1, 2005, through December 31, 2007, who completed formal resuscitation. Patients were resuscitated using the Parkland formula, adjusted to maintain urine output of 30 to 50 ml/hr. Patients who required greater amounts of fluid than expected were given a combination of 5% albumin and lactated Ringer's until fluid requirements normalized. Results were expressed as an hourly ratio (I/O ratio) of fluid infusion (ml/kg/%TBSA/hr) to urine output (ml/kg/hr). Predicted values for this ratio vary for individual patients but are usually less than 0.5 to 1.0. Fifty-two patients were reviewed, of whom 26 completed resuscitation using crystalloid alone, and the remaining 26 required albumin supplementation (AR). The groups were comparable in age, gender, weight, mortality, and time between injury and admission. AR patients had larger total and full-thickness burns and more inhalation injuries. Patients managed with crystalloid alone maintained mean resuscitation ratios from 0.13 to 0.40, whereas AR patients demonstrated progressively increasing ratios to a maximum mean of 1.97, until albumin was started. Administration of albumin produced a dramatic and precipitous return of ratios to within predicted ranges throughout the remainder of resuscitation. No patient developed abdominal compartment syndrome. Measuring hourly I/O ratios is an effective means of expressing and tracking fluid requirements. The addition of colloid to Parkland resuscitation rapidly reduces hourly fluid requirements, restores normal resuscitation ratios, and ameliorates fluid creep. This practice can be applied selectively as needed using predetermined algorithms.

▶ The use of colloid solutions for fluid resuscitation has been debated for many years. Most controversies centered around both the cost and risks of colloid administration. Colloid, whether given as plasma, albumin, or hetastarch, is significantly more expensive than crystalloid, and large-volume resuscitation with colloid can be expensive. A long-standing belief that colloid administration is associated with increased mortality among burn patients has also persisted from early studies. Although recent publications have reported the opposite, they have also failed to provide clear data that colloid improves survival. Lack of definitive studies on these issues has permitted the debate over the real value of colloid-based resuscitation to continue. The recent descriptions of fluid creep and a number of reports on abdominal compartment syndrome in burn patients developing during resuscitation prompt us to possibly reconsider other strategies to reduce fluid resuscitation volumes, particularly in patients with extensive burns. In this selection, the authors demonstrate a sharp decline in the I/O ratios in a group of patients who were demonstrating fluid creep and prompt return to normal resuscitation volumes. It is the author's practice to add colloid to the patients' resuscitation regimen when they are demonstrating evidence of increasing fluid requirements or the complications of excessive edema formation. By measuring the I/O ratio, the authors are able to better predict when the addition of colloid solutions would be predicted to markedly alter fluid infusion rates.

D. W. Mozingo, MD

High-frequency percussive ventilation and low tidal volume ventilation in burns: A randomized controlled trial
Chung KK, Wolf SE, Renz EM, et al (U.S. Army Inst of Surgical Res, Fort Sam Houston, TX; et al)
Crit Care Med 38:1970-1977, 2010

Objectives.—In select burn intensive care units, high-frequency percussive ventilation is preferentially used to provide mechanical ventilation in support of patients with acute lung injury, acute respiratory distress syndrome, and inhalation injury. However, we found an absence of prospective studies comparing high-frequency percussive ventilation with contemporary low-tidal volume ventilation strategies. The purpose of this study was to prospectively compare the two ventilator modalities in a burn intensive care unit setting.

Design.—Single-center, prospective, randomized, controlled clinical trial, comparing high-frequency percussive ventilation with low-tidal volume ventilation in patients admitted to our burn intensive care unit with respiratory failure.

Setting.—A 16-bed burn intensive care unit at a tertiary military teaching hospital.

Patients.—Adult patients ≥18 yrs of age requiring prolonged (>24 hrs) mechanical ventilation were admitted to the burn intensive care unit. The study was conducted over a 3-yr period between April 2006 and May 2009. This trial was registered with ClinicalTrials.gov as NCT00351741.

Interventions.—Subjects were randomly assigned to receive mechanical ventilation through a high-frequency percussive ventilation-based strategy (n = 31) or a low-tidal volume ventilation-based strategy (n = 31).

Measurements and Main Results.—At baseline, both the high-frequency percussive ventilation group and the low-tidal volume ventilation group had similar demographics to include median age (interquartile range) (28 yrs [23−45] vs. 33 yrs [24−46], $p =$ nonsignificant), percentage of total body surface area burn (34 [20−52] vs. 34 [23−50], $p =$ nonsignificant), and clinical diagnosis of inhalation injury (39% vs. 35%, $p =$ nonsignificant). The primary outcome was ventilator-free days in the first 28 days after randomization. Intent-to-treat analysis revealed no significant difference between the high-frequency percussive ventilation and the low-tidal volume ventilation groups in mean (± SD) ventilator-free days (12 ± 9 vs. 11 ± 9, $p =$ nonsignificant). No significant difference was detected between groups for any of the secondary outcome measures to include mortality except the need for "rescue" mode application ($p = .02$). Nine (29%) in the low-tidal volume ventilation arm did not meet predetermined oxygenation or ventilation goals and required transition to a rescue mode. By contrast, two in the high-frequency percussive ventilation arm (6%) required rescue.

Conclusions.—A high-frequency percussive ventilation-based strategy resulted in similar clinical outcomes when compared with a low-tidal volume ventilation-based strategy in burn patients with respiratory failure. However, the low-tidal volume ventilation strategy failed to achieve ventilation and oxygenation goals in a higher percentage necessitating rescue ventilation (Fig 2).

▶ High-frequency percussive ventilation (HFPV) is a pneumatically driven, pressure-limited, time-cycled mode of ventilation that delivers high-frequency

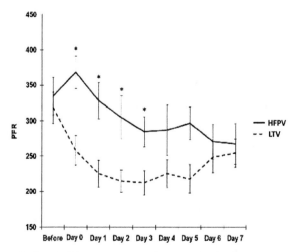

^HFPV denotes high frequency percussive ventilation, LTV denotes low-tidal volume ventilation, PFR denotes PaO₂/FiO₂ ratio.

FIGURE 2.—Comparison of the ratio of the partial pressure of arterial oxygen (Pa_{O_2}) to fraction of inspiratory oxygen (Fi_{O_2}). Data points are depicted as mean ± SEM *$p < .05$. (Reprinted from Chung KK, Wolf SE, Renz EM, et al. High-frequency percussive ventilation and low tidal volume ventilation in burns: a randomized controlled trial. *Crit Care Med.* 2010;38:1970-1977, with permission from the Society of Critical Care Medicine and Lippincott Williams & Wilkins).

bursts of gas superimposed on a biphasic inspiratory and expiratory pressure cycle set at 10 to 15 cycles per minute. After inhalation injury, the percussive airflow delivered by HFPV is believed to facilitate airway clearance of secretions and debris from epithelial sloughing, hemorrhage, and inflammation. Previous case-control studies demonstrated a decrease in the incidence of ventilator-associated pneumonia in patients with inhalation injury when supported with HFPV compared with conventional modes of ventilation. When compared with conventional ventilation, it has also been shown to improve gas exchange at lower peak and mean airway pressures in various patient populations. To date, only 1 prospective randomized controlled trial has been performed in adult burn patients involving 35 subjects with inhalation injury, which demonstrated improved oxygenation early during treatment, but no difference in later outcomes was realized. In this selection, the authors were the first to compare, in a randomized controlled fashion, HFPV with another low-tidal volume ventilation strategy in severely burned adult patients. By the intent-to-treat principle, there was no detectable difference in the primary end point of ventilator-free days in the first 28 days between an HFPV group and the low-tidal volume ventilation group. However, a large percentage of the low-tidal volume ventilation group required ventilation rescue by initiating other forms of ventilation, clouding the true results of the study.

D. W. Mozingo, MD

A randomized, controlled trial of immersive virtual reality analgesia, during physical therapy for pediatric burns

Schmitt YS, Hoffman HG, Blough DK, et al (Univ of Washington, Seattle; et al)
Burns 37:61-68, 2011

This randomized, controlled, within-subjects (crossover design) study examined the effects of immersive virtual reality as an adjunctive analgesic technique for hospitalized pediatric burn inpatients undergoing painful physical therapy. Fifty-four subjects (6—19 years old) performed range-of-motion exercises under a therapist's direction for 1—5 days. During each session, subjects spent equivalent time in both the virtual reality and the control conditions (treatment order randomized and counterbalanced). Graphic rating scale scores assessing the sensory, affective, and cognitive components of pain were obtained for each treatment condition. Secondary outcomes assessed subjects' perception of the virtual reality experience and maximum range-of-motion. Results showed that on study day one, subjects reported significant decreases (27—44%) in pain ratings during virtual reality. They also reported improved affect ("fun") during virtual reality. The analgesia and affect improvements were maintained with repeated virtual reality use over multiple therapy sessions. Maximum range-of-motion was not different between treatment conditions, but was significantly greater after the second treatment condition (regardless of treatment order). These results suggest that immersive virtual reality is an effective nonpharmacologic, adjunctive pain reduction technique in the pediatric burn population undergoing painful rehabilitation therapy. The magnitude of the analgesic effect is clinically meaningful and is maintained with repeated use.

▶ The results of this study suggest that immersive virtual reality is a useful and powerful adjunct for enhancing pain control during rehabilitation therapy in pediatric burn patients. When added to standard pharmacologic analgesia, virtual reality distraction therapy produced a statistically significant and clinically meaningful reduction in subjective patient pain ratings, as well as a significant increase in perceived fun. The concern for potential negative side effects of opioids in the pediatric population, as well as the widespread need for more effective nonpharmacologic adjuncts, supports continued research into the efficacy of virtual reality analgesia. Additional research is also warranted to investigate the mechanisms and ideal applications of virtual reality pain reduction techniques. There were several limitations in study design that may influence future studies. In this crossover design, both therapists and patients were aware of the treatment group assignment, and this may have influenced compliance and participation effort. If larger multicenter trials are considered, a between-group analysis might be helpful.

D. W. Mozingo, MD

Optimizing initial vancomycin dosing in burn patients
Elligsen M, Walker SAN, Walker SE, et al (Sunnybrook Health Sciences Centre, Toronto, Ontario, Canada)
Burns 37:406-414, 2011

Rationale.—Burned patients have altered vancomycin pharmacokinetics necessitating adjusted dosing. Published initial dosing recommendations to target troughs of 15—20 mg/L for this population are lacking.

Objective.—This study was conducted to develop initial vancomycin dosing recommendations based on the pharmacokinetics of vancomycin in acute burn patients.

Methods.—A retrospective chart review of 49 vancomycin treated burn patients was conducted. Mean pharmacokinetic parameters were determined and Monte Carlo Simulation was used to develop initial vancomycin dosing recommendations that target trough concentrations between 15 and 20 mg/L.

Results.—Vancomycin pharmacokinetic parameters were significantly ($p < 0.05$) different for vancomycin levels obtained 48 h to 14 days after burn versus >14 days after burn. Monte Carlo simulation indicated that the most commonly used empiric dosing regimen (1 g iv q12 h) attained targets with a probability of <10% in all burned patients. The probability of attaining targets was optimized to 20-25% by using 1.5 g iv q8 h, 1.75 g iv q8 h, 1 g iv q6 h, 1.25 g iv q6 h or 750 mg iv q4 h in patients 48 h to 14 days after burn and 1—1.25 g iv q8 h or 500 mg iv q4 h in patients >14 days after burn.

Conclusions.—This study provides initial vancomycin dosing recommendations for burned patients 48 h to 14 days after burn and patients >14 days after burn. However, because of the heterogeneity in pharmacokinetics and the observation that vancomycin pharmacokinetics change with time after burn, monitoring of vancomycin serum concentrations is required to ensure targets are met and maintained.

▶ Approximately half of the mortality seen in burns that survive initial resuscitation is related to the development of infectious complications. Clinical outcomes in critically ill patients with severe infection are worsened significantly when there is a delay in the administration of appropriate antimicrobial therapy, which would include inadequate dosing. Infections caused by *Staphylococcus aureus*, including methicillin-resistant strains, are particularly common in burn care, and treatment with vancomycin is often prescribed in this patient population. To optimize the probability of clinical cure in a patient with a serious infection caused by methicillin-resistant *S aureus*, vancomycin steady state serum trough concentrations between 15 and 20 mg/L are currently targeted. This selection was chosen because the authors point out the importance of assessing the day postburn when the treatment is to be initiated in helping to prescribe an appropriate initial dose. This selection offers practical advice yet provides detailed background information and pharmacokinetic analysis.

D. W. Mozingo, MD

Association Between Dietary Fat Content and Outcomes in Pediatric Burn Patients
Lee JO, Gauglitz GG, Herndon DN, et al (Univ of Texas Med Branch, Galveston)
J Surg Res 166:e83-e90, 2011

Background.—The aim of the study was to compare a low fat/high-carbohydrate diet and a high-fat diet on clinical outcomes by a retrospective cohort study.

Methods.—Nine hundred forty-four children with burns ≥ 40% of their total body surface area (TBSA) were divided into two groups: patients receiving Vivonex T.E.N. (low-fat/high-carbohydrate diet; $n = 518$) and patients receiving milk (high-fat diet; $n = 426$). Patient demographics, caloric intake, length of hospital stay, and incidence of sepsis, mortality, hepatic steatosis, and organomegaly at autopsy were determined.

Results.—Demographics and caloric intake were similar in both groups. Patients receiving Vivonex T.E.N. had shorter (intensive care unit) ICU stays (Vivonex T.E.N.: 31 ± 2 d; milk: 47 ± 2 d; $P < 0.01$), shorter ICU stay per % TBSA burn (Vivonex T.E.N.: 0.51 ± 0.02 d/%; milk: 0.77 ± 0.03 d/%; $P < 0.01$), lower incidence of sepsis (Vivonex T.E.N.: 11%; milk: 20%; $P < 0.01$), and lived significantly longer until death than those receiving milk (Vivonex T.E.N.: 20 ± 3 d; milk: 10 ± 2 d; $P < 0.01$). There was no difference in overall mortality between the two groups (Vivonex T.E.N.:15% versus milk: 13%; $P < 0.9$). Autopsies revealed decreased hepatic steatosis and decreased enlargement of kidney and spleen in patients receiving Vivonex T.E.N.

Conclusions.—The period with a low-fat/high-carbohydrate diet was associated with lower LOS, decreased incidence of organomegaly, infection, and hepatic steatosis post-burn compared with the period when a high-fat diet was used. These associations indicate the benefit of high carbohydrate/low fat nutrition; however, the findings in these time periods can also be likely due to the multifactorial effects of advances in burn care. We believe that these results have some relevance because high fat is associated with poorer outcomes compared with low fat.

▶ The metabolic consequences of severe burns are profound, and altering this response constitutes an ongoing challenge for successful burn outcomes. The release of inflammatory mediators and major hormonal changes lead to profound metabolic abnormalities postburn. Increased endogenous catecholamines cause increased rates of protein catabolism and accelerate muscle proteolysis as well as increase lipolysis.

Metabolic rates of burn patients can dramatically exceed those of other critically ill or traumatic patients and cause marked wasting of lean body mass within days after injury. This hypermetabolism and catabolism of muscle protein continues up to 6 to 9 months after a severe burn. Failure to meet the subsequent large calorie and protein requirements may result in impaired wound healing, organ dysfunction, susceptibility to infection, and death. Thus, adequate nutrition is imperative for the treatment of severely burned patients. The authors of this selection have previously shown that nutritional support of the hypermetabolic response in severely burned patients can abate the hypermetabolic response to a burn. Significant alterations in the metabolism of lipids, carbohydrates, and proteins determine the caloric makeup of the nutritional source to be provided to these patients. The authors have clearly demonstrated the importance of restricting fat in the provision of nutritional support to these complex patients. What was probably considered as multiple organ failure syndrome with hepatic dysfunction in the past was actually hepatic dysfunction due to overfeeding, as many severely burned patients developed fatty liver.

D. W. Mozingo, MD

Blood Product Transfusion: Does Location Make a Difference?
Palmieri TL, Sen S, Falwell K, et al (Shriners Hosp for Children Northern California and the Univ of California, Davis)
J Burn Care Res 32:61-65, 2011

Early blood product administration during acute blood loss may improve outcomes, yet blood product transfusion for anemia of critical illness has been associated with increased mortality. After major burn injury, patients have two sources of anemia: massive acute blood loss during excision and insidious losses in the intensive care unit (ICU). The purpose of this study was to assess the relationship between the administration of fresh frozen plasma (FFP), platelets, and cryoprecipitate and outcomes in children with major burn injury. This was a retrospective review of children admitted with >20% TBSA burn from 2006 to 2009. Parameters measured included demographics, injury characteristics, operations, blood product transfusions, and outcomes. A total of 143 children received a mean of 3342 ± 283 ml blood. Nonsurvivors had larger burns (62.1 ± 4.6% vs 41.0 ± 1.5% TBSA, $P < .001$) and received similar amounts of packed red blood cells (PRBCs) during hospitalization (12.8 ± 2.4 units vs 10.9 ± 1.0 units, $P = .5$) than survivors. Nonsurvivors received more total units of FFP during hospitalization than survivors (8.0 ± 1.7 units vs 3.1 ± 0.4 units, $P < .0001$) because of the FFP units transfused in the ICU (5.5 ± 1.2 units vs 1.1 ± 0.2 units, $P < .0001$). The overall FFP:PRBC transfusion ratio in survivors was 1:4, whereas mean FFP:PRBC volume ratio in nonsurvivors was 3:4 ($P < .0001$). Nonsurvivors received more platelets (3.4 ± 1.0 units vs 0.50 ± 0.1 units, $P < .001$) and cryoprecipitate (1.9 ± 0.9 units vs 0.3 ± 0.1 units, $P < .001$) than survivors, both in the operating room and in the ICU. Blood product use in children with severe burns is associated with increased mortality. Appropriate use of blood products may need to be different in the operating room (massive acute hemorrhage) vs the ICU (ongoing red cell senescence) (Table 4).

▶ Major burn injury frequently results in massive transfusion. A multicenter study reported that the mean number of packed red blood cell (PRBC) transfusions for patients with burn injury greater than 20% total body surface area (TBSA) was 10 units. Likewise, children also receive large numbers of blood transfusions during the course of burn care, particularly in the operating room. Excision of extremity and trunk burns in children results in the loss of approximately 2% blood volume/TBSA excised. Major burn excisions may require massive transfusion. Therapies that have shown improved outcomes in massive transfusion in other causes of hemorrhage, such as the early use of fresh frozen plasma (FFP) and other blood products, may very well benefit patients undergoing a major burn excision. The authors of this selection hypothesized that children receiving a higher ratio of FFP:PRBC or other

TABLE 4.—FFP:PRBC Ratio

	Survivors (n = 128)	Nonsurvivors (n = 15)
Total FFP:PRBC (ratio)	0.25 ± 0.03 (1:4)	0.75 ± 0.2* (3:4)
FFP:PRBC in OR (ratio)	0.25 ± 0.02 (1:4)	0.39 ± 0.07 (1:2.5)
FFP:PRBC in ICU (ratio)	0.23 ± 0.04 (1:4)	0.96 ± 0.23* (1:1)

OR, operating room; ICU, intensive care unit; FFP, fresh frozen plasma; PRBC, packed red blood cells.
*$P < .001$, survivors vs nonsurvivors.

blood products (cryoprecipitate or platelets) during periods of acute blood loss would receive fewer units of blood and have improved survival. However, patients receiving more FFP, platelets, and cryoprecipitate in this study had worse outcomes. Previous reports have cited an increased risk of mortality with increased FFP as well as with increased use of platelets and cryoprecipitate. This may be because of the increased severity of illness of nonsurvivors; however, it may also be because of the adverse effects of blood products in general. Recent studies in patients who experienced trauma suggest that the improvements seen with aggressive FFP use actually represent a survival bias based on the time frame chosen for the study as opposed to a true improvement. This suggests that a more aggressive approach to intraoperative repletion of coagulation factors may decrease subsequent need for FFP, platelet, and cryoprecipitate in the intensive care unit. This study confirms the detrimental effects of transfusion, but the optimal ratios will need to be defined in further studies.

D. W. Mozingo, MD

Colloid Normalizes Resuscitation Ratio in Pediatric Burns
Faraklas I, Lam U, Cochran A, et al (Univ of Utah Health Sciences Ctr, Salt Lake City)
J Burn Care Res 32:91-97, 2011

Fluid resuscitation of burned children is challenging because of their small size and intolerance to over- or underresuscitation. Our American Burn Association-verified regional burn center has used colloid "rescue" as part of our pediatric resuscitation protocol. With Institutional Review Board approval, the authors reviewed children with ≥15% TBSA burns admitted from January 1, 2004, to May 1, 2009. Resuscitation was based on the Parkland formula, which was adjusted to maintain urine output. Patients requiring progressive increases in crystalloid were placed on a colloid protocol. Results were expressed as an hourly resuscitation ratio (I/O ratio) of fluid infusion (ml/kg/%TBSA/hr) to urine output (ml/kg/hr). We reviewed 53 patients; 29 completed resuscitation using crystalloid alone (lactated Ringer's solution [LR]), and 24 received colloid supplementation albumin (ALB). Groups were comparable in age, gender, weight, and time from injury to admission. ALB patients had more inhalation injuries and larger total and full-thickness burns. LR patients maintained a median I/O of 0.17 (range, 0.08—0.31), whereas ALB patients demonstrated escalating ratios until the institution of albumin produced a precipitous return of I/O comparable with that of the LR group. Hospital stay was lower for LR patients than ALB patients (0.59 vs 1.06 days/% TBSA, $P = .033$). Twelve patients required extremity or torso escharotomy, but this did not differ between groups. There were no decompressive laparotomies. The median resuscitation volume for ALB group was greater than LR group (9.7 vs 6.2 ml/kg/%TBSA, $P = .004$). Measuring hourly I/O is a helpful means of evaluating fluid demands during burn shock

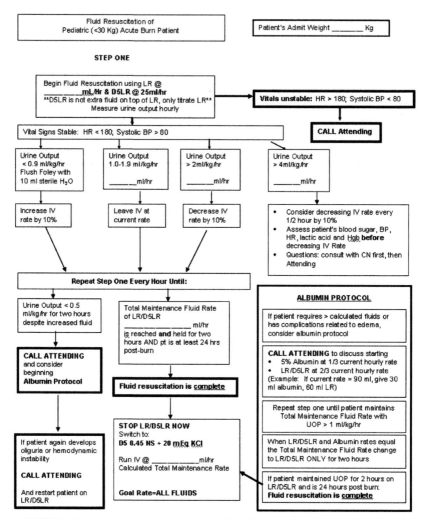

FIGURE 1.—Pediatric resuscitation protocol currently used in burn center. (Reprinted from Faraklas I, Lam U, Cochran A, et al. Colloid normalizes resuscitation ratio in pediatric burns. *J Burn Care Res.* 2011;32:91-97, with permission from the American Burn Association.)

resuscitation. The addition of colloid restores normal I/O in pediatric patients (Fig 1).

▶ Fluid creep, a term coined by Basil A. Pruitt Jr, MD, reflects the insidious tendency for burn patients to require increasing volumes of resuscitation fluid. This problem is likely multifactorial in nature and driven by increasing narcotic and benzodiazepine infusions during resuscitation and the ongoing oncotic dilution with aggressive crystalloid infusion. The authors of this selection have previously shown that using a ratio of the hourly fluid intake (I) to urine output (O) in burned adults, the occurrence of fluid creep could be detected more rapidly regardless of burn size. They also showed that adult patients who are difficult to resuscitate and experience fluid creep responded promptly to the introduction of colloids with a rapid return of the I/O ratio to normal, presumably preventing further complications. The authors of this selection have successfully integrated a similar approach in their pediatric burn population. Included in this review is Fig 1 from their article, which demonstrates their current clinical approach to pediatric burn fluid resuscitation.

D. W. Mozingo, MD

Adherence to Burn Center Referral Criteria: Are Patients Appropriately Being Referred?

Carter JE, Neff LP, Holmes JH IV (Wake Forest Univ Baptist Med Ctr, Winston-Salem, NC)
J Burn Care Res 31:26-30, 2010

The American Burn Association (ABA) has an established set of criteria for burn center referral to guide healthcare providers and improve patient outcomes. As U.S. healthcare becomes increasingly focused on improving quality of care (ie, pay-for-performance initiatives), assessing and monitoring the referral patterns to burn centers is critical in providing optimal burn care. Few studies have compared admission, treatment, and discharge patterns at burn centers and nonburn centers. Our goal was to compare practice and referral guidelines for patients with burn injuries by reviewing every discharge record in our state over a 2-year period. The study was conducted in a retrospective fashion using our state's hospital association patient database of International Classification of Diseases, 9th revision (ICD-9) discharge codes, querying 940.00 to 948.99, over the period of October 1, 2005, to September 30, 2007. Additional variables abstracted included the discharging hospital, outcome, race, gender, payor status, length of stay, procedures, and age. Adherence to referral criteria was established by comparing the discharge ICD-9 codes with the burn center referral criteria established by the ABA and American College of Surgeons Committee on Trauma in Guidelines for the Operation of Burn Centers. Injury patterns were analyzed using the 2 burn centers in our state and the remaining 107 nonburn centers providing care to burn patients. A total of 2036 adult patients aged 18 to 106 years sustained burn injuries requiring hospital admission, and 1416 (70%) met ABA referral criteria based on ICD-9 codes. Of the 1084 patients treated at burn centers, 88% met referral criteria. Of the 952 burns treated entirely at nonburn centers, 48% met referral criteria but were not transferred. The most common burns treated at nonburn centers included injuries to the hand, wrist, face, neck, and lower extremity. The mean number of criteria met by patients treated at nonburn centers was 1.5, and all deaths occurring at nonburn centers met referral criteria. A significantly higher percentage of patients with Medicare were not transferred from nonburn centers ($P \leq .00001$), and a significantly higher percentage of patients were discharged to nursing homes as opposed to home ($P = .01$) from nonburn centers. Forty-seven percent of the patients sustaining burn injuries in our state receive all of their acute inpatient care at nonburn centers, and almost half of these met ABA burn center referral criteria. Given the disparity in discharge placement and immediate availability of burn specialists in our state, all patients meeting ABA referral criteria should be referred to burn centers. More focused outreach and education for initial providers may help improve access and referral to burn centers.

▶ This selection was chosen since it demonstrates that a significant number of patients with burn injuries meeting the American Burn Association referral criteria are not referred to burn centers. Also, the data show that a significant portion of burn care is occurring at centers without the expertise of multidisciplinary burn care teams. Fig 1 in the original article demonstrates the breakdown on where patients receive care. The data also report a large number of the burn surgical procedures occurring at nonburn centers and performed on patients who do meet referral criteria for specialized burn care at a burn center. In this study, nonburn centers discharge a larger proportion of patients to skilled nursing facilities and a smaller proportion home than their burn center counterparts. For decades, the multidisciplinary team approach to burn care has been the cornerstone of improvements in this specialty. All cases of extensive burns and more complex patients are undoubtedly sent to burn centers but not until performance incentives or outcome metrics are applied to the care of thermally injured patients. Will all those patients who deserve this care be referred?

D. W. Mozingo, MD

Cultured Epithelial Autografts for Coverage of Large Burn Wounds in Eighty-Eight Patients: The Indiana University Experience

Sood R, Roggy D, Zieger M, et al (Indiana Univ School of Medicine, Indianapolis; et al)
J Burn Care Res 31:559-568, 2010

Since 1990, the authors have used a new technique for coverage of large burns, which begins with early tangential excision and coverage with cadaver allograft (A), followed by placement of cultured epithelial autograft (CEA) onto an allodermis base (CEA/A). They present their 18-year experience (1990–present) using CEA in 88 patients (20 children and 68 adults) with age range of 6 months to 73 years. A review of prospectively collected data was conducted on adult and pediatric patients grafted with CEA at the Indiana University Medical Center for definitive wound coverage (TBSA 28–98%). These patients were followed up for 3 to 90 months. Complications, take rates, and outpatient follow-ups were noted. The mean final take rate of CEA/A was 72.7%, and the overall patient survival rate was 91% (80 of 88 patients). Complications were classified as early and late, they included: (early) blistering and shearing (31%), pruritis and itching (4.7%), (late) CEA loss (2 patients, 2.3%), and wound contractures (66%). Contracture releases were performed on 32 patients (36%); of which, 18 were children (56%). Cultured keratinocytes provide an excellent alternative or adjunct to conventional split-thickness skin grafting in treating large burn wounds. A dedicated team of physicians, nurses, and therapists well rehearsed in CEA care are vital for success in keratinocyte grafting. The final graft take of 72.7% with a 91% overall survival rate gives much optimism for continuing to use CEA in critically burned patients (Table 6).

▶ This series of 88 patients treated with cultured epithelial autografts (CEAs) at Indiana University is the largest series published on this topic. Their 72.7% average final take rate of CEA and our 91% survival rate in 88 severely burned patients are impressive. This selection is included because it provides a thorough review of the topic and has many practical aspects of this technique outlined in the different sections. They identify a 7-stage plan of care that is included as Table 6. Also, they provide a list of nontoxic antimicrobials that may be useful for topical application when CEAs are used. The authors describe their preoperative, intraoperative,

TABLE 6.—CEA Patient Seven Stage Plan of Care

Stage A	Identify appropriate patient for CEA	>50% TBSA limited donor sites
Stage B	Obtain biopsy and send to laboratory	A 2 × 6-cm specimen of unburned tissue obtained sterically and placed in nutrient solution provided by the laboratory
Stage C	Wound preparation	Total excision completed by PBD 5–7. All wounds covered with thick cryopreserved allograft. Return to the operating room every 3–5 days to maximize engraftment of allograft. 3–4 days before CEA—obtain swab and quantitative cultures
Stage D	CEA placement	Remove allograft epidermis and reexcise wounds if necessary. Obtain swab/quantitative cultures of the wound bed. Place CEA. Dress with bridal veil and dry gauze—topicals if needed
Stage E	Postoperative care	CEA exposed to air 2 or more times/d. Topicals used as indicated. Therapy (OT/PT) held
Stage F	CEA takedown	Performed at the bedside (POD 7–10) Use Shur Clens to aid in removal of adherent backings
Stage G	Post-takedown	Initiate therapy (OT/PT). Resume hydrotherapy. If wound cultures are negative, then dry dressings. If wound cultures are positive, then topical antimicrobials

CEA, cultured epithelial autograft; *POD*, postoperative day; *PBD*, postburn day; *OT/PT*, occupational therapy/physiotherapy.

and postoperative care in a step-by-step manner. Their outcomes are well described and potential pitfalls and complications discussed.

D. W. Mozingo, MD

Patient Safety Measures in Burn Care: Do National Reporting Systems Accurately Reflect Quality of Burn Care?
Mandell SP, Robinson EF, Cooper CL, et al (Harborview Med Ctr, Seattle, WA; Harborview Med Ctr Quality Improvement, Seattle, WA)
J Burn Care Res 31:125-129, 2010

Recently, much attention has been placed on quality of care metrics and patient safety. Groups such as the University Health-System Consortium (UHC) collect and review patient safety data, monitor healthcare facilities, and often report data using mortality and complication rates as outcomes. The purpose of this study was to analyze the UHC database to determine if it differentiates quality of care across burn centers. We reviewed UHC clinical database (CDB) fields and available data from 2006 to 2008 for the burn product line. Based on the September 2008 American Burn Association (ABA) list of verified burn centers, we categorized centers as American Burn Association-verified burn centers, self-identified burn centers, and other centers that are not burn units but admit some burn patients. We compared total burn admissions, risk pool, complication rates, and mortality rates. Overall mortality was compared between the UHC and National Burn Repository. The UHC CDB provides fields for number of admissions, % intensive care unit admission, risk pool, length of stay, complication profiles, and mortality index. The overall numbers of burn patients in the database for the study period included 17,740 patients admitted to verified burn centers (mean 631 admissions/burn center/yr or per 2 years), 10,834 for self-identified burn centers (mean 437 admissions/burn center/yr or per 2 years), and 1,487 for other centers (mean 11.5 admissions/burn center/yr or per 2 years). Reported complication rates for verified burn centers (21.6%), self-identified burn centers (21.3%), and others (20%) were similar. Mortality rates were highest for self-identified burn centers (3.06%), less for verified centers (2.88%), and lowest for other centers (0.74%). However, these outcomes data may be misleading, because the risk pool criteria do not include burn-specific risk factors, and the inability to adjust for injury severity prevents rigorous comparison across centers. Databases such as the UHC CDB provide a potential to benchmark quality of care. However, reporting quality data for trauma and burns requires stringent understanding of injury data collection. Although quality measures are important for improving patient safety and establishing benchmarks for complication and mortality rates, caution must be taken when applying them to specific product lines.

▶ A huge emphasis has been placed on improving the quality of health care in the United States since the Institute of Medicine published their findings in

2001. Since that time, an increasing focus on monitoring and improving the quality of health care delivery has targeted performance at an institutional level. These monitoring agencies include governmental organizations, professional organizations, or private corporations evaluating and reporting quality care. Recently, medical specialties have begun to focus on quality improvement programs specific to their disciplines. The burn community has made the first step in this process by publishing a consensus article on the definition of infections and sepsis in burns, but a formal quality improvement program that is burn specific has yet to be established. The University Health-System Consortium (UHC) has been reporting burn-specific quality data for several years. Formed in 1984, the UHC is an alliance of 103 academic medical centers and 210 of their affiliated hospitals, representing approximately 90% of the nation's academic medical centers. The UHC currently sends reports to participating institutions rating quality of care in the burn product line. Care must be taken when using the UHC analysis since it includes verified burn centers, self-designated burn centers, and nonburn centers caring for burn patients (see Table 1 in the original article). Like institutions need to be compared when using these data. The authors of this selection have carefully reviewed the extent to which the UHC data are useful for burn center quality analysis. They point out a number of shortcomings associated with this approach, including the difficulty of obtaining outcome analysis other than mortality rates.

D. W. Mozingo, MD

Anemia of Thermal Injury: Combined Acute Blood Loss Anemia and Anemia of Critical Illness

Posluszny JA Jr, Gamelli RL (Loyola Univ Med Ctr Burn and Shock Trauma Inst, Maywood, IL)
J Burn Care Res 31:229-242, 2010

Background.—Severe burn injury is often complicated by anemia and the adverse events that accompany transfusion to treat the anemia. Interventions to manage anemia may be facilitated by dividing the anemia of thermal injury into acute blood loss anemia occurring early and related to surgical techniques, including tourniquets and epinephrine tumescence, and anemia of critical illness, which develops later, during wound healing and resolution of the critical injury.

Causes of Anemia.—Acute blood loss anemia results from surgical management of the burn wound, direct erythrocyte destruction, and increased red blood cell (RBC) sequestration. Estimated blood loss (EBL) varies with the techniques used, transfusion thresholds related to current standard practice, and individual preferences. Ways to determine EBL include combining differences in preoperative and postoperative hemoglobin concentrations with volume of transfusion, using surgical and anesthesia team estimates, measuring areas of grafting and debridement and dividing or multiplying by predetermined constants, using complex formulas based on patient age, weight, and area of excision, weighing laparotomy pads pre- and post-surgery, and using a swab washing machine to measure blood on gowns and drapes. Increased blood loss risk factors include excision surface area, percentage of third-degree burns, and longer time until first wound excision. Accurate preoperative EBLs help prepare for transfusion needs and avoid unnecessary cross matching, which is wasteful, costly, and time consuming.

Anemia of critical illness persists after the initial acute event resolves and results from the inability to produce enough RBCs to meet body needs. This multifactorial entity is an acute form of anemia of chronic disease and is related to wound care, phlebotomy, impaired nutrition and metabolism, blunted erythropoietin (EPO) production and/or response, and reprioritization of bone marrow cell production. Dressing change blood loss and laboratory sample collection contribute minimally. It can be difficult to incorporate the multiple techniques or therapies needed to achieve small reductions in blood loss into clinical practice, although these efforts can collectively reduce transfusion rates significantly. The mechanisms producing blunted erythropoiesis remain an enigma.

Transfusion Rates and Effects.—As burn size increases, the need for transfusion is more likely. Severe burn injuries require massive transfusions because of surgical blood loss from extensive excision and grafting and because of impaired erythropoiesis related to severe illness. Cardiac disease, acute respiratory distress syndrome, and age can also increase transfusion rates.

Blood products are transfused for acute anemia management, restoring hemoglobin concentration through the donor RBCs. The result is improved oxygen-carrying capacity, better cardiac function, and less cellular damage from hypoxia. However, packed RBC (pRBC) transfusions can transmit infectious diseases and produce an adverse immunomodulatory effect on patient morbidity and mortality, especially in critically ill patients. Transfusion-related acute lung injury (TRALI) can also occur. TRALI is defined as a new episode of acute lung injury (ALI) during or within 6 hours of a completed transfusion but not temporally related to a competing ALI. TRALI is not well-documented in burn patients and may require unique diagnostic clarifiers.

Reducing Transfusions.—Techniques to limit transfusions should diminish infectious complications and improve morbidity and mortality in burn patients without interfering with wound healing or organ perfusion. Administering exogenous recombinant human EPO (rhEPO) can augment the effects of endogenous EPO and increase RBC production. Tourniquet placement with and without previous limb exsanguination during excision and/or grafting, epinephrine tumescence, and the combination of these techniques can reduce transfusion requirements. Transfusions can be restricted with the goal of keeping hemoglobin concentration at 7 g/dl in burn patients.

Conclusions.—Severely burned patients require massive transfusions to manage the acute blood loss associated with surgery and the blunted erythropoiesis related to anemia of critical illness. Viewing anemia of thermal injury within this framework—as acute blood loss anemia initially and anemia of critical illness subsequently—will decrease transfusion rates and minimize adverse consequences.

▶ This selection was chosen not because it provides new information but because it is an extremely well written comprehensive review of the anemia associated with thermal injury. The distinction between acute blood loss anemia and anemia of critical illness is critical as we try to affect the need for blood transfusions in burn patients. Anemia resulting from burn injury is not strictly the result of acute blood loss or the critical illness, as there is some over-lap (Fig 1 in the original article). Transfusion-reducing strategies, such as eryth-ropoietin administration or lower transfusion thresholds, may have an even greater impact if studied within the context of either acute blood loss anemia or anemia of critical illness rather than being lumped together as anemia of thermal injury. Examining the contribution of both acute blood loss anemia and anemia of critical illness should bring to light the importance of this distinc-tion. Throughout this review, the authors highlight the advantages of using this distinction to improve patient care and research. Included is an exhaustive liter-ature review on the subject. This review is structured such that the mechanisms, trends, and treatments of anemia of thermal injury are defined and categorized to facilitate communication and further research on this topic.

D. W. Mozingo, MD

Outcomes with the Use of Recombinant Human Erythropoietin in Critically Ill Burn Patients

Lundy JB, Hetz K, Chung KK, et al (U.S. Army Inst of Surgical Res, Fort Sam Houston, TX; Brooke Army Med Ctr, Fort Sam Houston, TX)
Am Surg 76:951-956, 2010

Recent data demonstrate a possible mortality benefit in traumatically injured patients when given subcutaneous recombinant human erythropoi-etin (rhEPO). The purpose of this report is to examine the effect of rhEPO on mortality and transfusion in burn patients. We conducted a review of burn patients (greater than 30% total body surface area, intensive care unit [ICU] days greater than 15) treated with 40,000u rhEPO over an 18-month period (January 2007 to July 2008). Matched historical controls were identified and a contemporaneous cohort of subjects not adminis-tered rhEPO was used for comparison (NrhEPO). Mortality, transfusions, ICU and hospital length of stay were assessed. A total of 105 patients were treated (25 rhEPO, 53 historical control group, 27 NrhEPO). Hospital transfusions (mean 13,704 ± mL *vs* 13,308 ± mL; $P = 0.42$) and mortality (29.6 *vs* 32.0%; $P = 0.64$) were similar. NrhEPO required more blood transfusions (13,308 ± mL *vs* 6,827 ± mL; $P = 0.004$). No difference in mortality for the rhEPO and NrhEPO (32.0 *vs* 22.2%;

$P = 0.43$) was found. Thromboembolic complications were similar in all three groups. No effect was seen for rhEPO treatment on mortality or blood transfusion requirements in the severely burned.

▶ In thermally injured patients, the need for transfusion in critically ill patients is not only related to anemia associated with the inflammatory state but also related to large-volume blood loss during extensive burn wound excision and split-thickness skin grafting. The use of recombinant human erythropoietin (rhEPO) would have no impact on hemorrhage, hypovolemic shock, or the trigger to transfuse in this situation that is unique to critically ill burn patients. This selection failed to discern any difference in transfusion patterns in patients receiving rhEPO compared with those not receiving rhEPO. This report is retrospective and limited by the evaluation of a small number of patients. End points such as transfusion volumes are very heterogeneous as evidenced by large standard deviations. Dosing was also not standardized. When comparing rhEPO-treated patients with historical controls, the data do demonstrate a significant reduction in transfusion requirements in patients who develop acute kidney injury and require continuous venovenous hemofiltration. There appears to be no mortality benefit or reduction in transfusion requirements in any other subgroup or overall when rhEPO-treated patients are compared with historical and contemporaneous controls. The routine use of rhEPO in the treatment of severely burned patients to reduce hospital transfusion requirements or mortality is not substantiated.

D. W. Mozingo, MD

4 Critical Care

The Epidemiology of Sepsis in General Surgery Patients

Moore LJ, McKinley BA, Turner KL, et al (Methodist Hosp Res Inst/Weill Cornell Med College, Houston, TX; et al)

J Trauma 70:672-680, 2011

Background.—Sepsis is increasing in hospitalized patients. Our purpose is to describe its current epidemiology in a general surgery (GS) intensive care unit (ICU) where patients are routinely screened and aggressively treated for sepsis by an established protocol.

Methods.—Our prospective, Institutional Review Board-approved sepsis research database was queried for demographics, biomarkers reflecting organ dysfunction, and mortality. Patients were grouped as sepsis, severe sepsis, or septic shock using refined consensus criteria. Data are compared by analysis of variance, Student's t test, and χ^2 test ($p < 0.05$ significant).

Results.—During 24 months ending September 2009, 231 patients (aged 59 years $\pm$ 3 years; 43% men) were treated for sepsis. The abdomen was the source of infection in 69% of patients. Several baseline biomarkers of organ dysfunction (BOD) correlated with sepsis severity including lactate, creatinine, international normalized ratio, platelet count, and D-dimer. Direct correlation with mortality was noted with particular baseline BODs including beta natriuretic peptide, international normalized ratio, platelet count, aspartate transaminase, alanine aminotransferase, and total bilirubin. Most patients present with severe sepsis (56%) or septic shock (26%) each with increasing multiple BODs. Septic shock has prohibitive mortality rate (36%), and those who survive septic shock have prolonged ICU stays.

Conclusion.—In general surgery ICU patients, sepsis is predominantly caused by intra-abdominal infection. Multiple BODs are present in severe sepsis and septic shock but are notably advanced in septic shock. Despite aggressive sepsis screening and treatment, septic shock remains a morbid condition.

▶ Sepsis continues to be a common and serious problem among hospital inpatients. Previous epidemiologic studies have described sepsis within the general population in detail and have led to recent major initiatives to treating this serious problem, such as the Surviving Sepsis Campaign. Although these studies evaluated large numbers of patients, they used the International Classification of Disease, Ninth Edition, data from large state databases, which many investigators have recognized to be only moderately accurate, as they rely on hospital administrative discharge data predominately. In addition, surgical patients are rarely differentiated from medical patients in these studies. The authors of this selection, realizing that sepsis in surgical patients is different enough from that in nonsurgical patients, sought to assess this specific population. The modulation of immune function that occurs with surgery and anesthesia has been well described and is unlike that which occurs in the medical patient population, making comparisons of mixed populations inaccurate. Such populations need to be assessed separately. To date, there is a lack of epidemiologic data specifically addressing sepsis in the surgical patient, specifically ones that use clinical data sets, not administrative data sets. Although a recent study has identified that the need for emergency surgery is a risk factor for both the development of and death from sepsis and septic shock, other significant characteristics of the surgical sepsis population and their outcomes are not well described. In this study, a specific prospective description of the epidemiology of sepsis among surgical patients is described. Although the patient numbers are relatively small, this study sets the stage for comprehensive outcome studies in postsurgical sepsis and organ dysfunction syndromes.

D. W. Mozingo, MD

Systems Initiatives Reduce Healthcare-Associated Infections: A Study of 22,928 Device Days in a Single Trauma Unit

Miller RS, Norris PR, Jenkins JM, et al (Vanderbilt Univ Med Ctr, Nashville, TN)

J Trauma 68:23-31, 2010

Background.—"Implementation research" promotes the systematic conversion of evidence-based principles into routine practice to improve the quality of care. We hypothesized a system-based initiative to reduce nosocomial infection would lower the incidence of ventilator-associated pneumonia (VAP), urinary tract infection (UTI), and bloodstream infection (BSI).

Methods.—From January 2006 to April 2008, 7,364 adult trauma patients were admitted, of which 1,953 (27%) were admitted to the trauma intensive care unit and comprised the study group. Tight glycemic control was maintained using a computer algorithm for continuous insulin administration based on every 2-hour blood glucose testing. Centers for Disease Control and Prevention definitions of nosocomial infections were used. Evidence-based infection reduction strategies included the following: a VAP bundle (spontaneous breathing, Richmond Agitation-Sedation Scale, oral hygiene, bed elevation, and deep vein thrombosis/stress ulcer prophylaxis), UTI (expert insertion team and Foley removal/change at 5 days), and BSI (maximum barrier precautions, chlorhexidine skin prep, line management protocol). An electronic dashboard identified the at-risk population, and designated auditors monitored the compliance. Infection rates (events per 1,000 device days) were measured over time and compared annually using Fisher's exact test.

Results.—The study group had 22,928 device exposure days: 6,482 ventilator days, 9,037 urinary catheter days, and 7,399 central line days. Patient acuity, demographics, and number of device days did not vary significantly year-to-year. Annual infection rates declined between 2006 and 2008, and decreases in UTI and BSI rates were statistically significant ($p < 0.05$). These decreases pushed UTI and BSI rates below Centers for Disease Control and Prevention norms.

Conclusions.—Over 28 months, a systems approach to reducing nosocomial infection rates after trauma decreased nosocomial infections: UTI (76.3%), BSI (74.1%), and VAP (24.9%). Our experience suggests that infection reduction requires (1) an evidence-based plan; (2) MD and staff education/commitment; (3) electronic documentation; and (4) auditors to monitor and ensure compliance (Fig 9).

▶ Quality improvement initiatives can reduce hospital-acquired infections, costs, and mortality. Many randomized controlled clinical trials have helped to develop strategies to prevent hospital-acquired infections and form the basis for current evidence-based guidelines. These guidelines, standardized by the Centers for Disease Control and Prevention, are intended to help reduce or eliminate hospital-acquired infections in the intensive care unit population by the implementation of device-associated infection prevention bundles. These bundles are evidence-based sets of best practice guidelines designed to ensure optimal treatment, prevent or reduce complications, and improve outcome. They have been shown to be effective in reducing the incidence of hospital-acquired infections; however, they can be difficult to implement into clinical practice. This work describes development and implementation of an evidence-based practice to reduce health care—associated infections in critically injured patients. The system is reinforced with an online compliance monitoring system. The authors of this selection hypothesized that a system-based initiative to reduce hospital-acquired infections would lower the incidence of

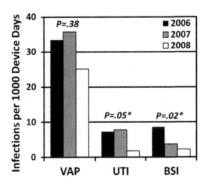

FIGURE 9.—Comparison of annual infection rates for pneumonia, UTIs, and BSIs; *p* values compare all three groups within each infection type. Not shown: pairwise comparisons (one-sided Fisher's exact test) were also statistically significant when comparing UTI rates in 2006 or 2007 to 2008 and comparing BSI rates in 2006 to 2007 or 2008. (Reprinted from Miller RS, Norris PR, Jenkins JM, et al. Systems initiatives reduce healthcare-associated infections: a study of 22,928 device days in a single trauma unit. *J Trauma.* 2010;68:23-31, with permission from Lippincott Williams & Wilkins.)

ventilator-associated pneumonia, catheter-associated urinary tract infections, and catheter-associated bloodstream infections. Their results are summarized in Fig 9, which is reproduced in this review. The selection was included because the text includes many examples of the actual online data tracking fields and examples of how the implementation of this plan markedly decreased their infection rate. It is an excellent template onto which other programs could be built or modeled.

D. W. Mozingo, MD

Duration of Red Cell Storage Influences Mortality After Trauma

Weinberg JA, McGwin G Jr, Vandromme MJ, et al (Univ of Tennessee Health Science Ctr, Memphis; Univ of Alabama at Birmingham)
J Trauma 69:1427-1432, 2010

Background.—Although previous studies have identified an association between the transfusion of relatively older red blood cells (RBCs) (storage ≥ 14 days) and adverse outcomes, they are difficult to interpret because the majority of patients received a combination of old and fresh RBC units. To overcome this limitation, we compared in-hospital mortality among patients who received exclusively old versus fresh RBC units during the first 24 hours of hospitalization.

Methods.—Patients admitted to a Level I trauma center between January 2000 and May 2009 who received ≥ 1 unit of exclusively old (≥ 14 days) vs. fresh (< 14 days) RBCs during the first 24 hours of hospitalization were identified. Risk ratios (RRs) and 95% confidence intervals (CIs) were calculated for the association between mortality and RBC age, adjusted for patient age, Injury Severity Score, gender, receipt of fresh frozen plasma or platelets, RBC volume, brain injury, and injury mechanism (blunt or penetrating).

Results.—One thousand six hundred forty-seven patients met the study inclusion criteria. Among patients who were transfused 1 or 2 RBC units, no difference in mortality with respect to RBC age was identified (adjusted RR, 0.97; 95% CI, 0.72−1.32). Among patients who were transfused 3 or more RBC units, receipt of old versus fresh RBCs was associated with a significantly increased risk of mortality, with an adjusted RR of 1.57 (95% CI, 1.14−2.15). No difference was observed concerning the mean number of old versus fresh units transfused to patients who received 3 or more units (6.05 vs. 5.47, respectively; $p = 0.11$).

Conclusion.—In trauma patients undergoing transfusion of 3 or more RBC units within 24 hour of hospital arrival, receipt of relatively older blood was associated with a significantly increased mortality risk. Reservation of relatively fresh RBC units for the acutely injured may be advisable.

▶ Current techniques for allogenic red cell preservation permit packed red blood cell (RBC) shelf life for up to 42 days. Certain morphologic and biochemical changes occur during storage before expiration, and these changes may worsen erythrocyte viability and function after transfusion. Despite a relatively large body of literature detailing the metabolic and structural deterioration that occurs during RBC storage, evidence for a significant detrimental clinical effect related to the transfusion of older blood remains less convincing, limited primarily to observations made in retrospective studies.

The association between the transfusion of relatively older blood and morbidity and mortality has been demonstrated in multiple retrospective studies of trauma patients using various study designs. It is notable, however, that a majority of patients in those studies received both fresh units and older stored units, making evaluation of the independent role of storage age on outcomes difficult. To overcome this limitation, the authors of this selection conducted a retrospective cohort study to evaluate the association between the age of transfused blood and in-hospital mortality among trauma patients who received exclusively old versus fresh packed RBCs during the first 24 hours of hospitalization.

The authors simplified the evaluation of storage age's effect on mortality by limiting the study population to those who received exclusively old versus fresh blood in the first 24 hours in a relatively large cohort.

In addition, as previous studies have been criticized for the lack of accounting for the confounding potential of the administration of blood products other than RBCs, they adjusted for the transfusion of fresh frozen plasma and platelets, as well. These results further support the notion that the transfusion of relatively older blood potentiates the risk of death after trauma.

D. W. Mozingo, MD

Ventilator-Associated Pneumonia is More Common and of Less Consequence in Trauma Patients Compared With Other Critically Ill Patients

Cook A, Norwood S, Berne J (East Texas Med Ctr, Tyler)
J Trauma 69:1083-1091, 2010

Background.—Ventilator-associated pneumonia (VAP) incidence is used as a quality measure. We hypothesized that patient and provider factors accounted for the higher incidence of VAP in trauma patients compared with other critically ill patients.

Methods.—We conducted a 2-year study of all intubated adult patients at our Trauma Center. VAP was identified according to the Centers for Disease Control and Prevention definition. Groups were compared for the incidence of VAP and outcomes.

Results.—The cohort of 2,591 patients included 511 trauma patients and 2,080 nontrauma patients. VAP occurred in 161 patients and more frequently in trauma patients (17.8% vs. 3.4%, $p < 0.001$). The overall death rate (17.4% vs. 9.8%, $p < 0.001$) and the death rate for VAP patients (31.4% vs. 11%, $p = 0.002$) was higher in the nontrauma group. Bronchoalveolar lavage was performed more frequently in the trauma patient group (22.1% vs. 8.9%, $p < 0.001$), and gram-negative organisms were isolated more commonly in trauma patients (65.9% vs. 30%, $p < 0.001$), respectively. VAP occurred earlier among the trauma group (mean 8.9 days vs. 14.1 days, $p < 0.001$). Trauma represented an odds ratio of 3.9 (95% confidence interval 2.4–6.3, $p < 0.001$) for the development of VAP.

Conclusion.—The incidence of VAP is greatest among trauma patients at our institution. The increased use of bronchoalveolar lavage, the earlier onset of VAP, and the higher incidence of gram-negative pneumonias suggest that both patient and provider factors may influence this phenomenon. VAP was associated with increased mortality in the nontrauma group only. These factors should be considered before VAP is applied as a quality indicator.

▶ In trauma patients, the aggressive identification and treatment of ventilator-associated pneumonia seem to diminish adverse outcomes and may represent the appropriate response to a frequent circumstance in this patient population. The authors of this selection have shown that the rates of ventilator-associated pneumonia are higher in trauma patients than in nontrauma patients as depicted in Fig 2 in the original article. Despite the higher incidence, outcomes were less affected than other patient populations. It is important to have a better understanding of the critical aspects of ventilator-associated pneumonia, specific to the population being treated, before the incidence rates of ventilator-associated pneumonia are applied as a metric of quality care. To benchmark the quality of care in critically ill trauma patients, one must measure those indicators specific to a given patient population. Prospective multi-institutional research will be needed to address the current issues associated with ventilator-associated pneumonia in trauma patients such that case-mix and risk stratification can be applied. Ventilator-associated pneumonia incidence rates should be evaluated in an observed-to-expected manner rather than simple rate per population analysis.

D. W. Mozingo, MD

Primary Fibrinolysis Is Integral in the Pathogenesis of the Acute Coagulopathy of Trauma

Kashuk JL, Moore EE, Sawyer M, et al (Penn State Hershey Med Ctr, PA)
Ann Surg 252:434-444, 2010

Background.—The existence of primary fibrinolysis (PF) and a defined mechanistic link to the "Acute Coagulopathy of Trauma" is controversial. Rapid thrombelastography (r-TEG) offers point of care comprehensive assessment of the coagulation system. We hypothesized that postinjury PF occurs early in severe shock, leading to postinjury coagulopathy, and ultimately hemorrhage-related death.

Methods.—Consecutive patients over 14 months at risk for postinjury coagulopathy were stratified by transfusion requirements into massive

(MT) >10 units/6 hours (n = 32), moderate (Mod) 5 to 9 units/6 hours (n = 15), and minimal (Min) <5 units/6 hours (n = 14). r-TEG was performed by adding tissue factor to uncitrated whole blood. r-TEG estimated percent lysis was categorized as PF when >15% estimated percent lysis was detected. Coagulopathy was defined as r-TEG clot strength = G < 5.3 dynes/cm^2. Logistic regression was used to define independent predictors of PF.

Results.—A total of 34% of injured patients requiring MT had PF, which was associated with lower emergency department systolic blood pressure, core temperature, and greater metabolic acidosis (analysis of variance, $P < 0.0001$). The risk of death correlated significantly with PF ($P = 0.026$). PF occurred early (median, 58 minutes; interquartile range, 1.2—95.9 minutes); every 1 unit drop in G increased the risk of PF by 30%, and death by over 10%.

Conclusions.—Our results confirm the existence of PF in severely injured patients. It occurs early (<1 hour), and is associated with MT requirements, coagulopathy, and hemorrhage-related death. These data warrant renewed emphasis on the early diagnosis and treatment of fibrinolysis in this cohort.

▶ Hemorrhagic shock and subsequent postinjury coagulopathy may be responsible for over half of deaths for patients presenting to a hospital following acute traumatic injury. This death rate has improved only slightly over the past 25 years despite the widespread adoption of damage control and other techniques. Previous studies from the authors of this selection as well as others have shown that among patients presenting with postinjury massive hemorrhage, the majority die from refractory coagulopathy even after surgical control of their wound has been obtained. The pathogenesis of the hemostatic derangements associated with these findings has remained elusive, in part because of limitations of conventional coagulation testing as well as a lack of rapid analysis of whole blood coagulation. Accordingly, only minimal advances have been made to directly address this issue. In this selection, the authors describe their recent experience with a rapid thrombelastography (r-TEG). They showed that fibrinolysis occurs early after injury and is associated with massive transfusion requirements, coagulopathy, and hemorrhage-related death. They did not obtain r-TEG studies immediately on arrival of patients in the emergency department, not permitting definition of the actual timing of onset of fibrinolysis in the injured patient. Also, most r-TEG values in this study were obtained after the initiation of resuscitation; therefore, the impact of such resuscitation on fibrinolysis remains to be seen. Future investigations are required to better ascertain the timing of onset of fibrinolysis, with the potential for early diagnosis and treatment.

D. W. Mozingo, MD

Postoperative Sepsis in the United States

Vogel TR, Dombrovskiy VY, Carson JL, et al (Robert Wood Johnson Med School, New Brunswick, NJ; Univ of Medicine and Dentistry of New Jersey, New Brunswick)
Ann Surg 252:1065-1071, 2010

Objectives.—To evaluate the incidence of postoperative sepsis after elective procedures, to define surgical procedures with the greatest risk for developing sepsis, and to evaluate patient and hospital confounders.

Background Data.—The development of sepsis after elective surgical procedures imposes a significant clinical and resource utilization burden in the United States. We evaluated the development of sepsis after elective procedures in a nationally representative patient cohort and assessed the effect of sociodemographic and hospital characteristics on the development of postoperative sepsis.

Methods.—The Nationwide inpatient sample was queried between 2002 and 2006 and patients developing sepsis after elective procedures were identified using the patient safety indicator "Postoperative Sepsis" (PSI-13). Case-mix adjusted rates were calculated by using a multivariate logistic regression model for sepsis risk and an indirect standardization method.

Results.—A total of 6,512,921 weighted elective surgical cases met the inclusion criteria and 78,669 cases (1.21%) developed postoperative sepsis. Case-mix adjustment for age, race, gender, hospital bed size, hospital location, hospital teaching status, and patient income demonstrated esophageal, pancreatic, and gastric procedures represented the greatest risk for the development of postoperative sepsis. Thoracic, adrenal, and hepatic operations accounted for the greatest mortality rates if sepsis developed. Increasing age, Blacks, Hispanics, and men were more likely to develop sepsis. Decreased median household income, larger hospital bed size, urban hospital location, and nonteaching status were associated with greater rates of postoperative sepsis.

Conclusions.—The development of postoperative sepsis is multifactorial and procedures, most likely to develop sepsis, did not demonstrate the greatest mortality after sepsis developed. Factors associated with the development of sepsis included race, age, hospital size, hospital location, and patient income. Further evaluation of high-risk procedures, populations, and environments may assist in reducing this costly complication.

▶ The development of sepsis creates a major health care burden. Somewhat limited epidemiologic information exists with regard to postoperative sepsis. Most major series describe nonsurgical patients or have only a small fraction of patients being studied as postsurgical patients. Some have recently shown that the incidence of sepsis and the number of sepsis-related deaths are increasing, although the overall mortality rate among patients with sepsis is declining. The National Healthcare Quality Reports estimate 11.6 cases of postoperative sepsis/1000 elective surgery discharges with a hospital length of stay of longer than 3 days. Other groups focusing on elective procedures have demonstrated that the rates of sepsis and severe sepsis have increased significantly over the last decade with little improvement in overall mortality. Sepsis remains one of the leading causes of death in the United States, and surgical patients account for approximately one-third of all sepsis cases. The objective of this study was to describe the epidemiology of postoperative sepsis in the United States after elective inpatient elective surgery by procedure type. Secondary aims included description of sociodemographic factors and hospital characteristics associated with the development of postoperative sepsis. The identification of high-risk groups, as identified in this selection, may assist in identifying opportunities for improvements in clinical care and resource use (Fig 1 in the original article) to reduce the incidence of sepsis.

D. W. Mozingo, MD

Centers for Medicare and Medicaid Services Quality Indicators Do Not Correlate With Risk-Adjusted Mortality at Trauma Centers
Shafi S, Parks J, Ahn C, et al (Univ of Texas Southwestern Med School, Dallas; et al)
J Trauma 68:771-777, 2010

Objectives.—The Centers for Medicare and Medicaid Services (CMS) publicly reports hospital compliance with evidence-based processes of care as quality indicators. We hypothesized that compliance with CMS quality indicators would correlate with risk-adjusted mortality rates in trauma patients.

Methods.—A previously validated risk-adjustment algorithm was used to measure observed-to-expected mortality ratios (O/E with 95% confidence interval) for Level I and II trauma centers using the National Trauma Data Bank data. Adult patients (≥ 16 years) with at least one severe injury (Abbreviated Injury Score ≥ 3) were included (127,819 patients). Compliance with CMS quality indicators in four domains was obtained from Hospital Compare website: acute myocardial infarction (8 processes), congestive heart failure (4 processes), pneumonia (7 processes), surgical infections (3 processes). For each domain, a single composite score was calculated for each hospital. The relationship between O/E ratios and CMS quality indicators was explored using nonparametric tests.

Results.—There was no relationship between compliance with CMS quality indicators and risk-adjusted outcomes of trauma patients.

Conclusions.—CMS quality indicators do not correlate with risk-adjusted mortality rates in trauma patients. Hence, there is a need to develop new trauma-specific process of care quality indicators to evaluate and improve quality of care in trauma centers.

▶ In this selection, the authors demonstrate a complete lack of relationship between publicly reported Centers for Medicare and Medicaid Services (CMS) quality indicators and risk-adjusted mortality in trauma patients. Therefore, compliance with the current CMS quality indicators does not reflect quality of care in the trauma patient population. Although compliance with these core measures has been associated with a decrease in overall hospital mortality from that expected, it appears that it need not be from the direct impact of those interventions. Compliance with measured quality indicators may simply be a marker for an institution that is dedicated to improving its overall quality of care for all patients. Most trauma centers are located within full-service acute care hospitals, and one would expect to see a correlation between compliance with CMS core measures for these hospitals and outcomes of their trauma patients. These findings suggest that potential benefits of compliance with CMS quality indicators do not extend to the trauma patient population. There are several possible explanations for these findings. Trauma patients represent a unique population group within these hospitals. It is known that most trauma patients are young and otherwise healthy with few comorbidities. Hence, they are not necessarily at risk for the diseases and complications that are targeted by CMS. For example, the incidence of coronary artery disease and congestive heart failure is very low in trauma patients. Although trauma patients are at risk of developing pneumonia, it is usually the hospital-acquired ventilator-associated type encountered in these patients, not the community-acquired pneumonia targeted by CMS. Similarly, in the case of surgical site infections, a large number of trauma patients do not require surgical intervention. Even when they do, the emergent nature of operations may not permit administration of prophylactic antibiotics before skin incision, appropriate hair removal, or perioperative use of β-blockers in certain patient populations, all of which are measured as CMS quality indicators for elective surgery. Prophylaxis against venous thromboembolism is another CMS core measure included in Surgical Care Improvement Project (SCIP). It is a common complication in trauma patients as well. Hence, compliance with SCIP measures should improve outcomes of trauma patients. A clear implication of these findings is that there needs to be a trauma-specific set of quality measures based on processes of care that ensure optimal care of the injured. These measures should be evidence based when possible and relevant to common injuries. Also, these quality measures would be best integrated into existing trauma registries for monitoring and reporting purposes since they represent a more clinically based nonadministrative data set.

D. W. Mozingo, MD

Jack A. Barney Resident Paper Award: Blood transfusions increase complications in moderately injured patients
Kopriva BM, Helmer SD, Smith RS (The Univ of Kansas School of Medicine - Wichita, KS; Virginia Tech Carilion School of Medicine, Roanoke)
Am J Surg 200:746-751, 2010

Background.—Previous assessments linked transfusions in trauma to increased respiratory and infectious complications. However, these studies included patients with severe trauma, brisk hemorrhage, and shock. Thus, the potentially harmful impact of transfusion was difficult to determine.

Methods.—A retrospective review of all trauma patients with an injury severity score (ISS) of 9 to 14 admitted to a Level 1 Trauma Center over a 5-year period was performed. Patients were stratified by transfusion history and injury severity.

Results.—Records of 2,332 patients were reviewed; 208 (8.9%) received at least 1 packed red blood cell transfusion. The incidence of complications was significantly higher in patients receiving transfusions (42.3% vs 9.0%; $P < .001$), and transfusion was a significant independent predictor of the development of a complication (odds ratio, 5.85; $P < .001$). Further, the association of transfusion with complications was dose-dependent. Transfusion was associated with a significantly increased hospital length of stay (10.6 vs 3.9 days; $P < .0001$).

Conclusions.—Moderately injured trauma patients receiving transfusions suffered significantly more complications. Indications for transfusion in this population should be reassessed carefully.

▶ There is still debate regarding the risks, benefits, and complications associated with blood transfusion therapy in trauma patients. The risks of acquiring blood-borne illnesses from transfusions are now very low. Most of these risks are related to the immune-modulating effects of blood transfusions, placing the trauma patient at higher risk for infections and lung injury. Many cohort studies have associated injured patients receiving packed red blood cell transfusions with an increased risk of respiratory and infectious complications. Most of these previous assessments of transfusion risk have included critically ill patients with severe trauma, significant blood loss, and shock.

This selection was chosen because the authors examined the impact of lesser volumes of blood transfusions on the outcomes of only moderately injured patients. Injury severity scores were between 9 and 14, and blood transfusions increased infectious complications nearly 5-fold. Considering the current trend toward using lesser volumes of crystalloid solutions and using resuscitation strategies that favor higher fresh frozen plasma to packed red blood cell ratios, one needs to be cautious of overusing the latter approach in moderately injured patients.

D. W. Mozingo, MD

Time and degree of glycemic derangement are associated with increased mortality in trauma patients in the setting of tight glycemic control
Corneille MG, Villa C, Wolf S, et al (Univ of Texas Health Science Ctr at San Antonio; et al)
Am J Surg 200:832-838, 2010

Background.—Tight glucose control (TGC) may reduce mortality in critically ill trauma patients. We hypothesize that euglycemia is beneficial, and a measure considering time and degree of hyperglycemia is most associated with mortality.

Methods.—We performed a review of intensive care unit trauma patients admitted for more than 3 days between January 2005 and December 2007 on a TGC protocol with a goal of 80 to 110 mg/dL. Hyperglycemic, hypoglycemic, and euglycemic time ranges, and area of interpolated curves above and below 80 to 110 mg/dL were assessed. Associations with mortality were based on logistic regression models adjusted for age, injury severity score, and admission Glasgow Coma Scale score.

Results.—A total of 546 patients were identified, and 68 (13%) died. Time spent as hyperglycemic ($P = .29$) and hyperglycemic area under the curve ($P = .58$) were not associated with mortality; hyperglycemic area/time ($P = .01$) was associated with mortality. Regarding hypoglycemia, area over the curve ($P = .009$) and time spent as hypoglycemic ($P = .002$) were associated with mortality.

Conclusions.—TGC prevents prolonged, high degrees of hyperglycemia; avoiding hypoglycemia likely provides mortality benefit for trauma patients (Fig 1).

▶ In surgery and critical care, few studies have had such immediate and far-reaching impact on practice as that of Van den Berghe and colleagues in 2001 where from a single-institution clinical trial, tight glucose control in the range of 80 to 110 g/dL became standard practice in intensive care units (ICUs) worldwide and was endorsed by numerous professional organizations. There remain some unresolved issues related to the optimal clinical setting, patient population, glucose control regimen, and target blood glucose range. Increased blood glucose levels above the normal range of 80 to 110 mg/dL are common in a wide variety of acute illnesses, irrespective of previously diagnosed diabetes. In an effort to mitigate the effects of hyperglycemia, tight glucose control protocols have been implemented in ICUs worldwide. Common to these protocols is the use of insulin to try to convert a hyperglycemic patient

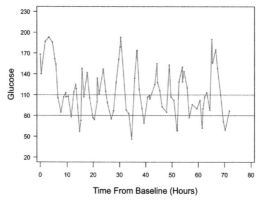

FIGURE 1.—A typical interpolated curve from which areas and times were calculated. (Reprinted from The American Journal of Surgery, Corneille MG, Villa C, Wolf S, et al. Time and degree of glycemic derangement are associated with increased mortality in trauma patients in the setting of tight glycemic control. *Am J Surg.* 2010;200:832-838. Copyright © 2010, with permission from Elsevier Inc.)

to a normoglycemic patient. There is wide inconsistency, however, in the methods used to describe glucose control and in the glucose end point, which showed a mortality or morbidity improvement. Based on their findings in this selection, the authors have suggested that the method of calculating the area under the curve, including both time and glucose measurement (both hypoglycemia and hyperglycemia), is a superior metric to assess glucose control and predict mortality in their patients. This study does not, however, conclude that hyperglycemia in itself can be determined to cause worse outcomes but only that there is an association between the 2.

D. W. Mozingo, MD

Challenging Issues in Surgical Critical Care, Trauma, and Acute Care Surgery: A Report From the Critical Care Committee of the American Association for the Surgery of Trauma
Napolitano LM, Fulda GJ, Davis KA, et al (Univ of Michigan, Ann Arbor)
J Trauma 69:1619-1633, 2010

Critical care workforce analyses estimate a 35% shortage of intensivists by 2020 as a result of the aging population and the growing demand for greater utilization of intensivists. Surgical critical care in the U.S. is particularly challenged by a significant shortfall of surgical intensivists, with only 2586 surgeons currently certified in surgical critical care by the American Board of Surgery, and even fewer surgeons (1204) recertified in surgical critical care as of 2009. Surgical critical care fellows (160 in 2009) represent only 7.6% of all critical care trainees (2109 in 2009), with the largest number of critical care fellowship positions in internal medicine (1472, 69.8%). Traditional trauma fellowships have now transitioned into Surgical Critical Care or Acute Care Surgery (trauma, surgical critical care, emergency surgery) fellowships. Since adult critical care services are a large, expensive part of U.S. healthcare and workforce shortages continue to impact our healthcare system, recommendations for regionalization of critical care services in the U.S. is considered. The Critical Care Committee of the AAST has compiled national data regarding these important issues that face us in surgical critical care, trauma and acute care surgery, and discuss potential solutions for these issues (Fig 1).

▶ This selection is included as it represents a comprehensive review of the current status of surgical critical care in the United States. The surgical intensivist still represents a minority of critical care providers in the United States (Fig 1), and the projected shortage of such specialists seems to unfortunately not have a solution on the horizon. Adult critical care services are a large expensive part of US health care, and workforce shortages continue to impact the health care system. Compared with some developed countries, the delivery of critical care services in the United States is fragmented and disorganized. There is little standardization of critical care services, and there is no regionalization of adult intensive care services as there are for neonatal services.

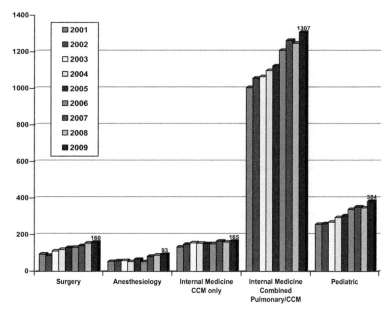

FIGURE 1.—Number of positions filled in critical care fellowship training programs in each specialty by year over the past decade. Data from http://www.acgme.org/adspublic/. Reports—Number of accredited programs and on-duty residents during academic year. (Reprinted from Napolitano LM, Fulda GJ, Davis KA, et al. Challenging issues in surgical critical care, trauma, and acute care surgery: a report from the critical care committee of the American association for the surgery of trauma. *J Trauma*. 2010;69:1619-1633, with permission from Lippincott Williams & Wilkins.)

Regionalization of critical care resources is not a new concept and has been discussed in various publications over the past 20 years as a way of assuring that all critically ill patients have access to critical care specialists. It is reasonable to consider such a strategy that would maximize resources, given the inevitable shortage of intensivists.

D. W. Mozingo, MD

Gender Differences in Glucose Variability after Severe Trauma

Mohr AM, Lavery RF, Sifri ZC, et al (UMDNJ-New Jersey Med School, Newark)

Am Surg 76:896-902, 2010

Gender differences in the physiological response to trauma can affect outcome. Both hyperglycemia and blood glucose (BG) variability predict a poor outcome after trauma. This study examined the hypothesis that both BG levels and the degree of BG variability after trauma are gender-specific and correlate with mortality and morbidity. A retrospective observational cohort study of 1915 trauma patients requiring critical care was performed. Admission BG as well as all BG values obtained during the first week while in the intensive care unit were analyzed. In each patient, the mean BG and the degree of BG variability were calculated. A total of 1560 males and 355 females were studied with an overall mortality rate of 12 per cent. Seventy-six per cent of deaths had a BG greater than 125 mg/dL on admission and as BG variability worsened, the mortality rate also increased. There was a significant difference in male BG variability when comparing survivors with nonsurvivors. Female BG variability did not predict mortality. Failed glucose homeostasis is an important marker of endocrine dysfunction after severe injury. Increased BG variability in males is associated with a higher mortality rate. In females, mortality cannot be predicted based on BG levels or BG variability. These data have significant implications for gender-related differences in postinjury management.

▶ The occurrence of hyperglycemia in patients who experienced trauma is well known, and until recently, an elevation of the blood glucose was largely considered a relatively unimportant component of the stress response after injury. However, recent studies have shown that admission hyperglycemia in trauma patients is associated with a worsened clinical outcome as well as persistent hyperglycemic response during the hospital stay. This failure of posttrauma glucose homeostasis may be a predictor of increased morbidity and mortality because the ability to maintain homeostasis in response to stress is thought to be a crucial survival mechanism. Recent data suggest that failed glucose homeostasis, as reflected in the variability of plasma glucose, is also associated with worse outcomes in critically ill patients. After trauma, fluctuations in glucose concentrations, reflected in glucose variability, may be a pathophysiological symptom or marker of postinjury endocrine dysfunction that is a component of ongoing multiple organ dysfunction. Although it was recognized that intensive insulin therapy led to a 34% relative reduction in mortality in a select surgical population in 2001, the benefits of insulin in acutely injured trauma patients remain undefined. Likewise, gender-specific differences have been well documented in experimental trauma-hemorrhage and sepsis studies. These gender differences, however, remain poorly understood and not well characterized clinically. In this selection, the 2 purposes were to investigate the effects of gender on the glycemic response to traumatic injury and to determine if glucose variability during the first week is of prognostic importance. The authors hypothesized that gender differences in glucose variability would occur and that the degree of glucose variability would correlate with morbidity and mortality. This study is the first to demonstrate that blood glucose variability was significantly different in male survivors as compared with nonsurvivors. The degree of variability was directly related to mortality in men. Women did not have the same clinical response to blood glucose variability, and this is another indication that men and women may respond differently following trauma.

D. W. Mozingo, MD

5 Transplantation

Introduction

This is an age of changes in health care. There have been recent legislative changes relating to health care delivery that will alter the delivery of transplant care to the population. In a 2-part article, Axelrod et al[1,2] review some of the potential impact of health care reform upon organ transplantation. While there are many unknowns in the process, the detailed transplant center data that are currently available within the public domain diminish the impact of certain elements of health care reform. Additionally, accountability for care has traditionally been an integral part of the transplant process, so it is probable that legislation will not have as significant impact on transplantation as other forms of surgery. However, increased access to care resulting from insurance reform is likely to exacerbate problems of organ availability to meet the needs of potential organ recipients.

The disparity in numbers of people awaiting organ transplantation and the numbers of available organs continues to grow. With more than 105 000 registrants on the national waitlist and only around 8000 deceased organ donors, the methodology for organ allocation is undergoing continued scrutiny. Modification of allocation algorithms raises the spectra of resource rationing. Indeed, the problems balancing optimal function and graft duration with values associated with equitable kidney allocation are being used to highlight difficulties associated with age and resource rationing.[3] The authors propose that the process be transparent, that rationing should occur only when the cost of not doing so is "too high," that they be able to discriminate outcomes between individuals of similar age, and finally that those affected by policy should have a voice in how the proposal is formulated. Solutions to the organ shortage have been difficult. One approach has been to use organs from individuals after death has occurred through circulatory rather than neurologic criteria, so called DCD (donation after cardiac death) organs. It has been queried whether these organs behave in a similar fashion as those from conventional, brain-dead, deceased organ donors. In a single-center review,[4] the ureteral complications after kidney transplantation were statistically similar irrespective of whether the kidney came from a living, neurologically heart beating deceased donor or a deceased donor declared through circulatory criteria. These results are in sharp contrast to the biliary tract strictures observed in livers retrieved from donors declared dead using circulatory criteria. While these biliary complications are well known, analysis of the

SRTR database[5] yielded some refinements and many expected results for DCD livers. Livers from older and heavier donors with longer time to circulatory death were less likely to function well. Recipients with a high MELD (Model for End-stage Liver Disease) score did not do as well with a DCD liver. There is much to learn regarding how to optimally use the organs that are available within the aggregate deceased-donor organ pool. A contentious issue in obtaining organs for transplantation has been a proposal to change the model to obtain organs from live individuals. A poll of 250 live organ donors found that almost half were favorable toward introducing some form of financial incentive for giving an organ, especially for those individuals that donate anonymously.[6] Certainly there will be much more discussion relating to the lack of organs for potential transplant recipients, and it will involve obtaining organs both from the living and the dead.

Improving transplant outcomes has been a long-term goal of the transplant community. The most common approach has been to use pharmacotherapy to overcome the host immune response to the transplanted organ. New products have been slow in recent development, but blockade of co-stimulatory proteins CD80/CD86 has been one of the more recent approaches to transplant immunosuppression.[7] The therapy appears durable, but where precisely it will be positioned within the spectrum of drugs remains somewhat uncertain. The path that an individual patient takes to a stable immunologic state with a transplanted organ has remained a source of interest. A study of stable kidney recipients (well defined) on monotherapy mTOR inhibitor or calcineurin inhibition demonstrated significantly different gene profiles within peripheral blood mononuclear cell phenotypes.[8] It is also becoming apparent that the spectrum of gene polymorphisms will affect drug metabolism and outcomes. In addition to understanding transplant outcomes, adverse events are also influenced by the gene profile. A multicenter group analyzed infections after pediatric heart transplantation[9] and found that distinct gene profiles were associated with greater likelihood of bacterial infections. In keeping with differences between individuals, the incidence of disease has been known to differ between ethnicities. The article by Lentine et al[10] assessed the impact of racial differences upon outcomes after live kidney donation. Not surprisingly, the development of hypertension, diabetes, and kidney dysfunction occurs at differing frequency according to ethnicity, suggesting the need for variable levels of follow-up appropriate for health.

Organ specific issues: kidney transplantation is the optimal form of therapy for many people with kidney failure. The processes that identify candidate individuals have evolved over time. Previous exclusion criteria included anyone identified as having HIV. As a chronic virus infecting immune cells and complicated by opportunistic infections, long-term immunosuppression was thought to be incompatible with the infection. However, with the advent of effective antiviral therapies, much has changed. A report from an NIH-sponsored multicenter trial[11] demonstrated that kidney transplantation can be successfully performed in patients with

HIV. Contrary to what would be suspected, this population was prone to early rejection and drug interactions, and monitoring was more complex but manageable. Outcomes were surprisingly good. Polyomavirus infects almost all people and the BK virus can occasionally produce serious transplant kidney dysfunction. Management strategies surrounding the BK virus have been uncertain. The Basel group[12] reported the major role that reduction of immunosuppression had in the treatment of BK virus nephropathy. Whether the addition of antiviral chemotherapy would serve as an adjunct remains controversial, although the results reported are very good.

The complications of portal hypertension play a significant role in the people seeking liver transplantation. The variable changes in portal flow characteristics between whole organ and live donation liver transplantation were assessed in a study by Jiang et al.[13] It was demonstrated that resolution of elevated pressures, spleen size, and collaterals was slower in recipients of "smaller" live donor grafts. This is an important consideration when one looks toward management strategies and discussions with patients. The impact of major surgery upon previously healthy individuals has been poorly studied.[14] Parikh et al assessed live liver donation on quality of life measurements. It is not surprising that surgery has a significant impact on the individual. Before live donation assumes a normative role in the care of end-stage liver failure, more understanding of the impact of morbidities is required.

While kidney and liver transplantation constitute the vast majority of procedures performed, other organs are also used very successfully. Pancreas transplantation has undergone significant technical improvements over the past several decades. With changes in immunosuppression, progressively improved outcomes had been observed. However, a more recent analysis[15] suggests that while early outcomes continue to improve, the long-term result after kidney/pancreas transplantation has hit a plateau. Reasons may be very diverse, but there is still room for better outcomes and understanding. Transplant outcome variability in relatively infrequently performed procedures has been a major a source of great debate. A study by Thabut et al[16] discusses outcome variation between centers that perform lung transplantation. Differences in outcomes attributed to surgical proficiency and judgment versus institutional resource availability were addressed and found to be difficult to dissect. While center volume has been demonstrated to influence outcomes, certainly there are many other variables that influence lung transplantation outcomes. The evolution of long-term lung dysfunction through bronchiolitis obliterans (BO) has been a problem for all lung transplant centers. A study by Bharat et al[17] assessed the effect of autoantibodies to collagen and tubulin, rather than alloantibodies, on the generation of BO. They demonstrated an increased likelihood of injury in those individuals that generate multiple antibody response, making us question the differences between immune responses to injury. One of the striking developments in transplantation has been the clinical application of vascularized composite allografts (hand and face most commonly) to the management of debilitating loss of limb or face. In the evolution of this technique, multiple technical, preservation, immunologic, and quality issues are discussed.[18] Composite allografts allow a special insight into potential application of organogenesis. A study by Delaere et al[19] discusses an instance where the recipient cells were allowed to repopulate the scaffolding of an allograft larynx, subsequently permitting a transplant without immunosuppression. This technology has much to diversify if it is to be used for other "self" organs, but it is quite exciting.

Transplantation affords for the persistent foreign antigen exposure to the recipient immune system. A study by Thaunat et al[20] reports that the immune response within the transplanted graft can differ from that of the circulating immunocytes. This is potentially a very important observation that may offer new strategies that address chronic rejection.

Many questions persist in transplantation biology. However, with the clinical successes achieved thus far, demand for organs is creating social pressures for more availability. Challenges for the future will involve increasing availability and understanding more of the immunobiology that will permit decreased morbidity for those most in need.

Timothy L. Pruett, MD

References

1. Axelrod DA, Millman D, Abbecassis DD. US Health Care Reform and Transplantation. Part I: overview and impact on access and reimbursement in the private sector. *Am J Transplant.* 2010;10:2197-2202.
2. Axelrod DA, Millman D, Abecassis MM. Health Care Reform and Transplantation, Part II: impact on the public sector and novel health care delivery systems. *Am J Transplant.* 2010;10:2203-2207.
3. Reese PP, Caplan AL, Bloom AD, Abt PL, Karlawish JH. How should we use age to ration health care? Lessons from the case of kidney transplantation. *J Am Geriatr Soc.* 2010;58:1980-1986.
4. Saeb-Parsy K, Kosmoliaptsis V, Sharples LD, et al. Donor type does not influence the incidence of major urologic complications after kidney transplantation. *Transplantation.* 2010;90:1085-1090.
5. Mathur AK, Heimbach J, Steffick DE, Sonnenday CJ, Goodrich NP, Merion RM. Donation after cardiac death liver transplantation: predictors of outcome. *Am J Transplant.* 2010;10:2512-2519.
6. van Buren MC, Massey EK, Maasdam L, et al. For love or money? Attitudes toward financial incentives among actual living kidney donors. *Am J Transplant.* 2010;10:2488-2492.
7. Vincenti F, Blancho G, Durrbach A, et al. Five-year safety and efficacy of belatacept in renal transplantation. *J Am Soc Nephrol.* 2010;21:1587-1596.
8. Brouard S, Puig-Pey I, Lozano JJ, et al. Comparative transcriptional and phenotypic peripheral blood analysis of kidney recipients under cyclosporin A or sirolimus monotherapy. *Am J Transplant.* 2010;10:2604-2614.
9. Ohmann EL, Brooks MM, Webber SA, et al. Association of genetic polymorphisms and risk of late post-transplantation infection in pediatric heart recipients. *J Heart Lung Transplant.* 2010;29:1342-1351.
10. Lentine KL, Schnitzler MA, Xiao H, et al. Racial variation in medical outcomes among living kidney donors. *N Engl J Med.* 2010;363:724-732.
11. Stock PG, Barin B, Murphy B, et al. Outcomes of kidney transplantation in HIV-infected recipients. *N Engl J Med.* 2010;363:2004-2014.

12. Schaub S, Hirsch HH, Dickenmann M, et al. Reducing immunosuppression preserves allograft function in presumptive and definitive polyomavirus-associated nephropathy. *Am J Transplant.* 2010;10:2615-2623.
13. Jiang SM, Zhang QS, Zhou GW, Huang SF, Lu HM, Peng CH. Differences in portal hemodynamics between whole liver transplantation and living donor liver transplantation. *Liver Transpl.* 2010;16:1236-1241.
14. Parikh ND, Ladner D, Abecassis M, Butt Z. Quality of life for donors after living donor liver transplantation: a review of the literature. *Liver Transpl.* 2010;16: 1352-1358.
15. Waki K, Terasaki PI, Kadowaki T. Long-term pancreas allograft survival in simultaneous pancreas-kidney transplantation by era: UNOS registry analysis. *Diabetes Care.* 2010;33:1789-1791.
16. Thabut G, Christie JD, Kremers WK, Fournier M, Halpern SD. Survival differences following lung transplantation among US transplant centers. *JAMA.* 2010;304:53-60.
17. Bharat A, Saini D, Steward N, et al. Antibodies to self-antigens predispose to primary lung allograft dysfunction and chronic rejection. *Ann Thorac Surg.* 2010;90:1094-1101.
18. Siemionow MZ, Kulahci Y, Bozkurt M. Composite tissue allotransplantation. *Plast Reconstr Surg.* 2009;124:e327-e339.
19. Delaere P, Vranckx J, Verleden G, De Leyn P, Van Raemdonck D. Tracheal allotransplantation after withdrawal of immunosuppressive therapy. *N Engl J Med.* 2010;362:138-145.
20. Thaunat O, Patey N, Caligiuri G, et al. Chronic rejection triggers the development of an aggressive intragraft immune response through recapitulation of lymphoid organogenesis. *J Immunol.* 2010;185:717-728.

US Health Care Reform and Transplantation. Part I: Overview and Impact on Access and Reimbursement in the Private Sector
Axelrod DA, Millman D, Abecassis MM (Dartmouth-Hitchcock Med Ctr, Lebanon, NH)
Am J Transplant 10:2197-2202, 2010

The Health Care Reform (HCR) legislation passed by Congress in 2010 will have significant impact on transplant centers, patients and health care professionals. The Act seeks to expand coverage, limit the growth in health care costs and reform the delivery and insurance systems. In Part I of this two part series, we provide an overview and perspective of changes in private health insurance resulting from HCR. Under the plan, all Americans will be required to purchase coverage through their employer or via an improved individual/small group market. This legislation limits abusive practices such as limitations on preexisting conditions, lifetime and annual coverage limitations and dropping of beneficiaries if they become sick. The legislation will also limit high-cost plans and regulate premium increases. Private sector reforms are likely to benefit our patients by increasing the number of patients with access to transplant services, since the use of 'preexisting' conditions will be eliminated. However without a concomitant increase in the organ supply, longer waiting times and greater use of marginal organs are likely to increase the cost of transplant. Furthermore, transplant providers will receive reduced reimbursement as a result of market consolidation and the growing power of large transplant networks.

▶ The impact of health care reform on organ transplantation will be important. The 2 articles by Axelrod and colleagues attempt to discern the impact of the new law on this form of care. The theme in the first article is about increased access to care as a consequence of insurance reform, removal of preexisting conditions as a reason for denial of insurance, and expansion of the population of insured. The downside of increased access is that it is unlikely to be associated with an increased number of organs. The societal cost of chronic organ failure is significant, and transplantation should not be a luxury. The process issues addressed by the Affordable Care Act are likely to pale next to the problems generated by insufficient availability of organs for those in need.

T. L. Pruett, MD

US Health Care Reform and Transplantation, Part II: Impact on the Public Sector and Novel Health Care Delivery Systems
Axelrod DA, Millman D, Abecassis MM (Dartmouth-Hitchcock Med Ctr, Lebanon, NH; Powers, Pyles, Sutter and Verville, P.C., Washington, DC; Northwestern Memorial Hosp, Chicago, IL)
Am J Transplant 10:2203-2207, 2010

The Patient Protection and Affordable Care Act passed in 2010 will result in dramatic expansion of publically funded health insurance coverage for low-income individuals. It is estimated that of the 32 million newly insured, 16 million will obtain coverage through expansion of the Medicaid Program, and the remaining 16 million will purchase coverage through their employer or newly legislated insurance exchanges. While the Act contains numerous provisions to improve access to private insurance as discussed in Part I of this analysis, public sector coverage will significantly be affected. The cost of health care reform will be borne disproportionately by Medicare, which faces nearly $500 billion in cuts to be identified by a new independent board. Transplant centers should be concerned about the impact of the reform on the financial aspects of transplantation. In addition, this legislation also utilizes the Medicare Program to drive reform of the health care delivery system, by encouraging the development of integrated Accountable Care Organizations, experimentation with new 'models' of health care delivery, and expanded support for Comparative Effectiveness Research. Transplant providers, including transplant centers and physicians/surgeons need to lead this movement, drawing on our experience providing comprehensive multidisciplinary care under global budgets with publically reported outcomes.

▶ The second article of the Axelrod series discusses the impact of the health care reform on governmental reimbursement for organ transplant services and the role of innovative approaches to care delivery that will allow care to be delivered more efficiently. The Accountable Care Organizations sound a lot like transplant programs when functioning effectively. Care for people with chronic organ failure demonstrates many options for care. It has been shown that there are markedly different outcomes with different types of therapy. It is possible to streamline care, reduce inefficiencies, and meet many of the goals of the Affordable Care Act. With change will come opportunity, but it is important to know the rules of the game.

T. L. Pruett, MD

How Should We Use Age to Ration Health Care? Lessons from the Case of Kidney Transplantation
Reese PP, Caplan AL, Bloom RD, et al (Univ of Pennsylvania, Philadelphia)
J Am Geriatr Soc 58:1980-1986, 2010

Competing visions for health reform in the United States and renewed interest in health technology assessment (HTA) have led to fierce national debates about the appropriateness of rationing. Because of a limited supply of organs, kidney transplantation has always required rationing and overt discussion of the ethics that guide it, but the field of transplantation has also contended recently with internal calls for a new rationing system. The aim of the Life Years from Transplantation (LYFT) proposal is to allocate kidneys to patients who obtain the greatest survival benefit from transplantation, which would lengthen the lives of kidney transplant recipients but restrict the ability of older Americans to obtain a transplant. The debate around the LYFT proposal reveals the ethical and policy challenges of identifying which patients should receive a treatment based on the results of cost-effectiveness and other HTA studies. This article argues that attempts to use HTA for healthcare rationing are likely to disadvantage older patients. Guiding principles to help ensure that resources such as kidneys are justly allocated across the life span are proposed.

▶ The current system of allocating organs does not discriminate by the quality of organ. As a consequence, organs are allocated to individuals irrespective of their age. The consequence has been that a number of older kidney transplant recipients have a functioning graft when they die. As available kidneys are in such short supply, losing kidneys that have many years of remaining function has been the subject of debate within the transplant community. The proposal to modify kidney allocation to match expected duration of recipient life with the amount of quality kidney function has raised many comments. The fact that this article appeared in the *Journal of the American Geriatric Society* speaks of the importance of the issue to the elderly. The arguments relating to the routine use of age as a major determinant for kidney allocation were cogently discussed within the article.

T. L. Pruett, MD

Donor Type Does Not Influence the Incidence of Major Urologic Complications After Kidney Transplantation

Saeb-Parsy K, Kosmoliaptsis V, Sharples LD, et al (Univ of Cambridge, UK; Inst of Public Health, Cambridge, UK; et al)

Transplantation 90:1085-1090, 2010

Background.—There has been a marked recent increase in the proportion of kidneys transplanted from live donors (LD) and donors after cardiac death (DCD) compared with donors after brain death (DBD). The purpose of this study was to compare the incidence of major urologic complications (MUCs: urinary leak and ureteric stenosis [US]) in kidney transplants procured from LD, DCD, and DBD and to identify the factors associated with MUCs.

Methods.—We studied 901 consecutive renal transplants (LD: 181, DCD: 198, and DBD: 522) performed in the Cambridge Transplant Centre during 1998 to 2008 by retrieving data from a prospective, cross-audited database, and detailed case note review. An ureteroneocystostomy over a double pigtail ureteric stent was performed in all transplants, and ureteric stents were removed after approximately 6 weeks. All ureteric stenoses were treated by surgical reconstruction.

Results.—Three patients developed urine leak, and 21 developed US. There was no significant difference in the incidence of US in kidneys retrieved from LD (2.8%), DBD (1.7%), or DCD (3.5%; $P=0.28$). Recipients with US had a higher incidence of acute rejection (48% vs. 27%; hazard ratio 3.2, $P=0.005$) and urinary tract infections before the diagnosis of US (48% vs. 19%; hazard ratio 3.0, $P=0.01$). The incidence of delayed graft function (38% vs. 26%), cold ischemia times (12.9 vs. 13.5 hr), and graft survival was not significantly associated with US.

Conclusions.—The incidence of MUCs is similar in kidneys transplanted from LD, DCD, and DBD. When complications do occur, they can be treated successfully by surgical reconstruction.

▶ A consequence of the organ shortage has been the increased use of categories of organ donors that were excluded in the past. The 2006 Institute of Medicine report on organ donation cited donation after circulatory cessation to be a significant source of organs for transplantation. There was concern that organs from these donors (subject to variable amounts of hypoperfusion and warm ischemia) would not function in equal fashion to conventional neurologically deceased organ donors. It has been demonstrated that such kidneys have similar function as those from neurologically dead donors except for more delayed graft function. However, there is concern that the ureter would suffer a similar fate as the bile duct seen with the donors after cardiac death liver. This article attempts to address urologic complications stratified by donor type: living, neurologic deceased, or circulatory deceased. A retrospective review did not demonstrate any significant differences, but the numbers were small. The authors did not discuss many of the significant perfusion issues (time from withdrawal to cessation of circulation, age, warm ischemic time, etc). While the article's conclusion is likely to be true, many issues remain to be clarified.

T. L. Pruett, MD

Donation after Cardiac Death Liver Transplantation: Predictors of Outcome
Mathur AK, Heimbach J, Steffick DE, et al (Univ of Michigan, Ann Arbor; Mayo Clinic, Rochester, MN; Arbor Res Collaborative for Health, Ann Arbor, MI)
Am J Transplant 10:2512-2519, 2010

We aimed to identify recipient, donor and transplant risk factors associated with graft failure and patient mortality following donation after cardiac death (DCD) liver transplantation. These estimates were derived from Scientific Registry of Transplant Recipients data from all US liver-only DCD recipients between September 1, 2001 and April 30, 2009 (n = 1567) and Cox regression techniques. Three years post-DCD liver transplant, 64.9% of recipients were alive with functioning grafts, 13.6% required retransplant and 21.6% died. Significant recipient factors predictive of graft failure included: age ≥ 55 years, male sex, African—American race, HCV positivity, metabolic liver disorder, transplant MELD ≥ 35, hospitalization at transplant and the need for life support at transplant (all, p ≤ 0.05). Donor characteristics included age ≥ 50 years and weight >100 kg (all, p ≤ 0.005). Each hour increase in cold ischemia time (CIT) was associated with 6% higher graft failure rate (HR 1.06, p < 0.001). Donor warm ischemia time ≥ 35 min significantly increased graft failure rates (HR 1.84, p = 0.002). Recipient predictors of mortality were age ≥ 55 years, hospitalization at transplant and retransplantation (all, p ≤ 0.006). Donor weight >100 kg and CIT also increased patient mortality (all, p ≤ 0.035). These findings are useful for transplant surgeons creating DCD liver acceptance protocols.

▶ Donation after cardiac death (DCD) liver transplant results have been disappointing. The development of late biliary strictures has been a significant morbidity leading to graft failure or retransplantation. In a review of the Scientific Registry of Transplant Recipients database, the DCD experience in the United States was analyzed. They confirmed that results after transplantation of DCD livers were not on par with livers from brain dead donors. DCD characteristics that were identified as resulting in inferior results were age older than 50 years, weight of more than 100 kg, and prolonged cold ischemia time. Multiple recipient characteristics were also identified. The variables that impact results after liver transplantation using DCD livers are wide and multifactorial. These livers do not perform on a level that yields consistent results.

T. L. Pruett, MD

For Love or Money? Attitudes Toward Financial Incentives Among Actual Living Kidney Donors

van Buren MC, Massey EK, Maasdam L, et al (Univ Med Ctr Rotterdam, the Netherlands)
Am J Transplant 10:2488-2492, 2010

Due to lengthening waiting lists for kidney transplantation, a debate has emerged as to whether financial incentives should be used to stimulate living kidney donation. In recent surveys among the general public approximately 25% was in favor of financial incentives while the majority was opposed or undecided. In the present study, we investigated the opinion of living kidney donors regarding financial incentives for living kidney donation. We asked 250 living kidney donors whether they, in retrospect, would have wanted a financial reward for their donation. We also investigated whether they were in favor of using financial incentives in a government-controlled system to stimulate living anonymous donation. Additionally, the type of incentive deemed most appropriate was also investigated. In general almost half (46%) of the study population were positive toward introducing financial incentives for living donors. The majority (78%) was not in favor of any kind of reward for themselves as they had donated out of love for the recipient or out of altruistic principles. Remarkably, 60% of the donors were in favor of a financial incentive for individuals donating anonymously. A reduced premium or free health insurance was the preferred incentive.

▶ There are not enough kidneys to meet the needs of people with end-stage renal disease. As such, kidneys obtained from live donors are a major source. In the United States, it is illegal to buy or provide fiscal incentives to obtain kidneys. However, there are many who feel that the law should be changed. This study from the Netherlands assessed attitudes from 250 live kidney donors regarding compensation. About half the donors felt that compensation would be proper, with an increased percentage favoring payment to donors of nondirected kidneys. Giving of oneself carries a significant risk and reward/incentive does not run counter to the sentiment of those having given. As long as there is a mismatch between numbers of organs available for transplantation and numbers of people waiting, the dialogue will continue about the role of incentives to help close the gap.

T. L. Pruett, MD

Five-Year Safety and Efficacy of Belatacept in Renal Transplantation

Vincenti F, Blancho G, Durrbach A, et al (Univ of California, San Francisco; Univ Hosp, Nantes, France; Paris-Sud Univ, Kremlin Bicetre, France; et al)
J Am Soc Nephrol 21:1587-1596, 2010

Belatacept is a first-in-class co-stimulation blocker in development for primary maintenance immunosuppression. A Phase II study comparing belatacept with cyclosporine (CsA) for prevention of acute rejection and protection of renal function in kidney transplant recipients demonstrated similar efficacy and significantly higher measured GFR at 1 year for belatacept, but the incidence of posttransplantation lymphoproliferative disorder was higher. Here, we present the results for the extension of this trial, which aimed to assess long-term safety and efficacy of belatacept. Seventy-eight of 102 patients who were receiving belatacept and the 16 of 26 who were receiving CsA completed the long-term extension period. GFR remained stable in patients who were receiving belatacept for 5 years, and the incidences of death/graft loss or acute rejection were low. The frequencies of serious infections were 16% for belatacept and 27% for CsA, and neoplasms occurred in 12% of each group. No patients who were treated with belatacept and one patient who was treated with CsA developed posttransplantation lymphoproliferative disorder during the follow-up period. Serious gastrointestinal disorders occurred more frequently with belatacept (12% belatacept *versus* 8% CsA), and serious cardiac disorders occurred more frequently with CsA (2% belatacept *versus* 12% CsA). Pharmacokinetic analyses showed consistent exposure to belatacept over time. CD86 receptor saturation was higher in patients who were receiving belatacept every 4 weeks (74%) compared with every 8 weeks (56%). In conclusion, this study demonstrated high patient persistence with intravenous belatacept, stable renal function, predictable pharmacokinetics, and good safety with belatacept over 5 years.

▶ There have been few new class immunosuppressive agents being developed. One of the few agents has been the antagonist of costimulatory signals, belatacept. Results have been encouraging. The current report speaks to the 5-year safety of the antibody. The side effects of belatacept were for the most part less frequent than cyclosporine A. This product should add another option for the treatment of people after organ transplantation.

T. L. Pruett, MD

Comparative Transcriptional and Phenotypic Peripheral Blood Analysis of Kidney Recipients Under Cyclosporin A or Sirolimus Monotherapy

Brouard S, Puig-Pey I, Lozano J-J, et al (Institut National de la Santé Et de la Recherche Médicale INSERM U643, France; Univ of Barcelona, Spain; Hosp Clinic, Mallorca, Barcelona, Spain; et al)
Am J Transplant 10:2604-2614, 2010

Due to its low level of nephrotoxicity and capacity to harness tolerogenic pathways, sirolimus (SRL) has been proposed as an alternative to calcineurin inhibitors in transplantation. The exact mechanisms underlying its unique immunosuppressive profile in humans, however, are still not well understood. In the current study, we aimed to depict the *in vivo* effects of SRL in comparison with cyclosporin A (CSA) by employing gene expression profiling and multiparameter flow cytometry on blood cells collected from stable kidney recipients under immunosuppressant monotherapy. SRL recipients displayed an increased frequency of CD4 + CD25highFoxp3 + T cells. However, this was accompanied by an increased number of effector memory T cells and by enrichment in NFkB-related pro-inflammatory expression pathways and monocyte and NK cell lineage-specific transcripts. Furthermore, measurement of a transcriptional signature characteristic of operationally tolerant kidney recipients failed to detect differences between SRL and CSA-treated recipients. In conclusion, we show here that the blood transcriptional profile induced by SRL monotherapy *in vivo* does not resemble that of operationally tolerant recipients and is dominated by innate immune cells and NFkB-related pro-inflammatory events. These data provide novel insights on the complex effects of SRL on the immune system in clinical transplantation.

▶ The role of immunosuppressive agents in maintenance of organ function is standard. It is often thought that once a stable state has been achieved, the immune response attains a common modality. This study is interesting as it studies stable recipients on either mammalian target of rapamycin (mTOR) inhibitor (sirolimus) or calcineurin inhibitor (CI) (cyclosporine) monotherapy. Gene profiling of peripheral blood mononuclear cells and fluorescence-activated cell sorter analysis demonstrated that in a stable immunologic condition, recipients on mTOR inhibitor monotherapy had a differing circulating cell phenotype profile and gene profile when contrasted to those on CI monotherapy. How much of the profile is related to the immune-stable condition versus the peculiar change by the drug remains unclear. It is possible that many immune profiles are associated with a stable/hyporesponsive condition or that the drug effect dominates the immune profile and the immunologic quiescent state is lost in the drug effect.

T. L. Pruett, MD

Association of genetic polymorphisms and risk of late post-transplantation infection in pediatric heart recipients

Ohmann EL, Brooks MM, Webber SA, et al (Univ of Pittsburgh, PA; et al)
J Heart Lung Transplant 29:1342-1351, 2010

Background.—Late infections are common causes of morbidity and mortality after pediatric heart transplantation. In this multicenter study from 6 centers, we investigated the association between genetic polymorphisms (GPs) in immune response genes and late post-transplantation infections in 524 patients.

Methods.—Late infection was defined as a clinical infectious process occurring >60 days after transplantation and requiring hospitalization, intravenous antimicrobial therapy, or a life-threatening infection requiring oral therapy. All patients provided a blood sample for GP analyses of 18

GPs in cytokine, growth factor, and effector molecule genes by single specific primer-polymerase chain reaction and/or sequencing. Significant associations in univariable analyses were tested in multivariable Cox regression models.

Results.—Late infection was common, with 48.7% of patients experiencing ≥1 late infection, 25.2% had ≥1 late bacterial infection, and 30.5% had ≥1 late viral infection. Older age at transplantation was a protective factor for late infection, both bacterial and viral (hazard ratio [HR] 0.89−0.92 per 1-year age increase, $p < 0.001$). Adjusting for age, race, and transplant etiology, late bacterial infection was associated with *HMOX1* A+326G AG and GG genotypes (HR, 2.41, 95% confidence interval [CI] 1.35−4.30; $p = 0.003$) and *GZMB* A−295G AA genotype (HR, 1.47; 95% CI; 1.03−2.1; $p = 0.036$). Late viral infection was associated with *FAS* A−670G GG genotype (HR, 1.42; 95% CI, 1.00−2.00; $p = 0.050$) in the adjusted model and with *CTLA4* A+49G AA and AG genotypes (HR, 1.49; 95% CI, 1.02−2.19; $p = 0.041$) in univariable analysis.

Conclusion.—We found an association between late bacterial infection and GP of *HMOX1*, which may control macrophage activation. A weaker association was also found between late viral infection and GP of *CTLA4*, a regulator of T-cell activation. This represents progress toward understanding the clinical and genetic risk factors of outcomes after transplantation.

▶ Some of the variations noted in the article by Brouard et al[1] are caused by genetic polymorphisms and differences in drug metabolism. Indeed, pharmacogenetics is demonstrating therapeutic outcome differences for various drugs, based on variations in gene sequences. This article demonstrates a different outcome; differing gene polymorphisms are associated with late infectious complications after pediatric heart transplantation. The diversity of the human genome will complicate efforts to understand the effect of immunosuppressive drugs and the sequelae of other facets of the immune response. It will get more complex before it gets clearer.

T. L. Pruett, MD

Reference

1. Brouard S, Puig-Pey I, Lozano JJ, et al. Comparative transcriptional and phenotypic peripheral blood analysis of kidney recipients under cyclosporin A or sirolimus monotherapy. *Am J Transplant.* 2010;10:2604-2614.

Racial Variation in Medical Outcomes among Living Kidney Donors

Lentine KL, Schnitzler MA, Xiao H, et al (Saint Louis Univ School of Med, MO; et al)
N Engl J Med 363:724-732, 2010

Background.—Data regarding health outcomes among living kidney donors are lacking, especially among nonwhite persons.

Methods.—We linked identifiers from the Organ Procurement and Transplantation Network (OPTN) with administrative data of a private U.S. health insurer and performed a retrospective study of 4650 persons who had been living kidney donors from October 1987 through July 2007 and who had post-donation nephrectomy benefits with this insurer at some point from 2000 through 2007. We ascertained post-nephrectomy medical diagnoses and conditions requiring medical treatment from billing claims. Cox regression analyses with left and right censoring to account for observed periods of insurance benefits were used to estimate absolute prevalence and prevalence ratios for diagnoses after nephrectomy. We then compared prevalence patterns with those in the 2005–2006 National Health and Nutrition Examination Survey (NHANES) for the general population.

Results.—Among the donors, 76.3% were white, 13.1% black, 8.2% Hispanic, and 2.4% another race or ethnic group. The median time from donation to the end of insurance benefits was 7.7 years. After kidney donation, black donors, as compared with white donors, had an increased risk of hypertension (adjusted hazard ratio, 1.52; 95% confidence interval [CI], 1.23 to 1.88), diabetes mellitus requiring drug therapy (adjusted hazard ratio, 2.31; 95% CI, 1.33 to 3.98), and chronic kidney disease (adjusted hazard ratio, 2.32; 95% CI, 1.48 to 3.62); findings were similar for Hispanic donors. The absolute prevalence of diabetes among all donors did not exceed that in the general population, but the prevalence of hypertension exceeded NHANES estimates in some subgroups. End-stage renal disease was identified in less than 1% of donors but was more common among black donors than among white donors.

Conclusions.—As in the general U.S. population, racial disparities in medical conditions occur among living kidney donors. Increased attention to health outcomes among demographically diverse kidney donors is needed. (Funded by the National Institute of Diabetes and Digestive and Kidney Diseases and others.)

▶ Ethnicity is certainly a factor in the genetic polymorphism story. The debate between nature and nurture has been a long-standing debate. This article discusses variations in outcomes after kidney donation as a function of ethnicity. While the article does not answer the question regarding causality, the differences are expected. Live organ donors have risks associated with not just the procedure but also during the follow-up period that extends the rest of their life.

T. L. Pruett, MD

Outcomes of Kidney Transplantation in HIV-Infected Recipients

Stock PG, Barin B, Murphy B, et al (Univ of California, San Francisco; EMMES Corporation, Rockville, MD; Mount Sinai School of Medicine, NY; et al)
N Engl J Med 363:2004-2014, 2010

Background.—The outcomes of kidney transplantation and immuno-suppression in people infected with human immunodeficiency virus (HIV) are incompletely understood.

Methods.—We undertook a prospective, nonrandomized trial of kidney transplantation in HIV-infected candidates who had CD4+ T-cell counts of at least 200 per cubic millimeter and undetectable plasma HIV type 1 (HIV-1) RNA levels while being treated with a stable antiretroviral regimen. Post-transplantation management was provided in accordance with study protocols that defined prophylaxis against opportunistic infection, indications for biopsy, and acceptable approaches to immunosuppression, management of rejection, and antiretroviral therapy.

Results.—Between November 2003 and June 2009, a total of 150 patients underwent kidney transplantation; survivors were followed for a median period of 1.7 years. Patient survival rates ($\pm$ SD) at 1 year and 3 years were 94.6 $\pm$ 2.0% and 88.2 $\pm$ 3.8%, respectively, and the corresponding mean graft-survival rates were 90.4% and 73.7%. In general, these rates fall somewhere between those reported in the national database for older kidney-transplant recipients ($\geq$65 years) and those reported for all kidney-transplant recipients. A multivariate proportional-hazards analysis showed that the risk of graft loss was increased among patients treated for rejection (hazard ratio, 2.8; 95% confidence interval [CI], 1.2 to 6.6; P=0.02) and those receiving antithymocyte globulin induction therapy (hazard ratio, 2.5; 95% CI, 1.1 to 5.6; P=0.03); living-donor transplants were protective (hazard ratio, 0.2; 95% CI, 0.04 to 0.8; P=0.02). A higher-than-expected rejection rate was observed, with 1-year and 3-year estimates of 31% (95% CI, 24 to 40) and 41% (95% CI, 32 to 52), respectively. HIV infection remained well controlled, with stable CD4+ T-cell counts and few HIV-associated complications.

Conclusions.—In this cohort of carefully selected HIV-infected patients, both patient- and graft-survival rates were high at 1 and 3 years, with no increases in complications associated with HIV infection. The unexpectedly high rejection rates are of serious concern and indicate the need for better immunotherapy. (Funded by the National Institute of Allergy and Infectious Diseases; ClinicalTrials.gov number, NCT00074386.)

► In the past, an individual with human immunodeficiency virus (HIV) was excluded from kidney transplantation if he/she presented with end-stage renal disease. The reasons for this are multiple. However, the advent of effective antiviral therapies has changed the discussion, as viral containment appears to be durable. In this setting, the National Institutes of Health—sponsored study for organ transplantation in patients with HIV has been conducted. This report summarizes the outcomes thus far for kidney transplants. The experience had some interesting observations. First, rather than being excessively immunosuppressed, the HIV+ population demonstrates a robust immune response against human alloantigens. The use of thymoglobulin resulted in a durable (years) diminution of CD4+ T cells. HIV nephropathy could be detected (2 cases) in the absence of HIV viremia. The results of the population demonstrated a patient and graft survival somewhere in between results of standard kidney recipients and transplanting individuals older than 65 years. In a population that had previously been deemed unsuitable for transplant therapy, this is an amazing outcome.

There were many controls in this study that do not apply to the average person with HIV. The reader should be aware of the restrictions that the study placed on potential recipients. However, this population should not be routinely excluded from transplant therapies. More information is needed, but the preliminary report is very important.

T. L. Pruett, MD

Reducing Immunosuppression Preserves Allograft Function in Presumptive and Definitive Polyomavirus-Associated Nephropathy
Schaub S, Hirsch HH, Dickenmann M, et al (Univ Hosp Basel, Switzerland)
Am J Transplant 10:2615-2623, 2010

Early detection of polyomavirus BK (BKV) viremia and reduction of immunosuppression is recommended for preventing polyomavirus-associated nephropathy (PyVAN), but systematic histological evaluations were not performed in previous studies. We routinely screen for decoy cells and, if positive, measure plasma BKV-loads. In a cohort of 203 consecutive renal transplantations performed from 2005–2008, 38 patients (19%) developed BKV-viremia and were treated with reduction of immunosuppression. Based on subsequent allograft biopsy results and peak BKV-viremia, patients were assigned to three groups: (i) definitive PyVAN (n = 13), (ii) presumptive PyVAN defined by plasma BKV-loads of $\geq 4 \log_{10}$ copies/ml (n = 17) and (iii) low BKV-viremia (n = 8). Clearance of BKV-viremia was achieved in 35/38 patients (92%) and subsequent clinical rejection occurred in 3/35 patients (8.6%), both without any difference among the groups. Patients with definitive PyVAN had higher peak plasma BKV-loads and required longer time for clearance (8.8 vs. 4.6 vs. 2.9 months; p = 0.001). However, allograft function remained stable from baseline to last follow-up at 34 months (range 18–60) in all three groups with median serum creatinine of 1.6 mg/dl, 1.6 mg/dl and 1.3 mg/dl, respectively. We conclude that screening for BKV-replication and reduction of immunosuppression is an effective strategy to preserve medium-term allograft function even in patients developing definitive PyVAN.

▶ Transplantation in the face of chronic viral infection is intriguing. In the article by Stock et al,[1] the outcome of immunosuppression and human immunodeficiency virus (HIV) was discussed. In this report, chronic viral infection with BK virus (BKV) is described. Unlike HIV, which causes systemic infection and immunodeficiency syndrome, the pathologic effect of BKV appears to be primarily limited to nephropathology. The Basel group report gives a bit of discipline to population management processes. In this process, urine cytology for decoy cells was done on routine protocol. When found, BKV was sought in the plasma. The authors describe a definitive, presumptive, and low BK viremia treatment strategy predicated upon reduction of immunosuppression. Nineteen percent of all kidney transplant recipients fell into one of the above categories. Ninety-two percent eventually cleared the viremia by reduction in immunosuppression alone. The numbers were too small, but kidney function appears to be maintained. This article makes several interesting points, but the most important centers around the need for routine evaluation of the kidney recipient and prompt action when infection in the kidney is detected.

T. L. Pruett, MD

Reference

1. Stock PG, Barin B, Murphy B, et al. Outcomes of kidney transplantation in HIV-infected recipients. *N Engl J Med*. 2010;363:2004-2014.

Differences in Portal Hemodynamics Between Whole Liver Transplantation and Living Donor Liver Transplantation

Jiang S-M, Zhang Q-S, Zhou G-W, et al (Guangxi Med Univ, Liuzhou, China)
Liver Transpl 16:1236-1241, 2010

The aim of this study was to investigate the differences in portal hemodynamics between whole liver transplantation and living donor liver transplantation (LDLT). Twenty patients who underwent LDLT (the L group) and 42 patients who underwent whole liver transplantation (the W group) were enrolled, and colored Doppler ultrasonography was performed preoperatively and on postoperative days (PODs) 1, 3, 5, 7, 30, and 90. The changes in the portal blood flow velocity (PBV) and portal blood flow volume (PBF) were monitored. The graft and spleen sizes were measured with angiographic computed tomography, and upper endoscopy was used to measure esophageal varices on PODs 14, 30, and 90. Although the portal venous pressure (PVP) decreased after graft implantation, it was higher in the L group with a smaller graft size ratio (25.7 ± 5.1 cm H_2O for the L group and 18.5 ± 4.6 cm H_2O for the W group, $P < 0.05$). PBF and PBV increased in both the W and L groups on POD 1 after transplantation; however, the PBF and PBV peaks were significantly higher in the W group. The postoperative PVP and graft volume were greatly related to PBF on POD 1. Grafts in the L group regenerated rapidly after the operation, and the volume increased from 704 ± 115 to 1524 ± 281 mL as early as 1 month after transplantation. A rapid improvement in splenomegaly was observed in both groups. An improvement in esophageal varices was observed in the W group on POD 14 after transplantation, whereas no change was observed in the L group. The portal venous flow in patients with portal hypertension showed a high perfusion state after LDLT, but in contrast to whole liver transplantation, the PVP elevation after LDLT postponed the closing time of the collateral circulation and affected the recovery from splenomegaly.

▶ The blood flow associated with live liver transplantation appears to be important for transplant outcomes. While this article does not discuss or analyze many of the issues relating to function, recovery, and outcome, it does give useful information relating to flow characteristics that distinguish live donor liver grafts from deceased/whole liver allografts. The smaller live donor grafts have higher resistance, lower flow, and higher portal pressures than the whole livers from deceased donors. Over time, flow characteristics normalize, volume of the live donor graft increases, and varices become less prominent. The authors describe 2 instances with a small-for-size syndrome effectively treated with anatomic manipulation (ligation of splenic artery) and pharmacologic treatment (somatostatin). The determinants of blood flow characteristics are not known. Learning more about intrahepatic control of portal blood flow will likely yield better understanding about how to minimize the small-for-size syndrome.

T. L. Pruett, MD

Quality of Life for Donors After Living Donor Liver Transplantation: A Review of the Literature
Parikh ND, Ladner D, Abecassis M, et al (Northwestern Univ, Chicago, IL)
Liver Transpl 16:1352-1358, 2010

Living donor liver transplantation (LDLT) decreases the shortage of liver grafts for patients in need of a liver transplant, but it involves 2 patients: a recipient and a living donor. Despite the magnitude of the procedure for LDLT donors, only a few studies have investigated the effect of LDLT on the quality of life (QOL) of donors. We performed a systematic search of the MEDLINE database to identify peer-reviewed articles assessing QOL in adults after LDLT donation. Nineteen studies describing 768 unique donors met our inclusion criteria for this review. The median number of donors enrolled in each study was 30 (range = 10-143), and the median follow-up period was 10.4 months (range = 3-51.3 months). Before donation, donor QOL was significantly better than that in control adult populations across all measured QOL domains. Within the first 3 months after donation, the physical domains of QOL were significantly worse than the predonation levels, but they returned to baseline levels within 6 months for the majority of patients (80%-93%). Mental domains of QOL remained unchanged throughout the donation process. Common donor concerns after LDLT included bloating, loss of muscle tone, poor body image, and fatigue. In conclusion, according to our review of the existing literature, most LDLT donors return to their baseline QOL within 6 months. However, there is a lack of long-term data on donor QOL after LDLT, and few standardized assessments include measures of common patient concerns. Additional studies are necessary to develop a comprehensive risk profile for LDLT that includes a rigorous assessment of donor QOL.

▶ The consequences of live organ donation are significant. Most studies about the psychosocial consequences of the process have focused on the kidney donor. Little work has been performed in the understanding of the liver donor. This report is a meta-analysis of studies surrounding quality-of-life assessments of live liver donors. There were only 19 studies found that related to the quality of life of liver donors. Not surprisingly, the live liver donor starts with an above-average quality of life before donation. After donation, things change. Unfortunately, long-term studies are not available. There is much to be learned about live donation.

T. L. Pruett, MD

Long-Term Pancreas Allograft Survival in Simultaneous Pancreas-Kidney Transplantation by Era: UNOS registry analysis
Waki K, Terasaki PI, Kadowaki T (Terasaki Foundation Laboratory, Los Angeles, CA; Univ of Tokyo, Japan)
Diabetes Care 33:1789-1791, 2010

Objective.—To determine whether short-term improvement in pancreas graft survival with simultaneous pancreas-kidney (SPK) transplants translated into improved long-term survival, then to examine the implications of that determination.

Research Design and Methods.—We analyzed data for 14,311 diabetic patients who received a first SPK transplant between October 1987 and November 2007, using Kaplan-Meier analysis for graft survival rates and Cox regression analysis for year-of-transplant effect.

Results.—Overall, from 1995 to 2004, 5-year pancreas graft survival stayed about the same (70−71%). Limiting analysis to grafts that survived more than 1 year, 5-year survival from 1987 to 2004 ranged from 80 to 84%. With 1987−1989 as reference, the adjusted hazard ratio for graft failure by year of transplant increased to 1.49 (95% CI 0.97−2.30) in 2000−2004.

Conclusions.—Long-term pancreas graft survival has remained unchanged despite the dramatic decreases in technical failures and early acute rejection rates that have contributed to prolonged SPK graft survival.

▶ Short-term results after kidney/pancreas transplantation have improved significantly over time. This has been the consequence of improvements in preservation techniques and immunosuppression. However, long-term outcomes have rarely been reported. This analysis of the national database demonstrates that despite early improvements in short-term pancreas function, the long-term trajectory of kidney/pancreas function has not changed despite differences in immunosuppression, reduction in rejection rates, and improvements in early results. These findings parallel those seen after kidney transplantation. The challenge for the community will be to understand the variables associated with this inexorable decline, discerning what is allospecific immune response and other active variables.

T. L. Pruett, MD

Survival Differences Following Lung Transplantation Among US Transplant Centers

Thabut G, Christie JD, Kremers WK, et al (Mayo Clinic College of Medicine, Rochester, MN; Univ of Pennsylvania, Philadelphia; et al)
JAMA 304:53-60, 2010

Context.—Although case loads vary substantially among US lung transplant centers, the impact of center effects on patient outcomes following lung transplantation is unknown.

Objective.—To assess variability in long-term survival following lung transplantation among US lung transplant centers.

Design, Setting, and Patients.—Analysis of data from the United Network for Organ Sharing registry for 15 642 adult patients undergoing lung transplantation between 1987 and 2009 in 61 US transplantation centers still active in 2008.

Main Outcome Measures.—Mixed-effect Cox models were fitted to assess survival following lung transplantation at individual centers.

Results.—In 2008, 19 centers (31.1%) performed between 1 and 10 lung transplantations; 18 centers (29.5%), from 11 to 25 transplantations; 20 centers (32.8%), from 26 to 50 transplantations; and 4 centers (6.6%), more than 50 transplantations. One-month, 1-year, 3-year, and 5-year survival rates among all 61 centers were 93.4% (95% confidence interval [CI], 93.0% to 93.8%), 79.7% (95% CI, 79.1% to 80.4%), 63.0% (95% CI, 62.2% to 63.8%), and 49.5% (95% CI, 48.6% to 50.5%), respectively. Characteristics of donors, recipients, and surgical techniques varied substantially among centers. After adjustment for these factors, marked variability remained among centers, with hazard ratios for death ranging from 0.70 (95% CI, 0.59 to 0.82) to 1.71 (95% CI, 1.36 to 2.14) for low- vs high-risk centers, for 5-year survival rates of 30.0% to 61.1%. Higher lung transplantation volumes were associated with improved long-term survival and accounted for 15% of among-center variability; however, variability in center performance remained significant after controlling for procedural volume ($P < .001$).

Conclusions.—Center-specific variation in survival following lung transplantation was only partly associated with procedural volume. However, other statistically significant sources of variability remain to be identified.

▶ Center effect has been recognized as an important factor in transplant outcomes. Typically, the number of transplants performed has been touted as the reason that practice makes perfect. By analyzing the national database, lung transplantation results demonstrate not only that greater center volume and experience are associated with better results but also that higher-than-expected survival was observed in many smaller programs. The findings suggest that by understanding center processes and professional skills, insights into those factors that yield superb clinical results may be gleaned. Similarly, those factors that do not affect significant clinical outcomes improvement may be realized. It is disappointing that analysis of best practices has not permitted sufficient understanding that permits overall system improvements.

T. L. Pruett, MD

Antibodies to Self-Antigens Predispose to Primary Lung Allograft Dysfunction and Chronic Rejection
Bharat A, Saini D, Steward N, et al (Washington Univ School of Med, St Louis, MO)
Ann Thorac Surg 90:1094-1101, 2010

Background.—Primary graft dysfunction (PGD) is a known risk factor for bronchiolitis obliterans syndrome (BOS) after lung transplantation. Here, we report that preformed antibodies to self-antigens increase PGD risk and promote BOS.

Methods.—Adult lung transplant recipients (n = 142) were included in the study. Primary graft dysfunction and BOS were diagnosed based on International Society for Heart and Lung Transplantation guidelines. Antibodies to self-antigens k-alpha-1 tubulin, collagen type V, and collagen I were quantitated using standardized enzyme-linked immunosorbent assays, and cytokines were analyzed using Luminex immunoassays (Biosource International, Camirillo, CA). Human leukocyte antigen (HLA) antibodies were measured using Flow-PRA (One Lambda, Canoga Park, CA).

Results.—Lung transplant recipients with pretransplant antibodies to self-antigens had increased risk of PGD (odds ratio 3.09, 95% confidence interval: 1.2 to 8.1, $p = 0.02$) compared with recipients without. Conversely, in patients with PGD, 34.7% were positive for pretransplant antibodies whereas in the PGD negative group, only 14.6% had antibodies ($p = 0.03$). Antibody positive patients demonstrated high levels of proinflammatory cytokines interleukin (IL)-1β (2.1-fold increase), IL-2 (3.0), IL-12 (2.5), IL-15 (3.0), and chemokines interferon-inducible protein-10 (3.9) and monocyte chemotactic protein-1 (3.1; $p < 0.01$ for all). On 5-year follow-up, patients without antibodies showed greater freedom from development of HLA antibodies compared with patients who had antibodies (class I: 67% versus 38%, $p = 0.001$; class II: 71% versus 41%, $p < 0.001$). Patients with pretransplant antibodies were found to have an independent relative risk of 2.3 (95% confidence interval: 1.7 to 4.5, $p = 0.009$) for developing BOS.

Conclusions.—Presence of antibodies to self-antigens pretransplant increases the risk of PGD immediately after transplant period and BOS on long-term follow-up. Primary graft dysfunction is associated with an inflammatory cascade that augments the alloimmune (anti-HLA) response that predisposes to BOS.

▶ Antibodies to alloantigens are an important variable in organ transplant outcomes. The role of autoantibodies has been associated with recurrent disease but not typically with primary graft outcomes. The findings were that patients with delayed graft (lung) function (DGF) had antibodies to self-antigens. In individuals with these antibodies, the odds ratio for the generation of DGF and chronic rejection is significantly higher. There are a plethora of variables that affect long-term outcomes after transplantation, many of which have not been part of our usual paradigms. Autoantibodies to collagens and tubulin are just not part of the usual screening modes. Whether the generation of such antibodies is the consequence of the initial lung disease or other traumas or unrelated is unclear. Such variables may be important in the gradual loss of function described in the article by Waki et al.[1] It will be interesting to discern how much of this chronic loss is innate immune response, self-response, allo-response, or unrelated to any immunologic component.

T. L. Pruett, MD

Reference

1. Waki K, Terasaki PI, Kadowaki T. Long-term pancreas allograft survival in simultaneous pancreas-kidney transplantation by era: UNOS registry analysis. *Diabetes Care.* 2010;33:1789-1791.

Composite Tissue Allotransplantation

Siemionow MZ, Kulahci Y, Bozkurt M (Cleveland Clinic, OH; Haydarpasa Training Hosp, Istanbul, Turkey; Dicle Univ Dept of Plastic and Reconstructive Surgery, Diyarbakır, Turkey)

Plast Reconstr Surg 124:327e-339e, 2009

Recently, composite tissue allotransplantation was introduced as a potential clinical treatment for complex reconstructive procedures, including tumor ablative operations, traumatic injuries, and extensive tissue loss secondary to burns. Composite tissue allotransplantations consist of heterogeneous tissues including skin, fat, muscle, nerves, lymph nodes, bone, cartilage, ligaments, and bone marrow, all presenting with different antigenicity. Thus, composite tissue allotransplantations are considered to elicit a stronger response compared with solid organ transplants. This article outlines different experimental models and current clinical applications of composite tissue allotransplantation.

▶ Over the past several years, vascularized composite allografts (VCAs) (face and hand) have begun to take their place in the clinical offerings of transplantation. The variables associated with successful VCAs are different from many of those associated with life-saving organs. Too few of these transplants have been performed to include an article comparing function, indication, complications, or immunosuppression optimization. However, the subject is important and represents an expansion of methods to care for people. This article is included as a summary of the long development of the processes that have finally arrived at clinical applicability. Over the next decade, it is likely that considerably more of these procedures will be performed.

T. L. Pruett, MD

Tracheal Allotransplantation after Withdrawal of Immunosuppressive Therapy
Delaere P, for the Leuven Tracheal Transplant Group (Univ Hosp Leuven, Belgium)
N Engl J Med 362:138-145, 2010

Reconstruction of long-segment tracheal defects requires a vascularized allograft. We report successful tracheal allotransplantation after indirect revascularization of the graft in a heterotopic position. Immunosuppressive therapy was administered before the operation, and the tracheal allograft was wrapped in the recipient's forearm fascia. Once revascularization was achieved, the mucosal lining was replaced progressively with buccal mucosa from the recipient. At 4 months, the tracheal chimera was fully lined with mucosa, which consisted of respiratory epithelium from the donor and buccal mucosa from the recipient. After withdrawal of immunosuppressive therapy, the tracheal allograft was moved to its correct anatomical position with an intact blood supply. No treatment-limiting adverse effects occurred.

▶ Transplantation will take on many faces in the future. Designing specific tissue and cell products (organs) is likely to become a reality. The report of tracheal reconstruction using a strategy that allowed repopulation of an allogeneic trachea with self-buccal mucosa, with subsequent transplantation without immunosuppression, is an intriguing first step. This is a remarkable endeavor that combines vascularized grafting techniques with repopulating cells onto a scaffold. If it can effectively be accomplished in this setting, it is feasible to repopulate other tissue scaffoldings with cells to recreate functional structures or organs. This is an exciting concept that can be hopefully replicated in the laboratory.

T. L. Pruett, MD

Chronic Rejection Triggers the Development of an Aggressive Intragraft Immune Response Through Recapitulation of Lymphoid Organogenesis

Thaunat O, Patey N, Caligiuri G, et al (Institut National de la Santé et de la Recherche Médicale, France; Assistance Publique Hopitaux de Paris, France; et al)
J Immunol 185:717-728, 2010

The unwarranted persistence of the immunoinflammatory process turns this critical component of the body's natural defenses into a destructive mechanism, which is involved in a wide range of diseases, including chronic rejection. Performing a comprehensive analysis of human kidney grafts explanted because of terminal chronic rejection, we observed that the inflammatory infiltrate becomes organized into an ectopic lymphoid tissue, which harbors the maturation of a local humoral immune response. Interestingly, intragraft humoral immune response appeared uncoupled from the systemic response because the repertoires of locally produced and circulating alloantibodies only minimally overlapped. The organization of the immune effectors within adult human inflamed tissues recapitulates the biological program recently identified in murine embryos during the ontogeny of secondary lymphoid organs. When this recapitulation was incomplete, intragraft B cell maturation was impeded, limiting the aggressiveness of the local humoral response. Identification of the molecular checkpoints critical for completion of the lymphoid neogenesis program should help develop innovative therapeutic strategies to fight chronic inflammation.

▶ The science behind the immune responses to chronic antigens (alloantigens and autoantigens) after organ transplantation is still unfolding. While systemic circulating cells from blood are often used to infer mechanisms relating to immune responses, this article provides evidence from human organs that significant compartmentalization may exist. In chronically rejected kidneys, organized aggregates of B cells were identified. The demonstration of diversity and apparent local differentiation is intriguing. There is the suggestion that targeted immunotherapy would have a differential benefit. Systemic administration of immunosuppressive agents may be less efficacious than geographically targeted therapies. There is certainly more to be learned regarding duration of exposure, intensity of exposure, prior immune events, and adequacy of antecedent immunosuppressive therapies, as it relates to the generation of locally differentiated immune responses.

T. L. Pruett, MD

6 Surgical Infection

Introduction

Despite years of research and considerable knowledge about the etiology of surgical infections, infections associated with surgical procedures continue to be a clinical problem. Vogel et al queried the National Inpatient Sample to analyze the outcomes of over 6 million surgical procedures.[1] While the study did not identify modalities to modulate the incidence of postoperative sepsis, it reported that this complication does not affect all peoples equally. African American and Hispanic ethnicity and public versus private insurance were associated with increased risk for life-threatening infection. This overview stresses the continued morbidity and mortality associated with generation of the most severe complication associated with surgical infections. In this light, the Surgical Care Improvement Project (SCIP) was initiated to reduce the rate of surgical complications in the United States, with a special area of emphasis on surgical infection. A series of procedures were recommended to participating institutions as a method to decrease the rate of surgical infections. A review of participating institutions[2] demonstrated that self-reported adherence to preventive practices did not result in an alteration of the rate of postoperative infections. Reasons for this observation are probably multiple, but it emphasizes the complexity of taking what is already known about individual factors and applying it meaningfully to population-based therapy. Also it gives credence to the reason that the YEAR BOOK continues to devote a chapter to papers published about surgical infections. While a resource expense and one that is typically addressed as a system issue, surgical site infections (SSIs) occur to individual people. A study by Andersson et al[3] reports on survey results of those inflicted by postoperative surgical infections. While limited in number and clarity, it reinforces that this adverse event has emotional and psychological consequences that go beyond the statistical and monetary associations. The long-term medical consequences of infection are also significant. A study by Moussavian et al[4] illustrates that over 50% of people with peritonitis will eventually develop an incisional hernia at the surgical site, independent of the methodology used for abdominal closure. The importance of surveillance is shown by an increased incidence of surgical site infections when techniques are changed. A study by Haessler et al[5] evaluates a rise in SSIs in a hospital and an association with inadequate adherence to hand-cleansing recommendations. Continual diligence is necessary, as many technological "improvements" can yield unintended adverse consequences.

Papers continue to be written about the application of single variable approaches to clinical practice with the goal to minimize the rate of surgical infection. While use of antimicrobial is relatively uncontroversial, several issues surrounding patient management continue to gain interest: glucose control, oxygenation and temperature control. While there are many confounders to this analysis, the importance of appropriate management during the perioperative period to influence outcomes is reemphasized. The role of glycemic control in the perioperative period has proven somewhat problematic. An article by Ata et al[6] demonstrated in colorectal and general surgery patients that the risk of SSI increased from 1.8% in people with perioperative blood glucose of 110 mg/dL or less to 17.7% in people with recorded glucose of greater than 220 mg/dL. Another variable known to be important for prevention of surgical infections is wound perfusion with oxygenated blood. In a study of colorectal patients undergoing elective resections, 23/116 patients developed SSIs.[7] Comparative perioperative upper arm tissue oxygen saturation was lower in people developing infections than those with an uneventful wound healing. Perioperative normothermia or hypothermia was assessed through the NSQIP data entries at a single institution.[8] Patient normothermia was not associated with altered risk for SSI, especially when compared to glucose control or intestinal surgery. The relative weight of these single variables is yet to be discerned along with any synergistic interactions.

Minimally invasive techniques are becoming normative in the conduct of surgical procedures. In fact, many surgeons and patients consider the performance of minimally invasive surgery the norm. Most studies have noted a decreased incidence of SSI when minimally invasive techniques are employed. A study by Kaafarani et al[9] reports the results of a trial in the VA system that compared laprascopic incisional/ventral hernia repair to open mesh repair. The results again demonstrated that the laprascopic approach is associated with a lesser rate of surgical site infection as compared to an open technique.[9] However, using the NSQIP database,[10] an analysis of almost 40 000 appendectomies demonstrated that while the incisional SSI was lower with a laprascopic (vs open) approach, organ space infections (intraperitoneal) were found to be significantly more common using the laprascopic technique. This finding was surprising as inspection and irrigation of the abdomen is much more accessible through a laparoscopic approach compared with the open technique through a small right lower quadrant incision. The study stresses that there are more issues to surgical procedures than that of skin wound infections.

Intriguingly, techniques that have been shown in the past to be efficacious continue to need justification. Oral antimicrobial agents in addition to fecal elimination was again studied in colon surgery.[11] Once again, the addition of intraluminal antimicrobial agents was demonstrated to be effective in reducing SSIs and organ space infections, as well as other benefits. This was true irrespective of whether intravenous antibiotics were administered. However, topical application of antibiotics has not achieved uniform benefit in reducing surgical infections. In a randomized protocol applying high doses of gentamicin into the subcutaneous wound after colon surgery,[12] the group with the gentamicin impregnated sponges had a higher a rate of SSI than the control (no sponge) group. This was observed despite the fact that all patients received antibiotics with an appropriate spectrum for colonic pathogens. Of course, there are other variables relevant to increased risks for surgical infections. A study of comorbidities in patients undergoing colorectal surgery for inflammatory bowel disease found an increasing risk for infection with weight loss, smoking, ASA class >2, and emergent procedure.[13] In this particular study, the rate of SSI varied from 15.5% in the lowest risk groups to over 36% in those patients with the highest risk.

There are many hypotheses in surgical care which have been the source of conjecture or belief. Bacterial translocation (finding enteric bacteria with mesenteric lymph nodes) has been an observed phenomenon with putative clinical relevance that has covered a wide spectrum. A report from Japan of bacterial products identified by polymerase chain reaction (PCR) before and after hepatobiliary surgery demonstrated a high correlation between a positive lymph node PCR and surgical infection.[14] This occurred even though the rate of culture positivity was minimal. While there is conjecture relating to causality, much is still speculation. Another position in surgery has been that prosthetic materials must be removed in the presence of established infection. A common scenario has been in orthopedic surgery with internal fixation. Under these circumstances, it is common practice to remove the foreign material. A study by Berkes et al[15] describes the consequences of "treating through" infection associated with internal fixation. Success with treatment of a closed fracture was about 80%, whereas successful healing associated with wound infection after repair of an open fracture was almost 60%. It must be noted that a significant percentage of patients had the hardware removed after bone union had occurred. Another example is in patients with peritoneal dialysis infection with enterococcus.[16] This infection should prove very difficult to eradicate because of the hardy constitution of the bacteria and the very difficult task of clearing infected plastic. It was surprising that durable control of symptoms was possible with a variety of antimicrobial therapies. Care of burns has been predicated on maintaining a low wound bacterial count, rapid wound excision, and coverage with some sort of biologic dressing (hopefully autologous skin). However, there should be concern within burn units that bacterial resistance to antimicrobials will lead to treatment failure. A study by Glasser et al[17] describes the efficacy and testing of antiseptics and antibiotics to treat drug-resistant bacteria. The discussion in this article is useful in explaining the differences in testing techniques. Surgical infections are a consequence of any surgical procedure. Even clean, rarely infected outpatient procedures such as Mohs surgery can have a surgical infection rate reduction. A rate of less than 1% was achieved with strict adherence to processes that have been demonstrated as efficacious.[18] Surgical infection is not inevitable, but the influencing factors may not be readily known. Often many think that only therapies directed specifically at either killing microbes or improving circulation and wound healing will diminish surgical infections. A retrospective review of clinical practice demonstrated that intraoperative administration of dexamethasone to prevent postoperative nausea was associated with an increased risk for surgical infection.[19] Preventing surgical infections reaches far into many aspects of medical care.

Surgical infection will continue to be a costly and morbid complication associated with surgery. To that end, continued understanding of risk-factor mitigation continues to be of importance to the practicing surgeon.

Timothy L. Pruett, MD

References

1. Vogel TR, Dombrovski VY, Carson JL, Graham AM, Lowry SF. Postoperative sepsis in the United States. *Ann Surg.* 2010;252:1065-1071.
2. Stulberg JJ, Delaney CP, Neuhauser DV, Aron DC, Fu P, Koroukian SM. Adherence to surgical care improvement project measures and the association with postoperative infections. *JAMA.* 2010;303:2479-2485.
3. Andersson AE, Bergh I, Karlsson J, Nilsson K. Patients' experiences of acquiring a deep surgical site infection: an interview study. *Am J Infect Control.* 2010;38:711-717.
4. Moussavian MR, Schuld J, Dauer D, et al. Long term follow up for incisional hernia after severe secondary peritonitis-incidence and risk factors. *Am J Surg.* 2010;200:229-234.
5. Haessler S, Connelly NR, Kanter G, et al. A surgical site infection cluster: the process and outcome of an investigation—the impact of an alcohol-based surgical antisepsis product and human behavior. *Anesth Analg.* 2010;110:1044-1048.
6. Ata A, Lee J, Bestle SL, Desemone J, Stain SC. Postoperative hyperglycemia and surgical site infection in general surgery patients. *Arch Surg.* 2010;145:858-864.
7. Govinda R, Kasuya Y, Bala E, et al. Early postoperative subcutaneous tissue oxygen predicts surgical site infection. *Anesth Analg.* 2010;111:946-952.
8. Lehtinen SJ, Onicescu G, Kuhn KM, Cole DJ, Esnaola NF. Normothermia to prevent surgical site infections after gastrointestinal surgery: holy grail or false idol? *Ann Surg.* 2010;252:696-704.
9. Kaafarani HM, Kaufman D, Reda D, Itani KM. Predictors of surgical site infection in laparoscopic and open ventral incisional herniorrhaphy. *J Surg Res.* 2010;163:229-234.
10. Fleming FJ, Kim MJ, Messing S, Gunzler D, Salloum R, Monson JR. Balancing the risk of postoperative surgical infections: a multivariate analysis of factors associated with laparoscopic appendectomy from the NSQIP database. *Ann Surg.* 2010;252:895-900.
11. Englesbe MJ, Brooks L, Kubus J, et al. A statewide assessment of surgical site infection following colectomy: the role of oral antibiotics. *Ann Surg.* 2010;252:514-519.
12. Bennett-Guerrero E, Pappas TN, Koltun WA, et al. Gentamicin-collagen sponge for infection prophylaxis in colorectal surgery. *N Engl J Med.* 2010;363:1038-1049.
13. Alavi K, Sturrock PR, Sweeney WB, et al. A simple risk score for predicting surgical site infections in inflammatory bowel disease. *Dis Colon Rectum.* 2010;53:1480-1486.

14. Mizuno T, Yokoyama Y, Nishio H, et al. Intraoperative bacterial translocation detected by bacterium-specific ribosomal RNA-targeted reverse-transcriptase polymerase chain reaction for the mesenteric lymph node strongly predicts postoperative infectious complications. *Ann Surg.* 2010;252:1013-1019.
15. Berkes M, Obremskey WT, Scannell B, Ellington JK, Hymes RA, Bosse M. Maintenance of hardware after early postoperative infection following fracture internal fixation. *J Bone Joint Surg Am.* 2010;92:823-828.
16. Sutherland SM, Alexander SR, Feneberg R, Schaefer F, Warady BA. Enterococcal peritonitis in children receiving chronic peritoneal dialysis. *Nephrol Dial Transplant.* 2010;25:4048-4054.
17. Glasser JS, Guymon CH, Mende K, Wolf SE, Hospenthal DR, Murray CK. Activity of topical antimicrobial agents against multidrug-resistant bacteria recovered from burn patients. *Burns.* 2010;36:1172-1184.
18. Martin JE, Speyer LA, Schmults CD. Heightened infection-control practices are associated with significantly lower infection rates in office-based Mohs surgery. *Dermatol Surg.* 2010;36:1529-1536.
19. Percival VG, Riddell J, Corcoran TB. Single dose dexamethasone for postoperative nausea and vomiting—matched case-control study of postoperative infection risk. *Anaesth Intensive Care.* 2010;38:661-666.

Postoperative Sepsis in the United States

Vogel TR, Dombrovskiy VY, Carson JL, et al (Robert Wood Johnson Med School, New Brunswick, NJ)
Ann Surg 252:1065-1071, 2010

Objectives.—To evaluate the incidence of postoperative sepsis after elective procedures, to define surgical procedures with the greatest risk for developing sepsis, and to evaluate patient and hospital confounders.

Background Data.—The development of sepsis after elective surgical procedures imposes a significant clinical and resource utilization burden in the United States. We evaluated the development of sepsis after elective procedures in a nationally representative patient cohort and assessed the effect of sociodemographic and hospital characteristics on the development of postoperative sepsis.

Methods.—The Nationwide inpatient sample was queried between 2002 and 2006 and patients developing sepsis after elective procedures were identified using the patient safety indicator "Postoperative Sepsis" (PSI-13). Case-mix adjusted rates were calculated by using a multivariate logistic regression model for sepsis risk and an indirect standardization method.

Results.—A total of 6,512,921 weighted elective surgical cases met the inclusion criteria and 78,669 cases (1.21%) developed postoperative sepsis. Case-mix adjustment for age, race, gender, hospital bed size, hospital location, hospital teaching status, and patient income demonstrated esophageal, pancreatic, and gastric procedures represented the greatest risk for the development of postoperative sepsis. Thoracic, adrenal, and hepatic operations accounted for the greatest mortality rates if sepsis developed. Increasing age, Blacks, Hispanics, and men were more likely to develop sepsis. Decreased median household income, larger hospital bed size, urban hospital location, and nonteaching status were associated with greater rates of postoperative sepsis.

Conclusions.—The development of postoperative sepsis is multifactorial and procedures, most likely to develop sepsis, did not demonstrate the greatest mortality after sepsis developed. Factors associated with the development of sepsis included race, age, hospital size, hospital location, and patient income. Further evaluation of high-risk procedures, populations, and environments may assist in reducing this costly complication.

▶ Infection that is associated with surgical procedures is a problem. This article analyzes the consequence of more than 6.5 million procedures and found that 1.2% were associated with postoperative sepsis, identified by *International Classification of Diseases, Ninth Revision* codes from a large database. The conclusions are predicable; this population had a high mortality rate, was more likely to have governmental rather than private insurance, and was more likely to be older, Hispanic,and African American. There are many other associated findings, but poor, sick, older males are more prone to develop postoperative sepsis. It is unquestionable that the cost of sepsis is significant, but the cost of surgical infection is even greater by virtue of its frequency. Depending on the class of wound, surgical site infections occur at 3- to 20-fold higher frequency. Efforts to minimize its occurrence are valid. Difficulties with this analysis are that data acquisition is imprecise because the event capture for the databases has a wide variance of definitions.

T. L. Pruett, MD

Adherence to Surgical Care Improvement Project Measures and the Association With Postoperative Infections
Stulberg JJ, Delaney CP, Neuhauser DV, et al (Case Western Reserve Univ, Cleveland, OH; Univ Hosps Case Med Ctr, Cleveland, OH)
JAMA 303:2479-2485, 2010

Context.—The Surgical Care Improvement Project (SCIP) aims to reduce surgical infectious complication rates through measurement and reporting of 6 infection-prevention process-of-care measures. However, an association between SCIP performance and clinical outcomes has not been demonstrated.

Objective.—To examine the relationship between SCIP infection-prevention process-of-care measures and postoperative infection rates.

Design, Setting, Participants.—A retrospective cohort study, using Premier Inc's Perspective Database for discharges between July 1, 2006 and March 31, 2008, of 405 720 patients (69% white and 11% black; 46% Medicare patients; and 68% elective surgical cases) from 398 hospitals in the United States for whom SCIP performance was recorded and submitted for public report on the Hospital Compare Web site. Three original infection-prevention measures (S-INF-Core) and all 6 infection-prevention measures

(S-INF) were aggregated into 2 separate all-or-none composite scores. Hierarchical logistical models were used to assess process-of-care relationships at the patient level while accounting for hospital characteristics.

Main Outcome Measure.—The ability of reported adherence to SCIP infection-prevention process-of-care measures (using the 2 composite scores of S-INF and S-INF-Core) to predict postoperative infections.

Results.—There were 3996 documented postoperative infections. The S-INF composite process-of-care measure predicted a decrease in postoperative infection rates from 14.2 to 6.8 per 1000 discharges (adjusted odds ratio, 0.85; 95% confidence interval, 0.76-0.95). The S-INF-Core composite process-of-care measure predicted a decrease in postoperative infection rates from 11.5 to 5.3 per 1000 discharges (adjusted odds ratio, 0.86; 95% confidence interval, 0.74-1.01), which was not a statistically significant lower probability of infection. None of the individual SCIP measures were significantly associated with a lower probability of infection.

Conclusions.—Among hospitals in the Premier Inc Perspective Database reporting SCIP performance, adherence measured through a global all-or-none composite infection-prevention score was associated with a lower probability of developing a postoperative infection. However, adherence reported on individual SCIP measures, which is the only form in which performance is publicly reported, was not associated with a significantly lower probability of infection.

▶ The Surgical Care Improvement Project (SCIP) was developed to diminish the risk of complications associated with surgical procedures. A variety of processes were recommended to improve outcomes, with several focused on prevention of surgical infections. In yet another analysis of a large database, 450 000 surgical discharges were analyzed and stratified by the self-reported adherence with the SCIP infection-prevention process-of-care measures. This self-reported compliance with individual elements of SCIP processes was not associated with reduction of infection, although a yes response to a binary response of general adherence to infection prevention was associated with a reduced risk of infection. Again, this analysis is subject to the same limitations of large databases. However, outcomes research is increasingly dependent on large pools of patient information that have been collected for other reasons. Self-reported compliance may or may not be accurately entered. However, assuming that the entries and data are reflective of care, despite each recommendation having level 1 reliability, other factors must be operative in the generation of surgical infections. The importance of systems must be assessed with reliably improved outcomes being the consequence.

T. L. Pruett, MD

Patients' experiences of acquiring a deep surgical site infection: An interview study

Andersson AE, Bergh I, Karlsson J, et al (Univ of Gothenburg, Göteborg, Sweden; Sahlgrenska Univ Hosp, Göteborg, Sweden)
Am J Infect Control 38:711-717, 2010

Background.—The negative impact of surgical site infection (SSI) in terms of morbidity, mortality, additional costs, and length of stay (LOS) in the hospital is well described in the literature, as are risk factors and preventive measures. Given the lack of knowledge regarding patients' experiences of SSI, the aim of the present study was to describe patients' experiences of acquiring a deep SSI.

Methods.—Content analysis was used to analyze data obtained from 14 open interviews with participants diagnosed with a deep SSI.

Results.—Patients acquiring a deep SSI suffer significantly from pain, isolation, and insecurity. The SSI changes physical, emotional, social, and economic aspects of life in extremely negative ways, and these changes are often persistent.

Conclusion.—Health care professionals should focus on strategies to enable early diagnosis and treatment of SSIs. The unacceptable suffering related to the infection, medical treatment, and an insufficient patient-professional relationship should be addressed when planning individual care, because every effort is needed to support this group of patients and minimize their distress. All possible measures should be taken to avoid bacterial contamination of the surgical wound during and after surgery to prevent the development of SSI.

▶ While the articles by Vogel et al and Stulberg et al[1,2] discussed outcomes from more than 2 million operative procedures, it must be remembered that while surgical infections occur after surgical interventions in a certain percentage of cases, the infections happen to individual people. In this article, 15 orthopedic patients with surgical infections were interviewed. Significant negative associations persisted for months or longer after developing wound infections. One would suspect that the negative psychological outcomes of infection may vary with the type of surgery. These outcomes should encourage the practicing surgeon to remember that the consequence of infection extends beyond antibiotics and wound care. It is important to talk with people and engage mental health specialists to facilitate adaptation and the person's ability to cope with adversity into the treatment strategy of the infectious complication.

T. L. Pruett, MD

References

1. Vogel TR, Dombrovskiy VY, Carson JL, Graham AM, Lowry SF. Postoperative sepsis in the United States. *Ann Surg.* 2010;252:1065-1071.
2. Stulberg JJ, Delaney CP, Neuhauser DV, Aron DC, Fu P, Koroukian SM. Adherence to surgical care improvement project measures and the association with postoperative infections. *JAMA.* 2010;303:2479-2485.

Long term follow up for incisional hernia after severe secondary peritonitis—incidence and risk factors
Moussavian MR, Schuld J, Dauer D, et al (Univ of Saarland, Homburg, Germany)
Am J Surg 200:229-234, 2010

Background.—In patients with secondary peritonitis, infections of the abdominal cavity might render the abdominal wall susceptible to secondary complications such as incisional hernia (IH).

Methods.—One hundred ninety-eight patients treated for secondary peritonitis underwent midline laparotomy. Ninety-two surviving patients accessible to clinical follow-up were examined for the occurrence of IH, and risk factors at the time of surgery or during follow-up were determined.

Results.—During a median follow-up period of 6 years, 54.3% of the patients developed IHs. A high body mass index, coronary heart disease, intense blood loss, requirement for intraoperative or postoperative transfusions, and small bowel perforation as a source of peritonitis were associated with IH.

Conclusions.—IH occurs quite frequently after surgery for secondary peritonitis. Preexisting risk factors for IH and intraoperative blood loss or requirement for blood transfusions were correlated with the development of IH. Interestingly, surgical technique was not correlated with the development of IH in this series.

▶ Diffuse peritonitis requires considerable surgical attention to achieve a favorable outcome. While many different techniques have been used in therapy, there are questions that arise about the long-term outcomes. In this study, 92 survivors of peritonitis had their abdominal incision examined. More than 50% of the patients were found to have incisional hernias on average of 6 years after resolution of infection. There was no association with multiplicity of procedures for initial control of peritonitis, such as running or interrupted closure, lavage, or other variable techniques used to control peritonitis. The consequence of surgical infection does not end with resolution of the infection and requires long-term follow-up to return a person to the maximal functional condition.

T. L. Pruett, MD

A Surgical Site Infection Cluster: The Process and Outcome of an Investigation—The Impact of an Alcohol-Based Surgical Antisepsis Product and Human Behavior
Haessler S, Connelly NR, Kanter G, et al (Baystate Med Ctr, Springfield, MA)
Anesth Analg 110:1044-1048, 2010

Background.—The institution of a process used to successfully execute a perioperative antibiotic administration system is but 1 component of preventing postoperative infections. Continued surveillance of infections is an important part of the process of decreasing postoperative infections. We recently experienced an increase in the number of postoperative infections in our patients. Using standard infection control methods of outbreak investigation, we tracked multiple variables to search for a common cause. We describe herein the process by which Quality Improvement methodology was used to investigate and manage this surgical site infection (SSI) cluster.

Methods.—As part of routine surveillance for SSI, the infection control division seeks out evidence of postoperative infections. Patients were defined as having an SSI according to National Healthcare Safety Network SSI criteria. SSI data are reviewed monthly and aggregated on a quarterly basis. The SSI rate was above our usual level for 3 consecutive quarters of 2007. This increase in the infection rate led to an internal outbreak investigation, termed a "cluster investigation." This investigation comprised multiple concurrent methods including manual chart review of all cases; review of microbiological data; and inspection of operating rooms, instrument processing facilities, and storage areas.

Results.—During 3 quarters, a trend emerged in our general surgical population that demonstrated that 4 surgical types had a sustained increase in SSI. The institutional antibiotic protocol was appropriate for prevention of the majority of these SSIs. As part of the investigation, direct observation of hand hygiene and surgical hand antisepsis technique was undertaken. At this time, there were 2 types of surgical hand preparation being used, at the discretion of the clinician: either a "standard" scrub with an antimicrobial soap or the application of a chlorhexidine gluconate and alcohol-based surgical hand antisepsis product. Observers noted improper use of this alcohol-based surgical hand antiseptic. This product was withdrawn from our operating rooms, and the SSI rate markedly decreased in the following 2 quarters.

Discussion.—In Conclusion, we report the results of a quality improvement process that investigated a 3-quarter increase in our SSI rate. An investigation was undertaken, and it was thought that the (mis)use of an alcohol-based hand antiseptic product was associated with the increased infection rate. Removing this product, along with reemphasizing the importance of infection control, was associated with a decrease in the infection rate to a level at or below our historical rate.

▶ Every institution is confronted with episodic outbreaks of infection. Infection control uses analysis of behavior and processes that can identify a practice that results in an increased rate of surgical infections. While Surgical Care Improvement Project practices are intended to diminish infection rates, contravening financial pressures have introduced new technologies to save time. One such change has been skin antiseptic preparation for surgical procedures. In this article, an outbreak of surgical site infections was traced to the failure to comply with adequate preparation of the skin. Such findings have been previously noted with time-saving processes in surgery. A combination of education and enforcement of policy resulted in a return to acceptable rates. Maintaining acceptable infection rates requires diligence.

T. L. Pruett, MD

Postoperative Hyperglycemia and Surgical Site Infection in General Surgery Patients
Ata A, Lee J, Bestle SL, et al (Albany Med College, NY)
Arch Surg 145:858-864, 2010

Hypothesis.—Postoperative hyperglycemia is an independent risk factor for postoperative surgical site infection (SSI).

Design.—Retrospective medical record review.

Setting.—Academic tertiary referral center.

Patients.—A total of 2090 general and vascular surgery patients in an institutional quality improvement database between November 1, 2006, and April 30, 2009.

Main Outcome Measure.—Postoperative SSI.

Results.—Postoperative glucose levels were available for 1561 patients (74.7.0%), of which 803 (51.4%) were obtained within 12 hours of surgery. The significant univariate predictors of SSI in general surgery patients were increasing age, emergency status, American Society of Anesthesiologists physical status classes P3 to P5, operative time, more than 2 U of red blood cells transfused, preoperative glucose level higher than 180 mg/dL (to convert to millimoles per liter, multiply by 0.0555), diabetes mellitus, and postoperative hyperglycemia. On multivariate adjustment, increasing age, emergency status, American Society of Anesthesiologists classes P3 to P5, operative time, and diabetes remained significant predictors of SSI for general surgery patients. After adjustment for postoperative glucose level, all these variables ceased to be significant predictors of SSI; only incremental postoperative glucose level remained significant. Subanalysis revealed that a serum glucose level higher than 140 mg/dL was the only significant predictor of SSI (odds ratio, 3.2; 95% confidence interval [CI], 1.4-7.2) for colorectal surgery patients. Vascular surgery patients were 1.8 times (95% CI, 1.3-2.5 times) more likely to develop SSI than were general surgery patients. Operative time and diabetes mellitus were the only significant univariate predictors of SSI among vascular surgery patients, and postoperative hyperglycemia was not associated with SSI.

Conclusions.—Postoperative hyperglycemia may be the most important risk factor for SSI. Aggressive early postoperative glycemic control should reduce the incidence of SSI.

▶ There are many variables that influence the rate of surgical infection. Aside from administration of appropriate prophylactic antibiotics, skin preparation, and wound contamination, there are other patient control variables that may influence surgical infections. In this article, the role of glycemic control was assessed.

The authors concluded that blood sugar levels greater than 140 mg/dL were incrementally associated with an increase of surgical site infection. While this is probably true, the information that was used to generate the information is interesting and somewhat confusing. A single blood sugar level measurement during the 12-hour postoperative period was assessed, and outcomes were associated with that measure of glycemic control. Amounts of insulin required, constant infusions, and intravenous injection versus subcutaneous administration were not addressed. Is it important to maintain serum glucose level of less than 140 mg/dL for the entire 12 perioperative hours or just some segment of it? At what time after surgery does the benefit of glycemic control attenuate? Certainly there are considerable issues that need to be clarified if we are to optimize application of tight control to the perioperative patient.

T. L. Pruett, MD

Early Postoperative Subcutaneous Tissue Oxygen Predicts Surgical Site Infection

Govinda R, Kasuya Y, Bala E, et al (Tufts Med Ctr, Boston, MA; Univ of Louisville, KY; Cleveland Clinic, OH)
Anesth Analg 111:946-952, 2010

Background.—Subcutaneous oxygen partial pressure is one of several determinants of surgical site infections (SSIs). However, tissue partial pressure is difficult to measure and requires invasive techniques. We tested the hypothesis that early postoperative tissue oxygen saturation (StO_2) measured with near-infrared spectroscopy predicts SSI.

Methods.—We evaluated StO_2 in 116 patients undergoing elective colon resection. Saturation was measured near the surgical incision, at the upper arm, and at the thenar muscle with an InSpectra™ tissue spectrometer model 650 (Hutchinson Technology Inc., Hutchinson, MN) 75 minutes after the end of surgery and on the first postoperative day. An investigator blinded to StO_2 assessed patients daily for wound infection. Receiver operating characteristic curves were used to analyze the performance of StO_2 measurements as a predictor of SSI.

Results.—In 23 patients ($\approx 20\%$), SSI was diagnosed 9 ± 5 days (mean $\pm$ SD) after surgery. Patients who did and did not develop an SSI had similar age (48 ± 14 vs 48 ± 15 years, respectively; $P = 0.97$) and gender (female:male, 15:8 vs 46:47, respectively), but patients who developed SSI weighed more (body mass index 32 ± 7 vs 27 ± 6 kg/m^2; $P < 0.01$). StO_2 at the upper arm was lower in patients who developed SSI than in those who did not develop SSI (52 ± 22 vs 66 ± 21; $P = 0.033$), and these measurements had a sensitivity of 71% and specificity of 60% for predicting SSI, using StO_2 of 66% as the cutoff point.

Conclusion.—StO_2 measured at the upper arm only 75 minutes after colorectal surgery predicted development of postoperative SSI, although the infections were typically diagnosed more than a week later. Although further testing is required, Sto_2 measurements may be able to predict SSI and thus allow earlier preventive measures to be implemented.

▶ An experimental variable that has been shown to increase the likelihood of surgical site infection (SSI) is tissue oxygen delivery. In experimental models, decreasing tissue oxygen saturation decreases the number of bacteria necessary to induce a recognizable soft tissue infection. Colonic surgery is associated with a certain degree of operative site bacterial contamination, which translates clinically into an increased frequency of SSI compared with clean surgery. This article confirms that factor known from laboratory science: a lower tissue oxygen tension is associated with a higher risk for wound infection. The risk for wound infection starts with the introduction of viable bacteria into the surgical wound. However, tissue oxygenation is perfusion and blood oxygenation dependent. It is unclear whether the study supports better perfusion or increased oxygenation. If the former is the case, a more direct measurement of tissue perfusion may be beneficial. Nevertheless, perioperative management of tissue oxygen delivery may yet prove to be an important quality metric. As with glycemic control, it will be important to discern the duration and strength of the association.

T. L. Pruett, MD

Normothermia to Prevent Surgical Site Infections After Gastrointestinal Surgery: Holy Grail or False Idol?

Lehtinen SJ, Onicescu G, Kuhn KM, et al (Med Univ of South Carolina (MUSC), Charleston; Med Univ Hosp Authority, Charleston, SC)
Ann Surg 252:696-704, 2010

Objective.—To analyze the association between perioperative normothermia (temperature $\geq 36°C$) and surgical site infections (SSIs) after gastrointestinal (GI) surgery.

Summary of Background Data.—Although active warming during colorectal surgery reduces SSIs, there is limited evidence that perioperative normothermia is associated with lower rates of SSI. Nonetheless, hospitals participating in the Surgical Care Improvement Project must report normothermia rates during major surgery.

Methods.—We conducted a nested, matched, case-control study; cases consisted of GI surgery patients enrolled in our National Surgical Quality Improvement Program database between March 2006 and March 2009 who developed SSIs. Patient/surgery risk factors for SSI were obtained from the National Surgical Quality Improvement Program database. Perioperative temperature/antibiotic/glucose data were obtained from medical records. Cases/controls were compared using univariate/random effects/logistic regression models. Independent risk factors for SSIs were identified using multivariate/random effects/logistic regression models.

Results.—A total of 146 cases and 323 matched controls were identified; 82% of patients underwent noncolorectal surgery. Cases were more likely to have final intraoperative normothermia compared with controls (87.6% vs. 77.8%, $P = 0.015$); rates of immediate postoperative normothermia were similar (70.6% vs. 65.3%, respectively, $P = 0.19$). Emergent surgery/higher wound class were associated with higher rates of intraoperative normothermia. Independent risk factors for SSI were diabetes, surgical complexity, small bowel surgery, and nonlaparoscopic surgery. There was no independent association between perioperative normothermia and SSI (adjusted odds ratio, 1.05; 95% confidence interval, 0.48–2.33; $P = 0.90$).

Conclusions.—Pay-for-reporting measures focusing on perioperative normothermia may be of limited value in preventing SSI after GI surgery. Studies to define the benefit of active warming after noncolorectal GI surgery are warranted.

▶ Maintenance of normal intraoperative body temperature is one of the Surgical Care Improvement Project (SCIP) objectives to reduce surgical complications. The literature on this variable has been closely intertwined with tissue perfusion and oxygen delivery to the surgical site as noted in the previous article. This study fails to find that normothermia is independently associated with reduction in risks for surgical site infection. It suffers in failing to address association with tissue perfusion. While normothermia may not be independently associated with reduced incidence of infection, it is important to discern clinically the relative contribution of body temperature to tissue perfusion in modest states of perioperative volume depletion. The negative results in this study do not conclusively negate the SCIP recommendations.

T. L. Pruett, MD

Predictors of Surgical Site Infection in Laparoscopic and Open Ventral Incisional Herniorrhaphy

Kaafarani HMA, Kaufman D, Reda D, et al (Tufts Med Ctr, Boston, MA; The Veterans Affairs Cooperative Studies Program Coordinating Ctr, Hines, IL; et al)
J Surg Res 163:229-234, 2010

Background.—Surgical site infection (SSI) after ventral incisional hernia repair (VIH) can result in serious consequences. We sought to identify patient, procedure, and/or hernia characteristics that are associated with SSI in VIH.

Methods.—Between 2004 and 2006, patients were randomized in four Veteran Affairs (VA) hospitals to undergo laparoscopic or open VIH. Patients who developed SSI within eight weeks postoperatively were compared to those who did not. A bivariate analysis for each factor and a multiple logistic regression analysis were performed to determine factors associated with SSI. The variables studied included patient characteristics and co-morbidities (e.g., age, gender, race, ethnicity, body mass index, ASA classification, diabetes, steroid use), hernia characteristics (e.g., size, duration, number of previous incisions), procedure characteristics (e.g., open *versus* laparoscopic, blood loss, use of postoperative drains, operating room temperature) and surgeons' experience (resident training level, number of open VIH previously performed by the attending surgeon). Antibiotic prophylaxis, anticoagulation protocols, preparation of the skin, draping of the wound, body temperature control, and closure of the surgical site were all standardized and monitored throughout the study period.

Results.—Out of 145 patients who underwent VIH, 21 developed a SSI (14.5%). Patients who underwent open VIH had significantly more SSIs than those who underwent laparoscopic VIH (22.1% *versus* 3.4%; $P = 0.002$). Among patients who underwent open VIH, those who developed SSI had a recorded intraoperative blood loss greater than 25 mL (68.4% *versus* 40.3%; $P = 0.030$), were more likely to have a drain placed (79.0% *versus* 49.3%; $P = 0.021$) and were more likey to be operated on by surgeons with less than 75 open VIH case experience (52.6% *versus* 28.4%; $P = 0.048$). Patient and hernia characteristics were similar between the two groups. In a multiple logistic regression analysis, the open surgical technique was associated with SSI (OR 8.03, 95% CI 2.03, 31.72; $P = 0.003$) while controlling for the VA medical center where the procedure was performed ($P = 0.041$).

Conclusion.—Open surgical technique and the medical center rather than patient co-morbidities or hernia characteristics are associated with the formation of postoperative SSI in VIH.

▶ Surgical technique is important in the prevention and generation of surgical site infection. As implied in the previous articles, it is commonly stated and accepted that laparoscopic procedures are associated with fewer surgical infections. In this study, individuals in need of ventral hernia repair at 4 Veteran Affairs hospitals were randomized between open and laparoscopic herniorrhaphy. The incidence of infection was strikingly lower when the laparoscopic technique was used. While this is certainly true for the average procedure, it is important to understand that multiple options are required to adequately care for the complex case. It was demonstrated in this series that experience is a key component in the risk of developing infections. Perhaps the routine ventral hernia should be approached laparoscopically, but judgment will have to discern when injury risk would override perceived benefit.

T. L. Pruett, MD

Balancing the Risk of Postoperative Surgical Infections: A Multivariate Analysis of Factors Associated With Laparoscopic Appendectomy From the NSQIP Database
Fleming FJ, Kim MJ, Messing S, et al (Univ of Rochester Med Ctr, NY)
Ann Surg 252:895-900, 2010

Objective.—To establish the relationship between operative approach (laparoscopic or open) and subsequent surgical infection (both incisional and organ space infection) postappendectomy, independent of potential confounding factors.

Background.—Although laparoscopic appendectomy has been associated with lower rates of incisional infections than an open approach, the relationship between laparoscopy and organ space infection (OSI) is not as clearly established.

Methods.—Cases of appendectomy were retrieved from the American College of Surgeons National Surgical Quality Improvement Program (NSQIP) database for 2005 to 2008. Patient factors, operative variables, and the primary outcomes of incisional infections and OSIs were recorded. Factors associated with surgical infections were identified using logistic regression models. These models were then used to calculate probabilities of OSI in clinical vignettes demonstrating varying levels of infectious risk.

Results.—A total of 39,950 appendectomy cases were included of which 30,575 (77%) were performed laparoscopically. On multivariate analysis, laparoscopy was associated with a lower risk of incisional infection [odds ratio (OR) 0.37, 95% confidence interval (CI) 0.32–0.43] but with an increased risk of OSI after adjustment for confounding factors (OR 1.44, 95% CI 1.21–1.73). For a low-risk patient, probability of OSI was calculated to be 0.3% and 0.4%, respectively, for open versus laparoscopic appendectomy, whereas for a high-risk patient, probabilities were estimated at 8.9% and 12.3%, respectively.

Conclusion.—Laparoscopy was associated with a decreased risk of incisional infection but with an increased risk of OSI. The degree of this increased risk varies depending on the clinical profile of a surgical patient. Recognition of these differences in risk may aid clinicians in the choice of operative approach for appendectomy.

▶ The article by Kaafarani et al[1] was convincing in demonstrating a diminution of surgical infections by using laparoscopic techniques. However, incisional infections are not the only type of infection that can occur. In this assessment of outcomes after appendectomy, the rate of incisional infection was indeed lower after laparoscopic appendectomy, but intra-abdominal abscess formation was more common after minimally invasive appendectomy. From a technique perspective, this article and the one by Kaafarani et al stress judgment and application. It is anticipated that the rate of intra-abdominal infection would have been diminished by more thorough abdominal inspection, irrigation, and reduction of residual contamination. While articles tend to make surgical decisions seem formulaic, it is crucial that the practitioner understand the reasons why some techniques have advantage over others.

T. L. Pruett, MD

Reference

1. Kaafarani HM, Kaufman D, Reda D, Itani KM. Predictors of surgical site infection in laparoscopic and open ventral incisional herniorrhaphy. *J Surg Res.* 2010;163: 229-234.

A Statewide Assessment of Surgical Site Infection Following Colectomy: The Role of Oral Antibiotics

Englesbe MJ, Brooks L, Kubus J, et al (Univ of Michigan, Ann Arbor; et al)
Ann Surg 252:514-520, 2010

Objective.—To determine the utility of adding oral nonabsorbable antibiotics to the bowel prep prior to elective colon surgery.

Summary Background Data.—Bowel preparation prior to colectomy remains controversial. We hypothesized that mechanical bowel preparation with oral antibiotics (compared with without) was associated with lower rates of surgical site infection (SSI).

Methods.—Twenty-four Michigan hospitals participated in the Michigan Surgical Quality Collaborative—Colectomy Best Practices Project. Standard perioperative data, bowel preparation process measures, and *Clostridium difficile* colitis outcomes were prospectively collected. Among patients receiving mechanical bowel preparation, a logistic regression model generated a propensity score that allowed us to match cases differing only in whether or not they had received oral antibiotics.

Results.—Overall, 2011 elective colectomies were performed over 16 months. Mechanical bowel prep without oral antibiotics was administered to 49.6% of patients, whereas 36.4% received a mechanical prep and oral antibiotics. Propensity analysis created 370 paired cases (differing only in receiving oral antibiotics). Patients receiving oral antibiotics were less likely to have any SSI (4.5% vs. 11.8%, $P = 0.0001$), to have an organ space infection (1.8% vs. 4.2%, $P = 0.044$) and to have a superficial SSI (2.6% vs. 7.6%, $P = 0.001$). Patients receiving bowel prep with oral antibiotics were also less likely to have a prolonged ileus (3.9% vs. 8.6%, $P = 0.011$) and had similar rates of *C. difficile* colitis (1.3% vs. 1.8%, $P = 0.58$).

Conclusions.—Most patients in Michigan receive mechanical bowel preparation prior to elective colectomy. Oral antibiotics may reduce the incidence of SSI.

▶ Surgical site infection is the result of the host's inability to contain/remove a bacterial load prior to the clinical manifestation of what we call an infection. Some of the clinical variables have been noted in the previous articles. However, the mainstay of minimization for risk of wound infection over the past several decades has been to kill the bacteria through the use of antimicrobial agents. It is interesting that the use of oral antibiotics is being revisited in prophylaxis after colonic surgery. In over 2000 colectomies, irrespective of the type of bowel preparation, the use of oral antibiotics was associated with a reduced rate of wound and organ space infections, shortened ileus, and a slightly increased risk of antibiotic-associated colitis. The authors made the necessary disclaimers about a retrospective study about inadvertent bias and unmeasured confounders. However, taken in totality of the surgical literature, fewer bacteria in the colon should be associated with diminished risk of infectious complications. Whether intravenous antimicrobials or topical antiseptics could induce a similar outcome is feasible but not conclusively addressed. The use of oral agents appears to widen the therapeutic window even when intravenous agents are used.

T. L. Pruett, MD

Gentamicin–Collagen Sponge for Infection Prophylaxis in Colorectal Surgery

Bennett-Guerrero E, for the SWIPE 2 Trial Group (Duke Univ Med Ctr, Durham, NC; Milton S. Hershey Med Ctr, PA; et al)
N Engl J Med 363:1038-1049, 2010

Background.—Despite the routine use of prophylactic systemic antibiotics, surgical-site infection continues to be associated with significant morbidity and cost after colorectal surgery. The gentamicin–collagen sponge, an implantable topical antibiotic agent, is approved for surgical implantation in 54 countries. Since 1985, more than 1 million patients have been treated with the sponges.

Methods.—In a phase 3 trial, we randomly assigned 602 patients undergoing open or laparoscopically assisted colorectal surgery at 39 U.S. sites to undergo either the insertion of two gentamicin–collagen sponges above the fascia at the time of surgical closure (the sponge group) or no intervention (the control group). All patients received standard care, including prophylactic systemic antibiotics. The primary end point was surgical-site infection occurring within 60 days after surgery, as adjudicated by a clinical-events classification committee that was unaware of the study-group assignments.

Results.—The incidence of surgical-site infection was higher in the sponge group (90 of 300 patients [30.0%]) than in the control group (63 of 302 patients [20.9%], P=0.01). Superficial surgical-site infection occurred in 20.3% of patients in the sponge group and 13.6% of patients in the control group (P=0.03), and deep surgical-site infection in 8.3% and 6.0% (P=0.26), respectively. Patients in the sponge group were more likely to visit an emergency room or surgeon's office owing to a wound-related sign or symptom (19.7%, vs. 11.0% in the control group; P=0.004) and to be rehospitalized for surgical-site infection (7.0% vs. 4.3%, P=0.15). The frequency of adverse events did not differ significantly between the two groups.

Conclusions.—Our large, multicenter trial shows that the gentamicin–collagen sponge is not effective at preventing surgical-site infection in patients who undergo colorectal surgery; paradoxically, it appears to result in significantly more surgical-site infections. (Funded by Innocoll Technologies; ClinicalTrials.gov number, NCT00600925.)

▶ With the premise that fewer bacteria result in a lower rate of wound infection and better healing, a study using topical delivery of antibiotic (gentamicin) in colon surgery was done. Collagen sponges impregnated with gentamicin were placed within the surgical wound after colon surgery and failed to diminish the rate of surgical site infection. This tactic, similar to adding antibiotic to wound irrigation, has been used in hundreds of thousands of instances. The reasons for these findings are likely to be multifactorial, but some would include the persistence of foreign material in the wound after the antibiotics have diffused away. Antimicrobial agents work but can be overcome by other surgical factors. This article is very illustrative of many of the factors that interplay in the generation of adverse clinical events.

T. L. Pruett, MD

A Simple Risk Score for Predicting Surgical Site Infections in Inflammatory Bowel Disease
Alavi K, Sturrock PR, Sweeney WB, et al (Univ of Massachusetts Med School, Worcester; et al)
Dis Colon Rectum 53:1480-1486, 2010

Purpose.—Patients with inflammatory bowel disease are often at highest risk for surgical site infections. We sought to define the predictors of surgical site infections and to develop a risk score for predicting those at highest risk.

Methods.—Patients undergoing a bowel resection for Crohn's disease or ulcerative colitis were identified from National Surgical Quality Improvement Program 2008. Univariate and multivariate analyses were conducted to identify predictors of surgical site infections. Clinically relevant prediction categories were developed and the predictive behavior of the model was validated by use of National Surgical Quality Improvement Program 2007. An integer-based scoring system risk score was created proportional to the logistic regression coefficients, grouping patients into categories of similar risk.

Results.—We identified 271,368 patients; 3981 of these patients underwent an operation for Crohn's disease (n = 2895) or ulcerative colitis (n = 1086). Nine hundred (22.6%) patients developed surgical site infections. Predictors included weight loss, smoking, emergent surgery, wound class, operative time (minutes), and an ASA score >2. A risk score was developed by stratifying patients into low (0–5), 15.6%; medium (6–8), 25.2%; and high (>8), 36.1% risk.

Conclusions.—Patients with inflammatory bowel disease are at high risk for surgical site infections. Preoperative factors including weight loss, smoking, emergent surgery and an ASA score >2 are strong predictors of surgical site infections. Operative time and wound class are important intraoperative predictors. A risk score, based on pre- and intraoperative variables, can be used to identify patients at highest risk of developing surgical site infections. This may allow for appropriate process measures to be implemented to prevent and lessen the impact of surgical site infections in this high-risk population.

▶ As a way to demonstrate the multiple variables associated with generation of infection, scoring systems have been developed to associate clinical conditions with proclivity to develop some adverse events after surgical interventions. This article uses the American College of Surgeons National Surgical Quality Improvement Program database to assess variables associated with the development of infection in patients undergoing surgery for inflammatory bowel disease. The population studied should have a significant bacterial contamination at the time of colectomy. The analysis confirms what years of clinical experience and prior articles have confirmed: that weight loss, smoking, emergency surgery, prolonged operative time, and American Society of Anesthesiologists class > 2 were associated with higher rates of infection. What is not clear is how much diminution of the risk occurs with cessation of smoking, nutrition, planned surgery, and shortened operative time. These sorts of studies demonstrate common factors but do little to help us understand how we should address them. We need to do better.

T. L. Pruett, MD

Intraoperative Bacterial Translocation Detected by Bacterium-Specific Ribosomal RNA-Targeted Reverse-Transcriptase Polymerase Chain Reaction for the Mesenteric Lymph Node Strongly Predicts Postoperative Infectious Complications After Major Hepatectomy for Biliary Malignancies
Mizuno T, Yokoyama Y, Nishio H, et al (Nagoya Univ Graduate School of Medicine, Japan; et al)
Ann Surg 252:1013-1019, 2010

Background.—There is little evidence indicating a causal linkage between bacterial translocation and postoperative infectious complication (POIC) in human studies.

Objective.—To investigate the correlation between the occurrence of bacterial translocation in the mesenteric lymph node (MLN) and POIC with a sensitive quantitative method using bacterium-specific ribosomal RNA (rRNA)-targeted reverse transcriptase—polymerase chain reaction (RT-qPCR).

Methods.—Patients who underwent major hepatectomy for biliary malignancies involving hepatic hilus were included in this study ($n = 65$). Mesenteric lymph nodes were harvested from the jejunal mesentery 2 times during the operation (MLN-1 harvested at laparotomy and MLN-2 harvested after tumor resection). Microorganisms were detected by a bacterium-specific rRNA-targeted RT-qPCR method. Perioperative factors and POIC were recorded prospectively.

Results.—Of 65 patients, 51 completed the study. Microorganisms were detected in MLN-1 and MLN-2 in 15 (29.4%) and 19 (37.3%) patients, respectively. The detection of microorganisms in MLN-1 was significantly correlated with the incidence of preoperative cholangitis ($P = 0.04$), whereas the detection of microorganisms in MLN-2 was significantly correlated with the incidence of POIC ($P = 0.002$). In multivariate analysis, a positive result for detection of microorganisms in MLN-2 was one of the independent predictive factors of POIC (odds ratio $= 26.1$).

Conclusions.—Intraoperative analysis of MLNs (especially MLN-2) by rRNA-targeted RT-qPCR can strongly predict the occurrence of POIC after hepatectomy for biliary malignancy. This method is more sensitive and faster at detection of microorganisms than the conventional culture method. Therefore, we can obtain the information of bacterial translocation immediately after the surgery and can select the group of patients with high risk for POIC.

▶ Bacterial translocation has been observed to occur for years. The variables associated with increased recovery of bacteria from mesenteric lymph nodes have been many, but typically, the more stress placed on the patient (animal in the experimental realm), the more bacterial translocation occurs. In this study, patients undergoing hepatic resections had mesenteric lymph nodes sampled before and after the major operative intervention. It was demonstrated that in those individuals with detection of bacteria after resection, a higher rate of wound infection was observed (odds ratio of 26, very significant). Whether this observation is causative (ie, the bacteria that translocate also cause wound infection) or associative (the stresses that facilitate bacterial translocation are also associated with an increased risk for wound infection) remains unclear and is not addressed in the article. What is certainly clear is that significant physiologic events occur during major surgical procedures, which extend well beyond those that meet the eye.

T. L. Pruett, MD

Maintenance of Hardware After Early Postoperative Infection Following Fracture Internal Fixation
Berkes M, Obremskey WT, Scannell B, et al (Hosp for Special Surgery, NY; Vanderbilt Univ Med Ctr, Nashville, TN; Carolinas Med Ctr, Charlotte, NC; et al)
J Bone Joint Surg Am 92:823-828, 2010

Background.—The development of a deep wound infection in the presence of hardware after open reduction and internal fixation presents a clinical dilemma, and there is scant literature to aid in decision-making. The purpose of the present study was to determine the prevalence of osseous union with maintenance of hardware after the development of postoperative infection within six weeks after internal fixation of a fracture.

Methods.—The present study included 121 patients from three level-I trauma centers, retrospectively identified from billing and trauma registries, in whom 123 postoperative wound infections with positive intraoperative cultures had developed within six weeks after internal fixation of acute fractures. The incidence of fracture union without hardware removal was calculated, and the parameters that predicted success or failure were evaluated.

Results.—Eighty-six patients (eighty-seven fractures; 71%) had fracture union with operative débridement, retention of hardware, and culture-specific antibiotic treatment and suppression. Predictors of treatment failure were open fracture (p = 0.03) and the presence of an intramedullary nail (p = 0.01). Several variables were not significant but trended toward an association with failure, including smoking, infection with Pseudomonas species, and involvement of the femur, tibia, ankle, or foot.

Conclusions.—Deep infection after internal fixation of a fracture can be treated successfully with operative débridement, antibiotic suppression, and retention of hardware until fracture union occurs. These results may be improved by patient selection based on certain risk factors and the specific bacteria and implants involved.

▶ Recommended approaches to the management of infected prosthetic devices vary by the observer and their background. The standard infectious diseases recommendation is to remove the device because once an inanimate material is contaminated, the environment precludes eradication of the infecting organisms. The approach from the clinician is often to attempt suppression of bacteria to a level that is clinically unrecognizable (irrelevant) and leave the device in place. While this is what is desirable, the patient's question becomes, when does such a practice become quixotic and when is it practical? This study attempts to address the problem by examining patients developing infections after open reduction and internal fixation of a fracture. The clinical end point is that which was desired by the patient: osseous healing of their fracture. It is surprising how little literature there is on the subject. This study demonstrates that it is possible to achieve osseous healing with retained hardware in most instances; however, there is still a significant failure rate (30%). It is still important that the practitioner gain insight into the individual factors and determine when the appropriate time is to give up and move toward removal of the device.

T. L. Pruett, MD

Enterococcal peritonitis in children receiving chronic peritoneal dialysis

Sutherland SM, For the International Pediatric Peritonitis Registry (IPPR) (Stanford Univ Med Ctr, CA; et al)
Nephrol Dial Transplant 25:4048-4054, 2010

Background.—Peritonitis is a common complication of chronic peritoneal dialysis (CPD) and can be associated with technique failure. Enterococcus is an uncommon peritoneal pathogen in children receiving CPD but represents a potential therapeutic challenge due to its innate resistance to cephalosporins and emerging resistance to glycopeptides.

Methods.—The International Pediatric Peritonitis Registry is a global consortium of 47 paediatric dialysis centres designed to address validation of the International Society for Peritoneal Dialysis paediatric peritonitis treatment guidelines. Between 2001 and 2004, peritonitis episodes were assessed in 392 participating children receiving CPD.

Results.—Among the 392 patients, 340 episodes of culture-positive peritonitis were evaluated. Twenty of these episodes were due to *Enterococcus* species (5.9%). There were no clinical characteristics uniquely associated with enterococcal peritonitis at presentation. After 3 days of therapy, 75% of patients were pain free, 95% had decreased effluent cloudiness and 90% were afebrile. Only one patient required a catheter exchange, and all patients experienced full functional recovery. Despite broad *in vitro* resistance to cephalosporins and 21% resistance to glycopeptides, neither *in vitro* resistance pattern nor choice of empiric antibiotic regimen affected short- or long-term outcomes.

Conclusions.—Enterococci are likely responsible for ~6% of culture-positive peritonitis episodes in children receiving CPD. Although it was not possible to identify patients with enterococcal peritonitis based on presentation, clinical response was not associated with *in vitro* resistance patterns, and patients who initially received a cephalosporin-based empiric regimen until culture results are available are likely to respond quickly and have full functional recovery.

▶ Along with indwelling intravenous catheters, peritoneal dialysis catheters tend to be one of the more common prosthetic materials to become infected. While relatively easy to remove, the consequences to the patient are so significant that many physicians resist. This article is fascinating in that it analyzes the outcomes of pediatric patients with infections caused by an organism that is quite resistant to antimicrobial agents. *Enterococcus* is very difficult to kill; β-lactam antibiotics are only bacterial static and cephalosporins rarely demonstrate any activity against the organism. However, in this experience, no patient received a regimen that was optimized for *Enterococcus* as first-line therapy. However, despite this observation, the patients did remarkably well with resolution of symptoms and clearance of the organism. The catheter was preserved in 19 of 20 instances. Clinical response should always be the final arbiter.

T. L. Pruett, MD

Activity of topical antimicrobial agents against multidrug-resistant bacteria recovered from burn patients
Glasser JS, Guymon CH, Mende K, et al (San Antonio Military Med Ctr, Fort Sam Houston, TX; US Army Inst of Surgical Res, Fort Sam Houston, TX)
Burns 36:1172-1184, 2010

Background.—Topical antimicrobials are employed for prophylaxis and treatment of burn wound infections despite no established susceptibility breakpoints, which are becoming vital in an era of multidrug-resistant (MDR) bacteria. We compared two methods of determining topical antimicrobial susceptibilities.

Methods.—Isolates of *Pseudomonas aeruginosa*, methicillin-resistant *Staphylococcus aureus* (MRSA), extended spectrum beta-lactamase (ESBL) producing *Klebsiella pneumoniae*, and *Acinetobacter baumanii-calcoaceticus* (ABC) from burn patients were tested using broth microdilution and agar well diffusion to determine minimum inhibitory concentrations (MICs) and zones of inhibition (ZI). Isolates had systemic antibiotic resistance and clonality determined. MDR included resistance to antibiotics in three or more classes.

Results.—We assessed 22 ESBL-producing *K. pneumoniae*, 20 ABC (75% MDR), 20 *P. aeruginosa* (45% MDR), and 20 MRSA isolates. The most active agents were mupirocin for MRSA and mafenide acetate for the gram-negatives with moderate MICs/ZI found with silver sulfadiazene, silver nitrate, and honey. MDR and non-MDR isolates had similar topical resistance. There was no clonality associated with resistance patterns.

Conclusion.—Despite several methods to test bacteria for topical susceptibility, no defined breakpoints exist and standards need to be established. We recommend continuing to use silver products for prophylaxis against gram-negatives and mafenide acetate for treatment, and mupirocin for MRSA.

▶ Antimicrobial resistance is a capacity that is common among bacteria retrieved from the hospital environment. This is an especially common occurrence in units with high-frequency use of antibiotics (intensive care units, burn units, etc) where it is sometimes common practice to use topical antimicrobial agents with the purpose to decrease risk for bacterial infection. The results of this report are not as interesting as the discussion and delineation of the issues in discerning adequate activity against resistant hospital organisms. This is especially true in the use of agents that are given topically to minimize wound contamination in burn patients. In vitro testing is certainly used to guide clinical practice. This article does an interesting job of sorting out many of the issues in antibiotic-resistant organisms.

T. L. Pruett, MD

Heightened Infection-Control Practices are Associated with Significantly Lower Infection Rates in Office-Based Mohs Surgery

Martin JE, Speyer L-A, Schmults CD (Univ of Texas Med Branch, Galveston; Brigham and Women's Hosp, Boston, MA)
Dermatol Surg 36:1529-1536, 2010

Background.—Reported infection rates for Mohs micrographic surgery (MMS) range from less than 1% to 3.5%.

Objective.—To determine whether lower infection rates are possible for MMS with a consistently applied infection-control regimen.

Methods.—A series of 832 consecutive patients with 950 tumors undergoing MMS formed the cohort for a retrospective study of infections before and after a program of heightened infection-control practices at a single-surgeon academic Mohs practice. The sterility upgrade included jewelry restrictions, alcohol hand scrub before stages and reconstruction, sterile gloves and (during reconstruction) sterile gowns for staff, and sterile towels and dressings for patients during Mohs stages.

Results.—Infection rate was 2.5% (9 infections/365 tumors) before the sterility upgrade and 0.9% (5 infections/585 tumors) after, a statistically significant difference (*p* = .04).

Conclusion.—MMS already has low rates of infection, but this study shows that rigorous infection-control practices can significantly affect infection rates.

▶ There has been a great deal of attention given to reducing surgical infections within the hospital setting. However, the practices associated with infection control and risk reduction for surgical patients are applicable across all settings. It is all too often that practices do not translate from one arena to another. This article discusses surgical site infection of a relatively minor clean procedure: Mohs micrographic surgery. It is performed in the outpatient environment and rarely has complications. In fact, during the control period before increased attention to sterile technique, 97.5% of the procedures were performed without infectious mishap. After introduction of techniques known to minimize introduction of bacteria into the wound, over 99% of the procedures were performed without infectious mishap. This study demonstrates 2 obvious facts: (1) any wound can become infected, and technique matters—Semmelweis taught us much about hygiene and the risk for infection—and (2) wounds will always become infected, either by human error or by endogenous contamination from the person being operated upon. Surgeons can alter the rate by innumerable technical components, but some people have such low threshold for infection that it will occur despite following all protocols.

T. L. Pruett, MD

Single dose dexamethasone for postoperative nausea and vomiting — a matched case-control study of postoperative infection risk
Percival VG, Riddell J, Corcoran TB (Royal Perth Hosp, Western Australia, Australia)
Anaesth Intensive Care 38:661-666, 2010

Dexamethasone is an effective prophylaxis against postoperative nausea and vomiting but is immunosuppressive and may predispose patients to an increased postoperative infection risk. This matched case-control study examined the association between the administration of a single intraoperative anti-emetic dose of dexamethasone (4 to 8 mg) and postoperative infection in patients undergoing non-emergency surgery in a university trauma centre. Cases were defined as patients who developed infection between one day and one month following an operative procedure under general anaesthesia. Controls who did not develop infection were matched for procedure, age and gender. Exclusion criteria included immunosuppressive medications, chronic glucocorticoid therapy, cardiac surgical and solid-organ transplantation procedures. Sixty-three cases and 172 controls were identified. Cases were more likely to have received dexamethasone intraoperatively (25.4 vs 11%, P=0.006), and less likely to have received perioperative antibiotic prophylaxis (60.3 vs 84.3%, P=0.001). Stepwise, multivariate conditional logistic regression confirmed these associations, with adjusted odds ratios of 3.03 (1.06 to 19.3, P=0.035) and 0.12 (0.02 to 0.7, P=0.004) respectively for the associations between dexamethasone and perioperative antibiotic prophylaxis, with postoperative infection. We conclude that intraoperative administration of dexamethasone for anti-emetic purposes may confer an increased risk of postoperative infection.

▶ Surgical infections occur in patients, and some clinical variables that we think are not relevant infection variables are mistaken. Treatments to minimize risk for postoperative nausea are common, and dexamethasone has proven quite useful in this regard. In this study, an association between dexamethasone administration and surgical site infection (SSI) was demonstrated. While this was true on multivariate analysis, it was also shown that perioperative antibiotics were less frequently given to those with SSI and dexamethasone. Chicken or egg? Variables associated with the development of clinical infection are enormous and likely to expand. Vigilance requires ongoing system assessments to identify and correct events associated with an increased incidence.

T. L. Pruett, MD

7 Endocrine

Adrenocortical carcinoma: is the surgical approach a risk factor of peritoneal carcinomatosis?
Leboulleux S, Deandreis D, Al Ghuzlan A, et al (Univ Paris Sud-XI, France)
Eur J Endocrinol 162:1147-1153, 2010

Context.—Peritoneal carcinomatosis (PC) is a rare site of distant metastases in patients with adrenocortical cancer (ACC). One preliminary study suggests an increased risk of PC after laparoscopic adrenalectomy (LA) for ACC.

Objective.—The objective of the study was to search for risk factors of PC including surgical approach.

Design.—This was a retrospective cohort study conducted in an institutional practice.

Patients.—Sixty-four consecutive patients with ACC seen at our institution between 2003 and 2009 were included. Mean tumor size was 132 mm. Patients had stage I disease in 2 cases, stage II disease in 32 cases, stage III disease in 7 cases, stage IV disease in 21 cases, and unknown stage disease in 2 cases. Surgery was open in 58 cases and laparoscopic in 6 cases.

Main Outcome.—The main outcome was the risk factors of PC.

Results.—PC occurred in 18 (28%) patients. It was present at initial diagnosis in three cases and occurred during follow-up in 15 cases. The only risk factor of PC occurring during follow-up was the surgical approach with a 4-year rate of PC of 67% (95% confidence interval (CI), 30-90%) for LA and 27% (95% CI, 15-44%) for open adrenalectomy (P=0.016). Neither tumor size, stage, functional status, completeness of surgery, nor plasma level of op'DDD was associated with the occurrence of PC.

Conclusion.—We found an increased risk of PC after LA for ACC. Whether this is related to an inappropriate surgical approach or to insufficient experience in ACC surgery should be clarified by a prospective program.

▶ Leboulleux et al analyze a group of 64 consecutive patients treated at their institution for more than 6 years for adrenocortical cancer for the development of peritoneal carcinomatosis (PC). They note that the only risk factor for the development of PC was a laparoscopic approach to the operation; 4 of 6 patients who underwent a laparoscopic approach developed PC versus 11 of 55 with an open approach. This study is included to demonstrate a classic example of referral bias. There is no attempt to determine what the denominator was for the patients referred with PC who were treated laparoscopically, and thus, the conclusion that the risk of PC is higher with a laparoscopic approach is invalid. As in the early days of laparoscopic colorectal surgery for cancer, port site recurrences proved ultimately to be the consequence of unskilled surgery, not an inherent danger in the laparoscopic approach.

T. J. Fahey III, MD

Laparoscopic Resection is Inappropriate in Patients with Known or Suspected Adrenocortical Carcinoma

Miller BS, Ammori JB, Gauger PG, et al (Univ of Michigan, Ann Arbor; et al)
World J Surg 34:1380-1385, 2010

Background.—Complete surgical resection is the mainstay of treatment for patients with adrenocortical cancer (ACC). Use of laparoscopy has been questioned in patients with ACC. This study compares the outcomes of patients undergoing laparoscopic versus open resection (OR) for ACC.

Methods.—A retrospective review (2003—2008) of patients with ACC was performed. Data were collected for demographics, operative and pathologic data, adjuvant therapy, and outcome. Chi-square analysis was performed.

Results.—Eighty-eight patients (66% women; median age, 47 (range, 18—81) years) were identified. Seventeen patients underwent laparoscopic adrenalectomy (LA). Median tumor size of those who underwent LA was 7.0 (range, 4—14) cm versus 12.3 (range, 5—27) cm for OR. Recurrent disease in the laparoscopic group occurred in 63% versus 65% in the open group. Mean time to first recurrence for those who underwent LA was 9.6 months (± 14) versus 19.2 months (± 37.5) in the open group ($p < 0.005$). Fifty percent of patients who underwent LA had positive margins or notation of intraoperative tumor spill versus 18% of those who underwent OR ($p = 0.01$). Local recurrence occurred in 25% of the laparoscopic group versus 20% in the open group ($p = 0.23$). Mean follow-up was 36.5 months (± 43.6).

Conclusions.—ACC continues to be a deadly disease, and little to no progress has been made from a treatment standpoint in the past 20 years. Careful and complete surgical resection is of the utmost importance. Although feasible in many cases and tempting, laparoscopic resection should not be attempted in patients with tumors suspicious for or known to be adrenocortical carcinoma.

▶ In this article, the Michigan group reports its experience with 88 patients with adrenocortical cancer (ACC) who presented to their multidisciplinary clinic over a 6-year period. Only 18 of the 88 patients had their surgery at Michigan, and all 17 of the laparoscopic adrenalectomies were performed at outside hospitals and seen postoperatively or at the time of recurrence. The laparoscopic group had smaller tumors but had higher rates of positive margins and/or intraoperative tumor rupture. On the basis of these data, the authors strongly condemn the use of laparoscopic adrenalectomy for known or suspected ACC.

Unfortunately, this study suffers from significant selection bias, as does the article from Leboulleux et al. Above what size would the authors recommend a laparoscopic approach be abandoned—4 cm (the size of the smallest ACC in their current series) or 6 cm? This editor strongly believes in the principles of surgical resection in ACC but does not agree that these cannot be achieved without going to an open resection of these tumors. There are ample data to suggest that properly conducted operations are the most important determinant of surgical outcome for this disease. As with so many surgical diseases, greater experience with the operation leads to better outcomes. This may be especially true for ACC, and thus surgeons with inadequate experience should not be permitted to approach adrenal masses known or suspected to be ACC. The choice of operative approach should be determined by the expert surgeon based on adequate data.

T. J. Fahey III, MD

Laparoscopic Versus Open Adrenalectomy for Adrenocortical Carcinoma: Surgical and Oncologic Outcome in 152 Patients
Brix D, German Adrenocortical Carcinoma Registry Group (Univ of Würzburg, Germany; et al)
Eur Urol 58:609-615, 2010

Background.—The role of laparoscopic adrenalectomy in the treatment of patients with adrenocortical carcinoma (ACC) is controversial.

Objective.—Our aim was to compare oncologic outcome in patients with ACC who underwent either open adrenalectomy (OA) or laparoscopic adrenalectomy (LA) for localised disease.

Design, setting, and participants.—We conducted a retrospective analysis of 152 patients with stage I–III ACC with a tumour ≤10 cm registered with the German ACC Registry.

Intervention.—Patients were stratified into two groups according to the surgical procedure (LA or OA). For comparison, we used both a matched pairs approach by selecting for each patient from the LA group ($n = 35$) one corresponding patient from the OA group ($n = 117$) and multivariate analysis in all 152 patients.

Measurements.—Disease-specific survival was chosen as the predefined primary end point. Secondary end points were recurrence-free survival, frequency of tumour capsule violation and postoperative peritoneal carcinomatosis, and incidence and reasons for conversion from LA to OA.

Results and Limitations.—LA and OA did not differ with regard to the primary end point using either the matched pairs approach (hazard ratio [HR] for death: 0.79; 95% confidence interval [CI], 0.36–1.72; $p = 0.55$) or multivariate analysis (HR for death: 0.98; 95% CI, 0.51–1.92; $p = 0.92$). Similarly, adjusted recurrence-free survival was not different between LA and OA (HR: 0.91; 95% CI, 0.56–1.47;

$p = 0.69$). Frequency of tumour capsule violation and peritoneal carcinomatosis were comparable between groups. In 12 of 35 patients of the LA group, surgery was converted to open surgery with no impact on the clinical outcome.

Conclusions.—For localised ACC with a diameter of ≤10 cm, LA by an experienced surgeon is not inferior to OA with regard to oncologic outcome (Fig 2).

▶ This article is a review of a multi-institutional database from the German Adrenocortical Carcinoma Registry and is the most balanced analysis of laparoscopic versus open adrenalectomies for adrenocortical carcinoma (ACC) to date. Although this does not take the place of a randomized prospective study, the authors used a matched-pair analysis to assess the impact of laparoscopic resection on disease-specific survival as well as recurrence-free survival and surgical missteps in tumors < 10 cm. Whether the comparison was performed as matched or versus the entire group of patients who underwent open adrenalectomy, there was no difference in either recurrence-free or overall survival between the 2 groups. Furthermore, as demonstrated in Fig 2 (included), there is no apparent detrimental effect of starting laparoscopically and having to convert to open. There were actually fewer tumor capsule violations in the laparoscopic group than in the open group (9% vs 15%), although this difference was not statistically significant.

The data suggest that well-conducted surgery can be performed either laparoscopically or as open for midsize ACC and that there is not an inherent danger in the laparoscopic approach if the surgeon has adequate experience. While this editor believes that there is no biologic reason to prevent the adaptation of laparoscopic adrenalectomy for ACC, this should not be interpreted as a green light for the occasional adrenal surgeon to attack an adrenal mass suspected to be

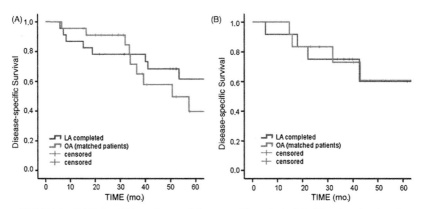

FIGURE 2.—(A) Kaplan-Meier estimates of disease-specific survival of the 23 patients in whom laparoscopic adrenalectomy (LA) was completed versus 23 matched patients with open adrenalectomy (OA). (B) Kaplan-Meier estimates of disease-specific survival of the 12 patients in whom LA was converted to OA versus 12 matched patients with OA. (Reprinted from Brix D, German Adrenocortical Carcinoma Registry Group. Laparoscopic versus open adrenalectomy for adrenocortical carcinoma: surgical and oncologic outcome in 152 patients. *Eur Urol.* 2010;58:609-615 with permission from European Association of Urology).

cancer laparoscopically. Because of the importance of a clean surgical resection, adrenalectomy for adrenal cancer, or suspected cancer, should be left to those with considerable experience in adrenal surgery.

T. J. Fahey III, MD

Recurrence of Adrenal Cortical Carcinoma Following Resection: Surgery Alone Can Achieve Results Equal to Surgery Plus Mitotane
Grubbs EG, Callender GG, Xing Y, et al (The Univ of Texas M.D. Anderson Cancer Ctr, Houston; et al)
Ann Surg Oncol 17:263-270, 2010

Background.—A recent nonrandomized interinstitutional study reported that adjuvant mitotane following surgery for adrenocortical carcinoma (ACC) was associated with decreased recurrence. Because of the limitations of this study, we investigated the influences of surgery and adjuvant mitotane in a large series of ACC patients evaluated and treated at a single referral center.

Study Design.—Retrospective evaluation of patients followed at a single institution after surgery for ACC.

Results.—218 patients with ACC underwent primary resection either at the index institution [surgery index (SI), $n = 28$] or an outside institution [surgery outside (SO), $n = 190$] and had a median follow-up of 88 months. SI patients had a superior disease-free survival compared with SO patients (median 25 versus 12 months, $P = 0.003$), and SI patients also had a superior overall survival compared with SO patients (median not reached versus 44 months, $P = 0.02$). Factors predicting increased risk of recurrence on multivariate analysis were surgery at an outside institution [hazard ratio (HR) 2.56, 95% confidence interval (CI) 1.44–4.53, $P = 0.001$] and no treatment with adjuvant mitotane (HR 1.95, 95% CI 1.06–3.59, $P = 0.03$), and those predicting a poorer survival were advanced stage at presentation ($P = 0.01$) and surgery at an outside institution (HR 2.62, 95% CI 1.31–5.25, $P = 0.007$).

Conclusions.—The recurrence rate of the index group (50%) in the current series, the overwhelming majority of whom did not receive adjuvant mitotane, is indistinguishable from that reported for those who received adjuvant mitotane (49%) in the recent interinstitutional report, emphasizing the importance of completeness of initial surgery in the management of patients with ACC.

▶ This article by Grubbs et al is an important addition to the literature in the debate over whether adjuvant mitotane is indicated in a patient with resected adrenocortical carcinoma. While the article does not present any data that refute the use of adjuvant mitotane, it makes a couple of very important points. First, adequate initial surgery is a critically important factor in the determination of recurrence rates. The authors note a recurrence rate of 50% in their own surgical experience versus 86% in patients referred from outside institutions. While one could argue that the patients referred from outside institutions are being referred because of recurrence, this recurrence rate is similar to that seen in the European series advocating the use of mitotane, and the benefit of mitotane in delaying recurrence may be more evident in patients with a higher risk of recurrence, ie, those with incomplete resection at the initial operation. This raises the question as to whether adjuvant mitotane is indicated in completely resected tumors with negative margins. Second, mitotane therapy is associated only with increased disease-free survival—but not overall survival—highlighting the need for further work in identifying new targets for therapy in adrenal cortical carcinoma.

T. J. Fahey III, MD

Improved quality of life, blood pressure, and biochemical status following laparoscopic adrenalectomy for unilateral primary aldosteronism
Sukor N, Kogovsek C, Gordon RD, et al (Univ of Queensland School of Medicine, Brisbane, Australia)
J Clin Endocrinol Metab 95:1360-1364, 2010

Context.—In 22 patients with unilateral primary aldosteronism (UPA), unilateral laparoscopic adrenalectomy (ADX) not only corrected hypokalemia and led to cure or improvement of hypertension, but also significantly improved quality of life (QOL).

Setting and Design.—In this pilot study, QOL was evaluated prospectively using SF-36 questionnaire before and 3 and 6 months after ADX in 22 patients [14 males] with UPA who underwent ADX within the Endocrine Hypertension Research Center, Greenslopes and Princess Alexandra Hospitals, between June 2007 and June 2008.

Results.—Eighty-six percent of patients were cured of hypertension, and the remainder improved. Plasma potassium normalized and, whereas renin concentration increased, plasma aldosterone, aldosterone/renin ratio, and number of antihypertensive agents decreased. Preoperatively, SF-36 scores for each QOL domain were lower for UPA patients than reported for the Australian general population, especially for physical functioning, role physical, vitality, and general health. Significant improvements were seen at 3 months in physical functioning, role physical, social functioning, role emotional, general health, mental health, and vitality and at 6 months in physical functioning, role physical, general health, role emotional, mental health, and vitality.

Conclusion.—Unilateral adrenalectomy had positive impacts not only on blood pressure and biochemical parameters, but also on QOL, which was impaired preoperatively but significantly improved by 3 months postoperatively.

▶ This article from the Queensland, Australia, hypertension group is a simple and straightforward study that documents that patients who undergo surgical treatment for primary hyperaldosteronism not only have resolution of their hypertension and hyperkalemia but also generally feel better. While this is not surprising, it has not been previously documented. The study would have greater impact if it had included a medically-only treated group. This may become more important as future generations of antihypertensives to combat hyperaldosterone states are introduced. Nevertheless, it adds another benefit to the surgical management of primary hyperaldosteronism, which makes the decision to recommend surgery easier for physicians and patients.

T. J. Fahey III, MD

Post-surgical hypocortisolism after removal of an adrenal incidentaloma: is it predictable by an accurate endocrinological work-up before surgery?
Eller-Vainicher C, Morelli V, Salcuni AS, et al (Univ of Milan, Italy; et al)
Eur J Endocrinol 162:91-99, 2010

Objective.—Few data are available regarding the need of steroid substitutive therapy after unilateral adrenalectomy for adrenal incidentaloma (AI). It is unknown whether, before surgery, the hypothalamic—pituitary—adrenal (HPA) axis secretion parameters can predict post-surgical hypocortisolism.

Aim.—This study aimed to evaluate whether, in AI patients undergoing unilateral adrenalectomy, postsurgical hypocortisolism could be predicted by the parameters of HPA axis function.

Design.—Prospective, multicenter.

Methods.—A total of 60 patients underwent surgical removal of AI (surgical indication: 29 subclinical hypercortisolism (SH); 31 AI dimension). Before surgery, SH was diagnosed in patients presenting at least three criteria out of urinary free cortisol (UFC) levels>60 mg/24 h, cortisol after 1-mg dexamethasone suppression test (1 mg-DST)>3.0 mg/dl, ACTH levels<10 pg/ml, midnight serum cortisol (MSC)>5.4 mg/dl.

Two months after surgery, HPA axis function was assessed by low dose ACTH stimulation test or insulin tolerance test when needed: 39 patients were affected (Group B) and 21 were not affected (Group A) with hypocortisolism. The accuracy in predicting hypocortisolism of pre-surgical HPA axis parameters or their combinations was evaluated.

Results.—The presence of >2 alterations among 1 mg-DST>5.0 mg/dl, ACTH<10 pg/ml, elevated UFC and MSC has the highest odds ratio (OR) for predicting post-surgical hypocortisolism (OR 10.45, 95% confidence interval, CI 2.54−42.95, P=0.001). Post-surgical hypocortisolism was predicted with 100% probability by elevated UFC plus MSC levels, but not ruled out even in the presence of the normality of all HPA axis parameters.

Conclusion.—Post-surgical hypocortisolism cannot be pre-surgically ruled out. A steroid substitutive therapy is indicated after unilateral adrenalectomy for SH or size of the adenoma (Table 3).

▶ This is an important article examining the ability to determine if a patient with an adrenal incidentaloma has subclinical hypercortisolism. While the conclusions of the article are in accordance with this editor's own experience that

TABLE 3.—Diagnostic Accuracy of Various Parameters and Combinations of Parameters of Pituitary—Adrenal Axis Activity in Predicting the Presence of Hypocortisolism After Surgery

Criterion	Parameters	Sensitivity	Specificity	PPV	NPV	Accuracy
I	A	79.5	23.8	66.0	38.5	60.0
II	B	59.0	52.4	69.7	40.7	56.0
III	C	33.3	85.7	81.3	40.9	51.6
IV	D	48.7	81.0	82.6	45.9	60.0
V	**E**	**64.1**	**81.0**	**86.2**	**54.8**	**70.0**
VI	F	64.1	38.0	65.8	36.4	55.0
VII	A+F	56.4	47.6	66.7	37.0	53.3
VIII	B+F	41.0	66.7	69.6	37.8	50.0
IX	C+F	30.8	85.7	80	40	50.0
X	A+D	33.3	81.0	76.5	39.5	50.0
XI	B+D	23.1	90.5	81.8	47.4	46.6
XII	C+D	10.3	90.5	66.7	35.2	38.3
XIII	**A+E**	**59.0**	**81.0**	**85.2**	**51.5**	**66.6**
XIV	B+E	48.7	85.7	86.4	47.4	61.6
XV	C+E	33.3	95.2	92.9	43.5	55.0
XVI	D+E	30.8	100.0	100.0	43.8	55.0
XVII	2 out of A, D, F	69.2	42.9	69.2	42.9	60.0
XVIII	2 out of B, D, F	56.4	61.9	73.3	43.3	58.3
XIX	2 out of C, D, F	48.7	81.0	82.6	45.9	60.0
XX	2 out of A, D, E, F	82.1	33.3	69.6	50.0	65.0
XXI	**2 out of B, D, E, F**	**74.4**	**57.1**	**76.3**	**54.5**	**68.3**
XXII	**2 out of C, D, E, F**	**69.2**	**76.2**	**84.4**	**57.1**	**71.7**
XXIII	3 out of A, D, E, F	56.4	76.2	81.5	48.5	63.3
XXIV	3 out of B, D, E, F	46.2	85.7	85.7	46.2	60.0
XXV	3 out of C, D, E, F	38.5	85.7	83.3	42.9	55.0
XXVI	1 out of A, D, E, F	97.4	9.5	66.7	66.7	66.0

Data are expressed as percentage, with the exception of *P* values. A, 1 mg-DST >1.8 mg/dl (50.0 nmol/l); B, 1 mg-DST >3.0 mg/dl (83 nmol/l); C, 1 mg-DST >5.0 mg/dl (138 nmol/l); D, elevated UFC >60.0 mg/24 h (65 nmol/24 h); E, midnight serum cortisol >5.4 mg/dl (149 nmol/l); F, ACTH <10 pg/ml (2.2 pmol/l). PPV, positive predictive value; NPV, negative predictive value. Criteria with at least 66% of accuracy are reported in bold.

postoperative hypocortisolism cannot be accurately ruled out based on preoperative testing, the methods used to reach this conclusion are somewhat questionable. All patients in the study were treated with full-dose cortisol replacement for 2 months postoperatively. This seems like an extraordinarily long period to get over the stress response and is not in accordance with what is known to be necessary to resolve a stress response. Furthermore, one has to wonder whether this was a long enough period to induce some mild adrenal insufficiency in some patients. So, while the parameters that can be used to help predict postoperative hypocortisolism are very useful, biochemical testing to determine the presence of postoperative hypocortisolism can be performed at a much earlier time point after surgery. Of note, the most useful test for detection of subclinical hypercortisolism appeared to be the midnight serum cortisol, a level that we virtually never obtain in the United States, as this would require hospital admission for establishing the diagnosis. Looking at the combinations reported in Table 3, it would appear that the combination of a 1-mg dexamethasone suppression test > 3.0 mg/dL + a urinary free cortisol level > 60 mg per 24 hours would be strongly predictive of subclinical hypercortisolism, and these are tests that we would routinely expect to have access to in the United States.

T. J. Fahey III, MD

Carcinoid Tumors of the Rectum: A Multi-institutional International Collaboration
Shields CJ, the International Rectal Carcinoid Study Group (Mater Misericordiae Univ Hosp and Dublin Academic Med Centre, Ireland; et al)
Ann Surg 252:750-755, 2010

Objective.—This study aims to describe recent experience with rectal carcinoids in European and North American centers.

Background.—While considered indolent, the propensity of carcinoids to metastasize can be significant.

Methods.—Rectal carcinoid patients were identified from prospective databases maintained at 9 institutions between 1999 and 2008. Demographic, clinical, and histologic data were collated. Median follow-up was 5 years (range, 0.5—10 years).

Results.—Two hundred two patients were identified. The median age was 55 years (range, 31—81 years). The majority of tumors were an incidental finding (n = 115, 56.9%). The median tumor size was 10 mm (range, 2—120 mm). Overall, 93 (49%) tumors were limited to the mucosa or submucosa, 45 (24%) involved the muscularis propria, 29 (15%) extended into the perirectal fat, and 6 (3%) reached the visceral peritoneum. The primary treatment modalities were endoscopic resection (n = 86, 43%) and surgical extirpation (n = 102, 50%). Forty-one patients (40%) underwent a high anterior resection, whereas 45 (44%) underwent anterior resection with total mesorectal excision. Seven patients (7%) underwent Hartman's procedure, 7 (7%) underwent abdomino-perineal resection, and 6 (6%) had transanal endoscopic microsurgery, whereas 4 (4%) patients underwent a transanal excision. Multiple variable logistic regression analysis demonstrated that tumor size greater than 10 mm and lymphovascular invasion were predictors of nodal involvement ($P = 0.006$ and < 0.001, respectively), whereas the presence of lymph node metastases and lymphovascular invasion was associated with subsequent development of distant metastases ($P = 0.033$ and 0.022, respectively). The presence of nodal metastases has a profound effect upon survival, with a 5-year survival rate of 70%, and 10-year survival of 60% for node positive tumors. Patients with distant metastases have a 4-year survival of 38%.

Conclusion.—Tumor size greater than 10 mm and lymphovascular invasion are significantly associated with the presence of nodal disease, rendering mesorectal excision advisable. Transanal excision is adequate for smaller tumors.

▶ Shields et al have put together a series of over 200 rectal carcinoid tumors from 8 institutions in Europe and 1 in the United States that gathered data prospectively. Of these, 100 underwent surgical excision (the remainder were excised endoscopically). The authors have nicely documented what has long been accepted: that carcinoid tumors less than 1 cm in size are generally indolent and can be cured via a transanal excision, as the risk of lymph node (LN) metastases is low (8%) and the risk of distant metastases in this group is 0. They also note that rectal carcinoids that do metastasize to LNs are associated with a significant drop in 5- and 10-year survival to 70% and 60%, respectively, and thus recommend that surgical treatment include mesorectal excision in this group. Unfortunately, there are no data presented to indicate that more aggressive resection results in better outcomes for these patients, and there are few data presented here or elsewhere to better stratify these tumors. Given the increase in the incidence of these tumors, studies analyzing molecular features of carcinoid tumors are needed.

T. J. Fahey III, MD

Clinicopathological Features of Pancreatic Endocrine Tumors: A Prospective Multicenter Study in Italy of 297 Sporadic Cases

Zerbi A, the members of the AISP-Network Study Group (San Raffaele Scientific Inst, Milan, Italy; et al)
Am J Gastroenterol 105:1421-1429, 2010

Objectives.—Information on pancreatic endocrine tumors (PETs) comes mostly from small, retrospective, uncontrolled studies conducted on highly selected patients. The aim of the study was to describe the clinical and pathological features of PETs in a prospective, multicenter study.

Methods.—Newly diagnosed, histologically proven, sporadic PETs observed from June 2004 to March 2007 in 24 Italian centers were included in a specific data set.

Results.—Two hundred ninety-seven patients (mean age 58.6 ± 14.7 years, females 51.2%, males 48.8%) were analyzed. In 73 cases (24.6%), the tumor was functioning (F) (53 insulinomas, 15 gastrinomas, 5 other syndromes) and in 232 (75.4%) it was non-functioning (NF); in 115 cases (38.7%), the diagnosis was incidental. The median tumor size was 20 mm (range 2−150). NF-PETs were significantly more represented among carcinomas ($P < 0.001$). Nodal and liver metastases were detected in 84 (28.3%) and 85 (28.6%) cases, respectively. The presence of liver metastases was significantly higher in the NF-PETs than in the F-PETs (32.1% vs. 17.8%; $P < 0.05$), and in the symptomatic than in the asymptomatic patients (34.6% vs. 19.1%; $P < 0.005$). At the time of recruitment, the majority of patients (251, 84.5%) had undergone surgery, with complete resection in 209 cases (83.3%).

Conclusions.—This study points out the high number of new cases of PETs observed in Italy, with a high prevalence of NF and incidentally discovered forms. The size of the tumor was smaller and the rate of metastasis was lower than usually reported, suggesting a trend toward an earlier diagnosis.

▶ This article reports a large contemporary series of pancreatic endocrine tumors registered prospectively and followed at 24 centers throughout Italy. The study highlights a couple of noteworthy trends that probably apply to pancreatic endocrine tumors (PETs) in the United States. First, nearly 40% of the cases were detected incidentally, and as might be expected, these tumors are smaller, bringing down the overall size of PETs encountered in clinical practice. Additionally, also secondary to the smaller size, the incidence of lymph node and liver metastases is lower than that seen in previous series—28% for each and a 41% overall rate of metastatic disease at the time of diagnosis. Finally, the authors demonstrate the importance of Ki67 staining in the characterization of PETs. Ki67 values correlated significantly with tumor size as well as nodal and liver metastases. Ki67 levels were also higher in nonfunctioning tumors than in functioning ones. This report serves as a nice barometer of the status of PETs as seen in current practice with a notable trend toward earlier diagnosis, which may present new dilemmas for the treating physicians.

T. J. Fahey III, MD

Survival following resection of pancreatic endocrine tumors: importance of R-status and the WHO and TNM classification systems
Pomianowska E, Gladhaug IP, Grzyb K, et al (Univ of Oslo, Norway; Rikshospitalet Univ Hosp, Oslo, Norway)
Scand J Gastroenterol 45:971-979, 2010

Objective.—The aim of this study was to delineate the clinical outcomes and pathological characteristics of surgically resected endocrine tumors of the pancreas and to determine the importance of the World Health Organization (WHO) and tumor-node metastasis (TNM) classifications, resection status, and Ki-67 expression for long-term survival.

Patients and Methods.—Sixty-nine patients underwent surgical tumor resection with curative intent during 1990–2007. Hospital records were reviewed retrospectively for medical, surgical, pathological, and radiological data.

Results.—Forty-one patients (59%) had non-functional tumors, 28 (41%) patients had functional tumors. Thirty-seven (54%) tumors were classified as WHO group 1 and the remaining 32 as WHO group 2. There were no poorly differentiated endocrine carcinomas. The overall R0-resection rate was 68%. Patients in whom all gross tumor was resected (R0/R1) had significantly better survival compared to patients with macroscopic residual disease (R2) ($p < 0.001$). There was no difference in survival between patients with R0 and R1 resections. Both the WHO ($p < 0.001$) and the TNM ($p < 0.001$) classifications significantly predicted five and 10-year survival after resection of the primary tumor. Survival analysis revealed significantly better outcome for patients with tumors with Ki-67 index < 2% ($p = 0.003$).

Conclusions.—Both WHO and TNM classifications reliably predict long-term survival in patients with resectable pancreatic endocrine tumors. R2 resection status predicted poor prognosis. R0 status did not improve prognosis relative to R1 status. Ki-67 index > 2% is a predictor of poor long-term survival.

▶ This article is a single-center report on the long-term outcome of patients undergoing treatment of pancreatic endocrine tumors (PETs). The authors document 5- and 10-year cancer-specific survival of 83% and 78%, respectively, and demonstrate that both the World Health Organization group classification and the TNM classification accurately predict outcome. Furthermore, the authors show that Ki-67 expression levels were highly predictive of outcome, and levels > 2% were correlated with the presence of liver metastases, larger tumors, and vascular invasion. Ki-67 levels < 2% were associated with a 95% cancer-free survival rate at 10 years. While this article does not add a new marker or test to the available armamentarium for the diagnosis and prognostication of PETs, it does confirm that either of the current staging systems can be used and that Ki-67 levels should be measured in PETs routinely.

T. J. Fahey III, MD

Parenchyma-Preserving Resections for Small Nonfunctioning Pancreatic Endocrine Tumors
Falconi M, Zerbi A, Crippa S, et al (Univ of Verona, Italy; Vita e Salute Univ, Milan, Italy)
Ann Surg Oncol 17:1621-1627, 2010

Background.—Parenchyma-preserving resections (PPRs), including enucleation and middle pancreatectomy (MP), are accepted procedures for insulinomas, but their role in the treatment of nonfunctioning pancreatic endocrine tumors (NF-PETs) is debated. The aim of this study was to evaluate perioperative and long-term outcomes after PPRs for NF-PETs.

Methods.—All patients who underwent PPRs for NF-PETs between 1990 and 2005 were included. Patients with multiple endocrine neoplasia type 1 were excluded.

Results.—Overall, 50 patients (23 men, 27 women, median age 59 years) underwent 26 enucleations and 24 MP. A total of 58% of NF-PETs were incidentally discovered. Median size of the tumors was 13.5 mm with no preoperative suspicion of malignancy in all patients. Overall morbidity and pancreatic fistula rates were 58 and 50%, respectively. Reoperation rate was 4%, with no mortality. Postoperative complications were higher in the MP group. At pathology, there were 34 (68%) benign lesions, 13 (26%) neoplasms of uncertain behavior, and 3 (6%) well-differentiated carcinomas. Forty-one patients (82%) had tumors ≤2 cm in size. Only eight patients (16%) had at least one lymph node removed. After a median follow-up of 58 months, no patient died of disease. Overall, four patients (8%) experienced tumor recurrence after a mean of 68 months. The incidence of exocrine/endocrine insufficiency was 8%.

Conclusions.—PPRs are generally safe and effective procedures for treating small NF-PETs. However, better selection criteria must be identified, and lymph node sampling should be performed routinely to avoid understaging. Long-term follow-up evaluation (>5 years) is of paramount importance given the possible risk of late recurrence.

▶ This article is an important follow-up to the previous 2 articles on pancreatic endocrine tumors. Given the increase in smaller nonfunctioning tumors that are being found incidentally, the question as to whether these tumors can be surgically managed with limited excisions as opposed to subjected to more extensive resections is an important one. The data presented in the article by Falconi et al suggest that this is indeed feasible and generally oncologically sound. The authors kept the limited restrictions to smaller tumors and therefore had a low recurrence rate (8%). Surprisingly, the authors recommend lymph node (LN) sampling in all cases—which the data they present do not really support. Practically this may be problematic—for a lesion in the head, what LNs should be resected? It would be more appropriate to attempt to determine a Ki-67 index on patients with tumors that might be considered for a limited resection. If the Ki-67 level was less than 2%, it would probably be reasonable to proceed with enucleation or a local resection such as a central pancreatectomy.

T. J. Fahey III, MD

Randomized clinical trial comparing open with video-assisted minimally invasive parathyroid surgery for primary hyperparathyroidism
Hessman O, Westerdahl J, Al-Suliman N, et al (Uppsala Univ, Sweden)
Br J Surg 97:177-184, 2010

Background.—Previous studies of video-assisted techniques for parathyroidectomy in patients with primary hyperparathyroidism have found similar or better results compared with bilateral neck exploration. The aim of the present study was to compare open minimally invasive parathyroidectomy with the video-assisted technique for primary hyperparathyroidism in a multicentre randomized trial.

Methods.—Some 143 patients were randomized to open (n = 75) or video-assisted (n = 68) parathyroidectomy after positive sestamibi scintigraphy. There were no differences in preoperative data. The open operation was performed through a 15-mm incision. The video-assisted techniques used were minimally invasive video-assisted parathyroidectomy (MIVAP) or video-assisted parathyroidectomy using the lateral approach (VAPLA). Data were collected prospectively including postoperative pain scoring.

Results.—The procedure was significantly quicker for the open compared to the video-assisted operations: mean(s.d.) 60(35) versus 84(47) min (P = 0.001). Both groups of patients had similar conversion rates and the same outcome, with comparable incision lengths, low scores for postoperative neck discomfort, high cosmetic satisfaction and low complication rates.

Conclusion.—Open minimally invasive parathyroidectomy for primary hyperparathyroidism was quicker than either video-assisted technique. Registration number: NCT00877981 (http://www.clinicaltrials.gov).

▶ The authors have put together a multicenter randomized prospective trial of open minimally invasive parathyroidectomy versus an endoscopic minimally invasive approach. The trial demonstrates essentially equivalent outcomes for all aspects of the surgery except for length of surgery time, which was significantly faster in the open group, 24 minutes faster on average. The authors do note that the surgeons may not have been truly expert in the art of endoscopic parathyroidectomy, a significant problem. Nevertheless, the trial does rather convincingly demonstrate that there is no real advantage to the endoscopic approaches. Buried in the article is the fact that in the study, which included a highly selected group of patients with primary hyperparathyroidism, sestamibi localization was incorrect in 25% and the need for bilateral exploration overall was 21%. Although the authors do not discuss this, these data argue for keeping the incision in a central location, not over the presumed site of the adenoma, in all cases.

T. J. Fahey III, MD

Recurrent hyperparathyroidism and forearm parathyromatosis after total parathyroidectomy

Melck AL, Carty SE, Seethala RR, et al (Univ of Pittsburgh School of Medicine, PA)
Surgery 148:867-875, 2010

Background.—In multiple endocrine neoplasia type I and renal failure, the type of initial parathyroidectomy for hyperparathyroidism may influence the operative risks and development of recurrence. We compared subtotal parathyroidectomy with total parathyroidectomy and immediate forearm autotransplantation (TPFA) in a large series with long-term follow-up.

Methods.—The data of patients treated from 1977 to 2009 by initial or reoperative TPFA or subtotal parathyroidectomy were examined for outcomes including the interval to sites and tissue patterns of recurrence.

Results.—Permanent hypoparathyroidism was rare and uninfluenced by disease type. Neither initial procedure nor underlying disease affected the mean time to reoperation for recurrent hyperparathyroidism. In renal failure, reoperation was more common after TPFA than subtotal parathyroidectomy (5/19, 26% vs 11/193, 6%; $P = .008$). Twelve patients required forearm reoperation after TPFA, which was often complicated by parathyromatosis (7/12, 58%). Further reoperative forearm surgery was more likely after explant excision than after en bloc resection (7/11 vs 0/8; $P = .01$) and occurred sooner in renal failure than in multiple endocrine neoplasia type I (mean 4.4 vs 9 years; $P = .04$). Permanent hypoparathyroidism was rare and uninfluenced by disease type.

Conclusion.—Because of frequent recurrence, TPFA should be abandoned as a treatment of renal hyperparathyroidism. In multiple endocrine neoplasia type I, subtotal parathyroidectomy has similar outcomes to TPFA. Forearm autotransplantation can be complicated by parathyromatosis, and surgeons should be prepared for reoperative en bloc resection.

▶ In this report, Dr Carty and her group at Pittsburgh identified a significant rate of forearm recurrence in patients who underwent a forearm transplant for renal hyperparathyroidism. Unfortunately, whether this rate is really representative of the true rate of recurrent hyperparathyroidism is difficult to ascertain from the study. One possibility is that patients who had recurrent hyperparathyroidism after a subtotal parathyroidectomy, leading to a neck recurrence, were less likely to undergo reoperative surgical treatment, which would artificially increase the percentage of recurrences in patients undergoing forearm transplant. While it makes sense that mincing up hyperplastic parathyroid tissue and placing it into any muscle pocket may lead to multiple foci of recurrent parathyroid tissue, the implications of this in renal hyperparathyroidism are that forearm reoperations are not uncommon. Finally, although the authors note that the surgeons doing total parathyroidectomy and forearm transplant were both very experienced, during the 33 years of the study, less than 1 forearm transplant was done per year (only 25 were done), raising the possibility that surgeon inexperience may have contributed to the high rate of recurrence after forearm transplant. However, other series in the literature have noted similar or higher rates of recurrence. While the conclusions of this study probably remain valid, the authors don't consider the third option for the surgical management of secondary renal hyperparathyroidism analyzed in the next article, total parathyroidectomy without autotransplantation.

T. J. Fahey III, MD

Total parathyroidectomy without autotransplantation for renal hyperparathyroidism
Coulston JE, Egan R, Willis E, et al (North Bristol NHS Trust, Bristol, UK)
Br J Surg 97:1674-1679, 2010

Background.—Parathyroidectomy is the standard treatment for renal hyperparathyroidism although controversy exists about the optimal surgical procedure. Total parathyroidectomy without either autotransplantation or thymectomy is one suggested approach. This study reviewed the medium- to long-term results of this procedure.

Methods.—A retrospective review was undertaken of patients undergoing total parathyroidectomy between August 2000 and March 2009. The procedure was performed by a single surgeon and median follow-up was 31 (range 1–120) months.

Results.—Data were obtained on 115 patients with no re-explorations for bleeding or clinical recurrent laryngeal nerve injuries. The rate of postoperative hypocalcaemia on the day after surgery was 15·7 per cent. Thirty-three patients (28·7 per cent) had an undetectable parathyroid hormone level at the end of follow-up. Fourteen patients (12·2 per cent) developed recurrent hyperparathyroidism with a median parathyroid hormone level of 35·4 (range 5·4–200·0) pmol/l. The reoperation rate was 3·5 per cent. Thymectomy tissue, taken if all four glands could not be identified, revealed no parathyroid glands.

Conclusion.—Total parathyroidectomy alone has minimal associated morbidity or mortality, and a good medium- to long-term clinical outcome with a low recurrence rate.

▶ There have been a number of series, largely from Europe, that have reported on total parathyroidectomy without autotransplantation. The data from these series, including this one, indicate that this is a viable alternative to either subtotal or total parathyroidectomy with forearm autotransplantation. The recurrence rate is low and comparable to that in the series reported by Melck et al.[1] It is interesting to note that two-thirds of patients in this study had their parathyroid hormone (PTH) level rise into the normal range during the course of follow-up. This confirms previous reports of a slow but modest rise in PTH even with a total parathyroid excision and is attributed to the presence of parathyroid rests. The strength of this study is the long-term follow-up, and while most patients have some persistent functioning parathyroid tissue, even those who do not have detectable PTH levels do not have long-term problems with bone disease. Renal physicians and endocrinologists in the United States—at least at the editor's institution—are wary of a total parathyroidectomy without auto-transplantation, and a prospective study to address the long-term concerns of a total parathyroidectomy would be highly desirable.

T. J. Fahey III, MD

Reference

1. Melck AL, Carty SE, Seethala RR, et al. Recurrent hyperparathyroidism and fore-arm parathyromatosis after total parathyroidectomy. *Surgery*. 2010;148:867-873.

The Effectiveness of Radioguided Parathyroidectomy in Patients With Negative Technetium Tc 99m—Sestamibi Scans
Chen H, Sippel RS, Schaefer S (Univ of Wisconsin, Madison)
Arch Surg 144:643-648, 2009

Background.—Many surgeons have shown that radioguided resection of parathyroid glands can facilitate intraoperative localization in selected patients with primary hyperparathyroidism, especially in the reoperative setting. However, in patients with negative technetium Tc 99m—sestamibi (hereafter referred to as "sestamibi") scans, the usefulness of the gamma probe is unclear. Thus, we were interested in determining the role of radio-guided techniques in patients with primary hyperparathyroidism and negative or nonlocalizing sestamibi scans.

Design.—Retrospective analysis of a prospective parathyroid database.

Setting.—Academic medical center.

Patients.—Seven hundred sixty-nine patients with primary hyperpara-thyroidism who had a sestamibi scan and underwent surgical invention by a single surgeon. All patients had radioguided parathyroidectomy using a handheld gamma probe.

Main Outcome Measures.—Radioactive counts, eucalcemia rate, and complications were compared between patients with positive and patients with negative sestamibi scans.

Results.—All enlarged parathyroid glands were localized with the gamma probe in patients with a negative or with a positive sestamibi scan with similar sensitivities. This occurred despite the fact that smaller parathryoid glands were present, on average, in patients with negative sestamibi scans (428 mg vs 828 mg, $P = .001$). Equivalent high post-operative eucalcemia rates (>98%) and low complication rates (0.5%) were achieved with radioguided techniques in both patient populations.

Conclusions.—Radioguided techniques are equally effective in patients with negative (nonlocalizing) sestamibi scans undergoing parathyroidectomy for primary hyperparathyroidism. Moreover, use of the gamma probe led to the detection of all parathyroid glands, including ectopically located ones. These data suggest that the gamma probe has an important role for localization of parathyroid glands in patients with negative preoperative sestamibi scans.

▶ Many endocrine surgeons have shunned the use of minimally invasive para-thyroidectomy (MIP) based on technetium Tc 99m sestamibi (MIBI) + gamma probe because MIBI scans localize disease in only 50% to 60% of patients with primary hyperparathyroidism (despite reports of successful localization in 70%-80%). This report by Chen suggests that a positive scan is not necessary for successful use of the probe intraoperatively. While the numbers reported seem quite convincing, it is not clear that the gamma probe is not simply being used to confirm an enlarged gland once it has been found surgically in these MIBI-negative cases, which is a substantially different use than using it to identify the offending gland. In other words, a 4-gland exploration by an expert parathyroid surgeon leads to high rate of success in MIBI-negative cases independent of the MIBI or the gamma probe, not because of the gamma probe.

T. J. Fahey III, MD

Analysis of the rising incidence of thyroid cancer using the Surveillance, Epidemiology and End Results national cancer data registry

Cramer JD, Fu P, Harth KC, et al (Univ Hosps Case Western Reserve Univ, Cleveland, OH; Case Western Reserve Univ, Cleveland, OH; Univ Hosp Case Med Ctr, Cleveland, OH)
Surgery 148:1147-1153, 2010

Background.—The incidence of thyroid cancer has more than doubled in recent decades. Debate continues on whether the increasing incidence is a result of an increased detection of small neoplasms or other factors.

Methods.—Using the Surveillance, Epidemiology and End Results database, we examined the overall incidence of thyroid cancer with variations based on tumor pathology, size, and stage, as well as the current surgical and adjuvant therapy of thyroid carcinoma.

Results.—Thyroid cancer incidence increased 2.6-fold from 1973 to 2006. This change can be attributed primarily to an increase in papillary thyroid carcinoma, which increased 3.2-fold ($P < .0001$). The increase in papillary thyroid carcinoma also was examined based on tumor size. Tumors ≤1 cm increased the most at a total of 441% between 1983 and 2006 or by 19.2% per year, the incidence of papillary thyroid carcinoma also increased at 12.3%/year in 1.1—2-cm tumors, 10.3%/year in 2.1—5-cm tumors, and 12.0%/year for >5-cm tumors (all $P < .0001$ by Cochran—Armitage trend test). We also demonstrated a positive correlation between papillary thyroid carcinoma tumor size and stage of disease (Spearman, $r = 0.285$, $P < .0001$). Operative treatment for thyroid cancer also has shifted with total thyroidectomy replacing partial thyroidectomy as the most common surgical procedure.

Conclusion.—Contrary to other studies, our data indicate that the increasing incidence of thyroid cancer cannot be accounted for fully by an increased detection of small neoplasms. Other possible explanations for the increase in clinically significant (>1 cm) well-differentiated thyroid carcinomas should be explored (Fig 2).

▶ This article is an important analysis of the increase in thyroid cancer in the United States over the past 3+ decades. While it documents that the vast majority of the increase is because of papillary microcarcinomas, as shown nicely in Fig 2, it also demonstrates that there was an impressive increase in larger cancers as well, even those greater than 5 cm. In the discussion of the

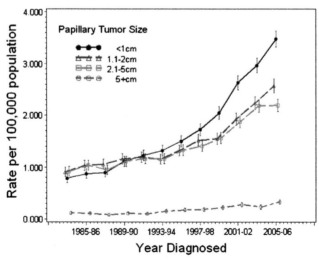

FIGURE 2.—PTC incidence rates by tumor size (1983—2006). Data are age-adjusted to the 2000 U.S. Census with 95% CI. (Reprinted from Cramer JD, Fu P, Harth KC, et al. Analysis of the rising incidence of thyroid cancer using the Surveillance, Epidemiology and End Results national cancer data registry. *Surgery.* 2010;148:1147-1153. Copyright 2010, with permission from Mosby, Inc.)

article, the authors note that the increase has been largely in the 45- to 60-year age group. The data suggest that while much of the increase may be secondary to more sensitive imaging techniques, there exists a strong possibility that there is also a component of real increase that must be explained. Is there an underlying environmental explanation that needs to be addressed? This question will be extraordinarily difficult to tease out until we know more about the underlying molecular changes that are responsible for the initiation of papillary thyroid cancer and its variants.

T. J. Fahey III, MD

Mild hypercalcitoninaemia and sporadic thyroid disease
Cherenko M, Slotema E, Sebag F, et al (Univ Hosp Marseilles, France)
Br J Surg 97:684-690, 2010

Background.—Not operating on patients with mild hypercalcitoninaemia (MHCT) and sporadic thyroid disease carries the risk of omitting curative surgery for medullary thyroid cancer, but systematic surgery would result in unnecessary treatment of benign pathology. This study reviewed the management of MCHT and non-hereditary thyroid disease in one centre.

Methods.—MCHT was defined as an increase in basal and stimulated calcitonin levels not exceeding 30 and 200 pg/ml respectively. Over 15 years, 125 patients who presented with MCHT and sporadic thyroid disease were followed. Surgery was indicated only if there were local pressure symptoms or suspicious histomorphological changes in solitary nodules.

Results.—Fifty-five patients underwent total thyroidectomy and 18 unilateral total lobectomy. Histological examination revealed medullary microcarcinoma in six patients (two women and four men). C-cell hyperplasia was found in 54 patients (74 per cent) and 13 (18 per cent) harboured no C-cell pathology. Calcitonin levels stabilized after lobectomy and became undetectable following thyroidectomy. They normalized during follow-up in a third of patients who did not have surgery.

Conclusion.—Not all patients with MHCT and sporadic thyroid disease require surgery.

▶ Calcitonin testing is a standard part of thyroid nodule evaluation in many centers in Europe. While this can identify patients with unsuspected medullary thyroid carcinoma (MTC), it also (perhaps with equal frequency in unselected patients) leads to the identification of patients with minimally elevated calcitonin levels. It is these patients who sometimes lead to difficult decisions regarding thyroidectomy. Cherenko et al provide a series with long-term follow-up and help to delineate who can be safely watched. Of the 125 patients with mild hypercalcitoninemia, 73 ultimately underwent surgery. The authors repeated the basal test in all cases, and if elevation remained, then a pentagastrin-stimulated calcitonin was obtained. Six patients had MTC, but unfortunately, in most cases the degree of elevation of the basal and stimulated calcitonin did not differentiate those who needed surgery from those who could have been safely observed. Surgery was performed for indications other than the elevation of calcitonin. Though the authors do not explicitly state it, it would be safe to conclude that minimal elevations in basal calcitonin should be investigated by repeat calcitonin testing, including obtaining a stimulated calcitonin level, and then continued observation—with surgery reserved only for those patients who have additional indications for thyroid surgery or a rise in calcitonin on follow-up (though this did not appear to happen in this series).

T. J. Fahey III, MD

Shear Wave Elastography: A New Ultrasound Imaging Mode for the Differential Diagnosis of Benign and Malignant Thyroid Nodules

Sebag F, Vaillant-Lombard J, Berbis J, et al (La Timone Univ Hosp, Marseille, France; Laboratory of Clinical Epidemiology, Marseille, France; et al)
J Clin Endocrinol Metab 95:5281-5288, 2010

Context.—Elastography uses ultrasound (US) to assess elasticity. Shear wave elastography (SWE) is a new technique that estimates tissue stiffness in real time and is quantitative and user independent.

Objectives.—The aim of the study was to assess the efficiency of SWE in predicting malignancy and to compare SWE with US.

Design.—Ninety-three patients and 39 control subjects were included in the study. Predictive value of SWE was assessed by correlation between elasticity, US parameters, and histology. Elasticity index (EI) was first analyzed alone. Scores have been constructed with echographic parameters, i.e. vascularity, hypoechogenicity, and microcalcifications (Score 1 = US Score), and with the same parameters plus EI (Score 2 = US + SWE Score). For statistical analysis, univariate and multivariate analysis and receiver operating characteristic curves were used.

Results.—A total of 146 nodules from 93 patients were analyzed. Twenty-nine nodules (19.9%) were malignant. Mean ($\pm$SD) EI was 150 ± 95 kPa (range, 30–356) in malignant nodules vs. 36 ± 30 (range, 0–200) kPa in benign nodules ($P < 0.001$, Student's t test). For a positive predictive value of at least 80%, characteristics of tissue elasticity (cutoff, 65 kPa) were: sensitivity = 85.2%, and specificity = 93.9%. Characteristics of the US Score were: sensitivity = 51.9% [95% confidence interval (CI), 33.1; 70.7], and specificity = 97% (95% CI, 93.6; 1). Characteristics of the US + SWE Score were: sensitivity = 81.5% (95% CI, 66.9; 96.1), and specificity = 97.0% (95% CI, 93.6; 1).

Conclusion.—Promising results have been obtained with SWE. This technique may be applied to multinodular goiters. Larger prospective studies are needed to confirm these results and to define the respective places of SWE, US, and FNA.

▶ Improving the initial evaluation of thyroid nodules has become an interest of many basic and clinical scientists around the globe. While many have focused on the addition of molecular techniques to fine-needle aspiration, the group from La Timone University has turned to a novel technique for ultrasound. The results appear promising, and certainly further study is warranted. However, the data presented suffer through the apparent omission of one of the most difficult groups in which to characterize thyroid nodules—those patients with Hashimoto thyroiditis. From the data presented, it would appear that patients with Hashimoto thyroiditis would present a difficult group on which to apply shear wave elastography because the entire thyroid can take on the density of a malignant nodule. I look forward to seeing more thorough testing of this new modality.

T. J. Fahey III, MD

Impact of Proto-Oncogene Mutation Detection in Cytological Specimens from Thyroid Nodules Improves the Diagnostic Accuracy of Cytology

Cantara S, Capezzone M, Marchisotta S, et al (Univ of Siena, Italy)

J Clin Endocrinol Metab 95:1365-1369, 2010

Context.—Fine-needle aspiration cytology (FNAC) is the gold standard for the differential diagnosis of thyroid nodules but has the limitation of inadequate sampling or indeterminate lesions.

Objective.—We aimed to verify whether search of thyroid cancer-associated protooncogene mutations in cytological samples may improve the diagnostic accuracy of FNAC.

Study Design.—One hundred seventy-four consecutive patients undergoing thyroid surgery were submitted to FNAC (on 235 thyroid nodules) that was used for cytology and molecular analysis of BRAF, RAS, RET, TRK, and PPRγ mutations. At surgery these nodules were sampled to perform the same molecular testing.

Results.—Mutations were found in 67 of 235 (28.5%) cytological samples. Of the 67 mutated samples, 23 (34.3%)were mutated by RAS, 33 (49.3%) by BRAF, and 11 (16.4%) by RET/PTC. In 88.2% of the cases, the mutation was confirmed in tissue sample. The presence of mutations at cytology was associated with cancer 91.1% of the time and follicular adenoma 8.9% of the time. BRAF or RET/PTC mutations were always associated with cancer, whereas RAS mutations were mainly associated with cancer (74%) but also follicular adenoma (26%). The diagnostic performance of molecular analysis was superior to that of traditional cytology, with better sensitivity and specificity, and the combination of the two techniques further contributed to improve the total accuracy (93.2%), compared with molecular analysis (90.2%) or traditional cytology (83.0%).

Conclusions.—Our findings demonstrate that molecular analysis of cytological specimens is feasible and that its results in combination with cytology improves the diagnostic performance of traditional cytology.

▶ Molecular analysis of fine-needle aspiration (FNA) cytology specimens is now being recognized as a valuable adjunct to traditional cytology. Here

Pacini's group has presented a large surgical series of FNA cytology results with surgical follow-up. The results are impressive and indicate that using a mutation panel that includes analysis of 3 genes, *BRAF, RET-PTC*, and Ras, improved both the sensitivity and specificity of thyroid FNA. Fig 1 in the original article details the data. It is interesting to note that mutation analysis picked up a significant number of malignancies even in the benign group, which is somewhat counterintuitive. Traditionally accepted rates of malignancy in nodules deemed benign by FNA cytology are in the range of 1% to 3%, yet the data here demonstrate that 25% of these benign nodules should have had surgery (10% cancers and 15% follicular adenomas), a number that is inconsistent with a benign classification on cytology. The results for indeterminate nodules are more in line with accepted rates of malignancy and importantly indicate that only 1 patient might have been faced with a completion thyroidectomy. This number also seems too good to be true, as most malignancies in indeterminate nodules in other series have not been associated with identifiable known mutations. Nevertheless, molecular analysis has come of age in thyroid nodule diagnosis. All that remains to be determined is what will be the most cost-effective tests to apply and to what cytology diagnoses should molecular analysis be applied.

T. J. Fahey III, MD

Correlation between the *BRAF* V600E Mutation and Tumor Invasiveness in Papillary Thyroid Carcinomas Smaller than 20 Millimeters: Analysis of 1060 Cases

Basolo F, Torregrossa L, Giannini R, et al (Univ of Pisa, Italy)
J Clin Endocrinol Metab 95:4197-4205, 2010

Context.—Evaluation of the degree of neoplastic infiltration beyond the thyroid capsule remains a unique parameter that can be evaluated by histopathological examination to label a papillary thyroid carcinoma (PTC) of 20 mm or less in size as a pT1 or pT3 tumor.

Objective.—We correlated the *BRAF* V600E mutation with both clinical-pathological features and the degree of neoplastic infiltration to redefine the reliability of the actual system of risk stratification in a large selected group of PTCs smaller than 20 mm.

Design.—The presence of *BRAF* mutations was examined in 1060 PTCs less than 20 mm divided into four degrees of neoplastic infiltration: 1) totally encapsulated; 2) not encapsulated without thyroid capsule invasion; 3) thyroid capsule invasion; and 4) extrathyroidal extension.

Results.—The overall frequency of the *BRAF* V600E mutation was 44.6%. In both univariate and multivariate analyses, *BRAF* mutations showed a strong association with PTC variants (classical and tall cell), tumor size (11–20 mm), multifocality, absence of tumor capsule, extrathyroidal extension, lymph node metastasis, higher American Joint Commission on Cancer stage, and younger patient age. In PTCs staged as pT1 with thyroid capsule invasion, the frequency of *BRAF* mutations was significantly higher than in pT1 tumors that did not invade the thyroid capsule (67.3 *vs.* 31.8%, respectively; *P* < 0.0001). No statistically significant difference in *BRAF* alterations was found between pT1 tumors with thyroid capsule invasion and pT3 tumors (67.3 and 67.5%, respectively).

Conclusion.—We suggest that evaluation of *BRAF* status would be useful even in pT1 tumors to improve risk stratification and patient management, although follow-up data are necessary to confirm our speculations.

▶ This study from the group at Pisa is an excellent analysis of the incidence of *BRAF* mutations in small thyroid cancers. The data show that similar to larger papillary thyroid cancers, *BRAF* mutations are found more commonly in tumors with more aggressive features. In the 578 microcarcinomas included in the study, the incidence of *BRAF* mutations in tumors with extrathyroidal extension or American Joint Commission on Cancer stage III or IV was essentially identical to that seen in the 11- to 20-mm tumors. This is an important observation and supports an article we wrote several years ago suggesting that the size of the carcinoma did not really matter while the pathologic features did—the presence of extrathyroidal extension being perhaps the most important.[1] The data presented by Basolo's group solidify *BRAF* as an important molecular marker of prognosis even in the smallest papillary thyroid cancers.

T. J. Fahey III, MD

Reference

1. Arora N, Turbendian HK, Kato MA, Moo TA, Zarnegar R, Fahey TJ III. Papillary thyroid carcinoma and microcarcinoma: is there a need to distinguish the two? *Thyroid.* 2009;19:473-477.

Influence of prophylactic central lymph node dissection on postoperative thyroglobulin levels and radioiodine treatment in papillary thyroid cancer
Hughes DT, White ML, Miller BS, et al (Univ of Michigan, Ann Arbor; Saint Joseph's Hosp, Ann Arbor, MI)
Surgery 148:1100-1107, 2010

Background.—Prophylactic central lymph node dissection with total thyroidectomy (TT) for the treatment of papillary thyroid cancer (PTC) is controversial because of the possibility of increased morbidity with uncertain benefit. The purpose of this study is to determine whether prophylactic central neck dissection provides any advantages over TT alone.

Methods.—Retrospective cohort study of patients with PTC without preoperative evidence of lymph node involvement undergoing either TT or TT with bilateral central lymph node dissection (TT + BCLND).

Results.—From 2002 to 2009, 143 patients with clinically node-negative PTC underwent either TT (*n* = 65) or TT + BCLND (*n* = 78). The groups were similar in age, gender, tumor size, multifocality, angioinvasion, and metastasis/age/completeness-of-resection/invasion/size score. The presence of involved central neck lymph nodes upstaged 28.6% of patients in the TT + BCLND group to stage III disease, which resulted in higher radioactive iodine ablation doses. Stimulated serum thyroglobulin levels and the number of patients with undetectable stimulated thyroglobulin levels before and 1 year after radioactive iodine ablation were equivalent.

Conclusion.—The addition of routine central lymph node dissection to TT for the treatment of PTC upstages nearly one third of patients over the age of 45 thereby changing the dose of radioactive iodine ablative therapy, but does not change postoperative thyroglobulin levels after completion of radioiodine treatment.

▶ The role of prophylactic central neck dissection (CND) continues to be debated by surgeons treating patients with papillary thyroid cancer.[1] Here the Michigan group analyzes its experience over the greater part of the first decade of the 21st century. Like we reported in 2009, the authors note an increase in the incidence of postoperative temporary hypoparathyroidism along with a higher incidence of parathyroids found in the specimen and an increased need to autotransplant parathyroids. This did not lead to an increase in permanent complications (either recurrent laryngeal nerve injury or permanent hypoparathyroidism). It also did not result in a difference in local recurrence in the central neck between the groups; however, the patients who underwent CND had a 2.5-fold higher incidence of extrathyroidal extension. This is a substantial difference in what is probably the most significant risk factor for recurrence in tumors of this size. So while the authors conclude that there was no difference in postoperative thyroglobulin levels, this could be viewed as looking at the data as the glass is half empty. In reality, the expected recurrence rate for the group that underwent CND should be 2 to 5 times higher than the group that just had total thyroidectomy, suggesting that the CND and the higher radioactive iodine dose received in those patients were effective in reducing recurrence.

T. J. Fahey III, MD

Reference

1. Moo TA, Umunna B, Kato M, et al. Ipsilateral versus bilateral central neck lymph node dissection in papillary thyroid carcinoma. *Ann Surg.* 2009;250:403-408.

Central Neck Lymph Node Dissection for Papillary Thyroid Cancer: Comparison of Complication and Recurrence Rates in 295 Initial Dissections and Reoperations
Shen WT, Ogawa L, Ruan D, et al (Univ of California, San Francisco)
Arch Surg 145:272-275, 2010

Background.—The American Thyroid Association recently changed its management guidelines for papillary thyroid cancer (PTC) to include routine central neck lymph node dissection (CLND) during thyroidectomy. We currently perform CLND during thyroidectomy only if enlarged central nodes are detected by palpation or ultrasonography; we perform CLND in the reoperative setting for recurrence in previously normal-appearing or incompletely resected nodes. Critics of this approach argue that reoperative CLND has higher complication and recurrence rates than initial CLND. We sought to test this argument, using it as our hypothesis.

Design.—Retrospective review.

Setting.—University hospital.

Patients.—All patients undergoing CLND for PTC between January 1, 1998, and December 31, 2007.

Interventions.—Thyroidectomy and CLND.

Main Outcome Measures.—Complications (neck hematoma, recurrent laryngeal nerve injury, and hypoparathyroidism) and recurrence of PTC.

Results.—Altogether, 295 CLNDs were performed: 189 were initial operations and 106 were reoperations. The rate of transient hypocalcemia (41.8%vs23.6%) was significantly higher in patients undergoing initial CLND compared with those undergoing reoperative CLND. Rates of neck hematoma (1.1% vs 0.9%), transient hoarseness (4.8% vs 4.7%), permanent hoarseness (2.6% vs 1.9%), and permanent hypoparathyroidism (0.5% vs 0.9%) were not different between initial and reoperative CLND. In addition, recurrence rates in the central (11.6% vs 14.1%) and lateral (21.7% vs 17.0%) compartments were not different between the 2 groups.

Conclusions.—Reoperative CLND for PTC has a lower rate of temporary hypocalcemia, the same rate of other complications, and the same rate of recurrence compared with initial CLND. Choosing to observe non-enlarged central neck lymph nodes for PTC does not result in increased complications or recurrence if reoperation is required.

▶ This article examining the role of central neck dissection (CND) in the management of patients with papillary thyroid cancer compares a group of patients who underwent CND at the initial operation versus those who had recurrence in the central neck. The authors' practice is to perform CND only in cases where there is evidence for lymph node (LN) metastases, either by preoperative ultrasonography or by palpation or inspection at the time of surgery. The authors' hypothesis was that CND performed as a reoperative endeavor would be associated with a higher complication rate and in fact did not find that there was any difference in complication rate between the 2 groups.

This study is heavily flawed for several reasons. First, while the authors' surgical complication rate is laudable, it is contrary to other reports in the literature. It would be wrong to conclude that a reoperative CND performed by a wide range of surgeons would have similar low rates of surgical morbidity. Second, a recurrence rate of 14% after a reoperative CND is excessively high if you have removed the group of patients who are most likely to recur in the first place—those who presented with central or lateral neck LN metastases at initial presentation. The patients who underwent reoperation should have a very low rate of recurrence, as these theoretically had less aggressive disease to begin with, thus suggesting that the opportunity to cure them was missed with the initial surgical and postoperative radioactive iodine treatments. Finally, it would have been very useful to have serum thyroglobulin data available to adequately compare the 2 groups. Much further work needs to be done to come to the conclusions drawn in this article.

T. J. Fahey III, MD

Iodine Biokinetics and Radioiodine Exposure after Recombinant Human Thyrotropin-Assisted Remnant Ablation in Comparison with Thyroid Hormone Withdrawal

Taïeb D, Sebag F, Farman-Ara B, et al (Centre Hospitalo-Universitaire de la Timone, Marseille, France; et al)
J Clin Endocrinol Metab 95:3283-3290, 2010

Context.—A few prospective studies have evaluated the use of recombinant human TSH (rhTSH) for radioiodine remnant ablation.

Objective.—Our objective was to compare the effects of the both TSH regimens on iodine biokinetics in the thyroid remnant, dosimetry, and radiation protection.

Design.—We conducted a prospective randomized study.

Materials and Methods.—Eighty-eight patients were enrolled for radioiodine ablation to either the hypothyroid or rhTSH arms. A whole-body scan was performed at 48 and 144 h after therapy. Dose rates were assessed at 24, 48, and 144 h. Urinary samples were obtained during the first 48 h. Thyroglobulin was assessed before and after therapy. Iodine biokinetics in the remnants were calculated from γ-count rates. Radiation-absorbed dose was calculated using OLINDA software. Exposure estimation was based on a validated model.

Results.—The effective half-life in the remnant thyroid tissue was significantly longer after rhTSH than during hypothyroidism ($P = 0.01$), whereas 48-h ^{131}I uptakes and residence times were similar. After therapy, thyroglobulin release (a marker of cell damage) was lower in the rhTSH arm. The mean total-body effective half-life and residence time were shorter in patients treated after rhTSH. Residence time was also lower for the colon and stomach. Absorbed dose estimates were lower in the rhTSH arm for the lower large intestine, breasts, ovaries, and the bone marrow. Dose rates at the time of discharge were lower in the rhTSH group with a reduction in cumulative radiation exposure to contact persons.

Conclusions.—In comparison with thyroid hormone withdrawal, rhTSH is associated with longer remnant half-life of radioactive iodine while also reducing radiation exposure to the rest of the body and also to the general public who come in contact with such patients.

▶ This is a well-designed randomized study comparing thyroid hormone withdrawal prior to radioactive iodine (RAI) ablation versus recombinant human thyrotropin (rhTSH) stimulation. The major findings are that the RAI uptake into the remnant is similar between the groups, but the retention of RAI in the remnant is significantly longer in the rhTSH group. Perhaps more important—since the dose of RAI delivered to the remnant appears to be similar—is that the excess RAI is cleared more rapidly in the rhTSH group, leading to a reduced exposure to the patient and potentially therefore to people close to the patient. As awareness of radiation doses with diagnostic tests and therapeutic radiation treatments becomes more widespread, the reduction in the total body dose of RAI is a compelling argument to use rhTSH as the method to prepare the patient rather than thyroid hormone withdrawal.

T. J. Fahey III, MD

Does Postoperative Thyrotropin Suppression Therapy Truly Decrease Recurrence in Papillary Thyroid Carcinoma? A Randomized Controlled Trial
Sugitani I, Fujimoto Y (Cancer Inst Hosp, Koto-ku, Tokyo, Japan)
J Clin Endocrinol Metab 95:4576-4583, 2010

Context.—TSH suppression therapy has been used to decrease thyroid cancer recurrence. However, validation of effects through studies providing a high level of evidence has been lacking.

Objective.—This single-center, open-label, randomized controlled trial tested the hypothesis that disease-free survival (DFS) for papillary thyroid carcinoma (PTC) in patients without TSH suppression is not inferior to that in patients with TSH suppression.

Design.—Participants were randomly assigned to receive postoperative TSH suppression therapy (group A) or not (group B). Before assignment, patients were stratified into groups with low- and high-risk PTC according to the AMES (age, metastasis, extension, size) risk-group classification.

Interventions and Outcome Measures.—For patients assigned to group A, L-T$_4$ was administered to keep serum TSH levels below 0.01 μU/ml. TSH levels were adjusted to within normal ranges for patients assigned to group B. Recurrence was evaluated by neck ultrasonography and chest computed tomography.

Results.—Eligible participants were recruited from 1996—2005, with 218 patients assigned to group A and 215 patients to group B. Analysis was performed on an intention-to-treat basis. DFS did not differ significantly between groups. The 95% confidence interval of the hazard ratio for recurrence was 0.85—1.27 according to Cox proportional hazard modeling, within the margin of 2.12 required to declare 10% noninferiority.

Conclusions.—DFS for patients without TSH suppression was not inferior by more than 10% to DFS for patients with TSH suppression. Thyroid-conserving surgery without TSH suppression should be considered for patients with low-risk PTC to avoid potential adverse effects of TSH suppression.

▶ This interesting study compares 2 groups of patients with papillary thyroid carcinoma treated with thyroid hormone for thyrotropin (TSH) suppression or, if needed, to keep the TSH in the normal range. Initial treatment was purely surgical—no patient received radioactive iodine—and most patients had a hemi-thyroidectomy and ipsilateral central neck dissection. The authors included patients with both low-risk and high-risk tumors in the analysis, though the majority had low-risk tumors. Given this treatment algorithm, the authors demonstrate that there is no difference in outcomes for patients who had TSH suppression versus those who did not. This did not appear to hold true for patients with high-risk tumors who had lower disease-free survival rates at 10 years than those who were suppressed.

While the data are somewhat difficult to apply to US patients because of the differences in initial treatment, they do support the contention that TSH suppression is unnecessary in low-risk patients. One can conclude that TSH suppression can be reserved for patients with evidence for persistent life-threatening disease, such as pulmonary metastases, and that even patients with mild elevation in thyroglobulin can be successfully maintained on thyroid hormone doses that keep the TSH in the lower normal range.

T. J. Fahey III, MD

Empiric High-Dose 131-Iodine Therapy Lacks Efficacy for Treated Papillary Thyroid Cancer Patients with Detectable Serum Thyroglobulin, but Negative Cervical Sonography and ^{18}F-Fluorodeoxyglucose Positron Emission Tomography Scan
Kim WG, Ryu J-S, Kim EY, et al (Univ of Ulsan College of Medicine, Seoul, Korea; et al)
J Clin Endocrinol Metab 95:1169-1173, 2010

Context.—Some patients with elevated serum thyroglobulin (Tg) but a negative diagnostic whole body scan (WBS) after initial therapy for differentiated thyroid carcinoma may benefit from empirical radioactive iodine (RAI) therapy. However, previous studies enrolled patients with negative diagnostic WBS, regardless of neck ultrasonography (USG) and/or ^{18}F-fluorodeoxyglucose positron emission tomography (FDG-PET), which have become the preferred diagnostic procedures in such patients.

Objective.—The aim of this study was to evaluate the usefulness of empirical RAI therapy in patients with elevated stimulated Tg level and negative USG/FDG-PET findings after initial therapy for papillary thyroid carcinoma (PTC).

Design.—This comparative study enrolled 39 patients with elevated stimulated Tg, negative diagnostic WBS, and negative USG/FDG-PET 1 yr after initial treatment. Empirical RAI therapy was performed in 14 patients (treatment group), whereas 25 patients were followed up without therapy (control group).

Results.—There was no significant between-group difference in basal clinicopathological parameters. None of the 14 patients in the treatment group showed iodine uptake on posttreatment WBS. Five of 14 patients (36%) in the treatment group and eight of 25 (32%) in the control group had recurrence during the median 37 months of follow-up ($P = 0.99$). Changes in serum stimulated Tg concentrations did not differ between the two groups.

Conclusion.—Empirical RAI therapy and posttreatment WBS were not useful diagnostically or therapeutically in patients with positive serum stimulated Tg if such patients had negative USG and negative FDG-PET findings after initial treatment of PTC.

▶ Like the previous study, this study argues against old treatment patterns that are slowly becoming obsolete. The study provides evidence that should relegate empiric treatment with radioactive iodine (RAI) for an elevated thyroglobulin level to the history books. While the study is not a randomized prospective study and has flaws, it is clear that empiric treatment with RAI does not reduce clinical recurrences and provides no advantage in disease-free survival. Criticism can be directed at the way patients ended up in the treatment group versus the nontreatment group—the patients selected whether to be treated or not, which could potentially introduce substantial bias—but the 2 groups matched up very well with regard to the pathologic characteristics of the tumors. Specifically, there were no differences in extrathyroidal extension, lymph node metastases, or standard staging systems. Taken together, the study provides support for those who do not favor empiric treatment with RAI, myself included.

T. J. Fahey III, MD

Long-Term Efficacy of Lymph Node Reoperation for Persistent Papillary Thyroid Cancer

Al-Saif O, Farrar WB, Bloomston M, et al (The Ohio State Univ, Columbus)
J Clin Endocrinol Metab 95:2187-2194, 2010

Objective.—The objective of the study was to determine the outcome of surgical resection of metastatic papillary thyroid cancer (PTC) in cervical lymph nodes after failure of initial surgery and I^{131} therapy.

Design.—This was a retrospective clinical study.

Setting.—The study was conducted at a university-based tertiary cancer hospital.

Patients.—A cohort of 95 consecutive patients with recurrent/persistent PTC in the neck underwent initial reoperation during 1999–2005. All had previous thyroidectomy ($\pm$nodal dissection) and I^{131} therapy. Twenty-five patients with antithyroglobulin (Tg) antibodies were subsequently excluded.

Main Outcome Measures.—Biochemical complete remission (BCR) was stringently defined as undetectable TSH-stimulated serum Tg.

Results.—A total of 107 lymphadenectomies were undertaken in these 70 patients through January 2010. BCR was initially achieved in 12 patients (17%). Of the 58 patients with detectable postoperative Tg, 28 had a second reoperation and BCR was achieved in five (18%), seven had a third reoperation, and none achieved BCR. No patient achieving BCR had a subsequent recurrence after a mean follow-up of 60 months (range 4–116 months). In addition, two more patients achieved BCR during long-term follow-up without further intervention. In total, 19 patients (27%) achieved BCR and 32 patients (46%) achieved a TSH-stimulated Tg less than 2.0 ng/ml. Patients who did not achieve BCR had significant reduction in Tg after the first ($P < 0.001$) and second ($P = 0.008$) operations. No patient developed detectable distant metastases or died from PTC.

Conclusions.—Surgical resection of persistent PTC in cervical lymph nodes achieves BCR, when most stringently defined, in 27% of patients, sometimes requiring several surgeries. No biochemical or clinical recurrences occurred during follow-up. In patients who do not achieve BCR, Tg levels were significantly reduced. The long-term durability and impact of this intervention will require further investigation.

▶ Two other studies[1,2] have provided evidence against empiric medical treatment of papillary thyroid cancer (PTC) (thyrotropin [TSH] suppression) and empiric treatment with radioactive iodine (RAI) for thyroglobulin (Tg)-positive patients having undergone initial surgical and RAI treatment of PTC. This study provides evidence that surgical treatment also has its limits in the management of patients with persistent Tg elevation after appropriate initial treatment for PTC. While it is clear that surgery is effective at clearing gross disease in the neck that is documented in recurrence, the ability to return the Tg to undetectable levels is actually low—only approximately a quarter of patients will achieve a biochemical complete response. Additional surgical interventions to try to get the Tg to undetectable levels are largely futile. While the long-term outcome in patients with persistent low-level elevations of Tg is not well studied, these patients can be expected to do well and surgery should be reserved for the management of well-documented disease, not the pursuit of a biochemical cure.

T. J. Fahey III, MD

References

1. Kim WG, Ryu JS, Kim EY, et al. Empiric high-dose 131-iodine therapy lacks efficacy for treated papillary thyroid cancer patients with detectable serum thyroglobulin, but negative cervical sonography and 18F-fluorodeoxyglucose positron emission tomography scan [published online ahead of print January 15, 2010]. *J Clin Endocrinol Metab.* 2010;96:1169-1173.
2. Sugitani I, Fujimoto Y. Does postoperative thyrotropin suppression therapy truly decrease recurrence in papillary thyroid carcinoma? A randomized controlled trial [published online ahead of print July 21, 2010]. *J Clin Endocrinol Metab.* 2010;95:4576-4583.

Serum Thyroid-Stimulating Hormone Concentration and Morbidity from Cardiovascular Disease and Fractures in Patients on Long-Term Thyroxine Therapy

Flynn RW, Bonellie SR, Jung RT, et al (Univ of Dundee, UK; Edinburgh Napier Univ, UK)
J Clin Endocrinol Metab 95:186-193, 2010

Context.—For patients on T_4 replacement, the dose is guided by serum TSH concentrations, but some patients request higher doses due to adverse symptoms.

Objective.—The aim of the study was to determine the safety of patients having a low but not suppressed serum TSH when receiving long-term T_4 replacement.

Design.—We conducted an observational cohort study, using data linkage from regional datasets between 1993 and 2001.

Setting.—A population-based study of all patients in Tayside, Scotland, was performed.

Patients.—All patients taking T_4 replacement therapy (n = 17,684) were included.

Main Outcome Measures.—Fatal and nonfatal endpoints were considered for cardiovascular disease, dysrhythmias, and fractures. Patients were categorized as having a suppressed TSH ($\leq$0.03 mU/liter), low TSH (0.04–0.4 mU/liter), normal TSH (0.4–4.0 mU/liter), or raised TSH (>4.0 mU/liter).

Results.—Cardiovascular disease, dysrhythmias, and fractures were increased in patients with a high TSH: adjusted hazards ratio, 1.95 (1.73–2.21), 1.80 (1.33–2.44), and 1.83 (1.41–2.37), respectively; and patients with a suppressed TSH: 1.37 (1.17–1.60), 1.6 (1.10 –2.33), and 2.02 (1.55–2.62), respectively, when compared to patients with a TSH in the laboratory reference range. Patients with a low TSH did not have an increased risk of any of these outcomes [hazards ratio: 1.1 (0.99 –1.123), 1.13 (0.88 –1.47), and 1.13 (0.92–1.39), respectively].

Conclusions.—Patients with a high or suppressed TSH had an increased risk of cardiovascular disease, dysrhythmias, and fractures, but patients with a low but unsuppressed TSH did not. It may be safe for patients treated with T_4 to have a low but not suppressed serum TSH concentration.

▶ The final study reviewed relating to thyroid cancer completes the theme of the articles discussed here; we as surgeons and physicians treating thyroid cancer need to be wary of overtreatment. This article provides solid evidence that overexuberant suppression of thyroid-simulating hormone (TSH) can be dangerous and increases both cardiovascular morbidity as well as risk of fracture. Interestingly and somewhat surprisingly, the authors also documented that there was an increased risk of cardiovascular disease and fractures in patients with a high TSH level, a finding that is somewhat counterintuitive. It is unclear what underlies the increased risk associated with an elevated TSH level, although I would suspect that this is related to other social and medical factors and not to the direct effects of elevated TSH. While the study did not find an association between mild decreases in serum TSH level and risks of cardiac morbidity or fractures, further study of this group is necessary, as prior studies have identified potential adverse effects of mild decreases in TSH level below normal.

T. J. Fahey III, MD

8 Nutrition

Effect of early enteral nutrition on morbidity and mortality in children with burns

Khorasani EN, Mansouri F (Kermanshah Univ of Med Sciences, Mashhad, Khorasan, Iran)

Burns 36:1067-1071, 2010

Burns increase the metabolic demands of the body and can lead to severe weight loss and increased risk of death.

Early enteral support is believed to improve gastrointestinal, immunological, nutritional and metabolic responses to critical injury; however, this premise is in need of further substantiation by definitive data. This research aimed to examine the effectiveness and safety of early enteral feeding in paediatric patients suffering from burns.

Materials and Methods.—This clinical trial was carried out with a total number of 688 children with burns hospitalised in the Burn Department across a 2-year period (September 2002–September 2004). The subjects were randomised into two groups.

A total of 322 patients received only intravenous resuscitation, in accordance with current treatment protocols, in the first 48 h and were considered as the late enteral nutrition group (LEN group); 366 patients were nourished early enteral nutrition group (EEN group), such that both groups received similar amounts of fluid in the first 48 h. Initiation of enteral nutrition commenced between 3 and 6 h following the burn. The patients were kept in the unit until they were discharged. Wound management did not vary between groups.

Results.—In our study, the mean age was 5 ± 3 years in the LEN group and 5 ± 3.5 years in the EEN group. Hot liquids were the most common cause of burns in both groups. The mean percentage of burn was reported as 20 ± 13 in the LEN group and 22 ± 15 in the EEN group. Mean duration of hospitalisation was 16.4 ± 3.7 days in the LEN group and 12.6 ± 1.3 in the EEN group for cured patients ($P < 0.05$). A total of 40 patients (12%) in the LEN group and 31 patients (8.5%) in the EEN group expired ($P < 0.05$).

Conclusion.—Our research showed that EEN decreases duration of hospitalisation and mortality in children with burns.

▶ Burns are a devastating injury marked by prolonged hypermetabolism with catabolism of muscle and fat as the individual struggles to maintain homeostasis. In adults, Alexander et al demonstrated that early enteral nutrition

171

improved outcome compared with standard care. It is intuitive that the application of enteral nutrition would be beneficial, but it is not proven that early onset of enteral nutrition would be more beneficial than the later onset of such nutrition. This prospective randomized trial showed statistically lower hospital length of stay and mortality in 688 pediatric burn patients who received early enteral nutrition that started within 48 hours of the injury compared with those who received standard intravenous resuscitation and enteral nutrition after 48 hours.

This is a very important clinical trial, as it consisted of a large group of patients with well-defined outcomes. The use of early enteral nutrition should become standard as part of the clinical care of pediatric burn patients.

J. M. Daly, MD

Early enteral nutrition reduces mortality in trauma patients requiring intensive care: A meta-analysis of randomised controlled trials
Doig GS, Heighes PT, Simpson F, et al (Univ of Sydney, New South Wales, Australia; Royal North Shore Hosp, St Leonards, New South Wales, Australia)
Injury 42:50-56, 2011

Introduction.—To determine whether the provision of early standard enteral nutrition (EN) confers treatment benefits to adult trauma patients who require intensive care.

Materials and Methods.—MEDLINE and EMBASE were searched. Hand citation review of retrieved guidelines and systematic reviews was undertaken and academic and industry experts were contacted.

Methodologically sound randomised controlled trials (RCTs) conducted in adult trauma patients requiring intensive care that compared the delivery of standard EN, provided within 24 h of injury, to standard care were included.

The primary analysis was conducted on clinically meaningful patient-oriented outcomes, which included mortality, functional status and quality of life. Secondary analyses considered vomiting/regurgitation, pneumonia, bacteraemia, sepsis and multiple organ dysfunction syndrome. Meta-analysis was conducted using an analytical method known to minimise bias in the presence of sparse events. The impact of heterogeneity was assessed using the I^2 metric.

Results.—Three RCTs with 126 participants were found to be free from major flaws and were included in the primary analysis. The provision of early EN was associated with a significant reduction in mortality (OR = 0.20, 95% confidence interval 0.04–0.91, $I^2 = 0$). No other outcomes could be pooled. A sensitivity analysis and a confirmatory analysis conducted using a different analytical method confirmed the presence of a mortality reduction.

Conclusion.—Although the detection of a statistically significant reduction in mortality is promising, overall trial quality was low and trial size was small. The results of this meta-analysis should be confirmed by the conduct of a large multi-center trial.

▶ Decades ago, Alexander and others demonstrated that the use of early enteral nutrition in burn patients significantly reduced complications and seemed to improve healing as well as immunologic outcomes. Subsequently, many trials have been conducted to evaluate the use of enteral nutrition in trauma patients as a means to improve outcomes. The studies have been described in patients after blunt and penetrating trauma and with or without head injury. Scoring systems such as Injury Severity Scores have been used to improve the randomization of patients into control and experimental groups. Studies have also evaluated the use of enteral versus parenteral nutrition in this clinical setting. Finally, the term early has been debated relative to the timing of nutritional intervention. This meta-analysis attempts to combine clinical studies that have been conducted properly. Their results indicate that early nutrition is beneficial in trauma patients. However, they call for further studies to improve the power of observation and rigor of scientific inquiry.

J. M. Daly, MD

Enteral nutrition with or without *N*-acetylcysteine in the treatment of severe acute alcoholic hepatitis: A randomized multicenter controlled trial
Moreno C, Langlet P, Hittelet A, et al (Université Libre de Bruxelles, Brussels, Belgium; Brugmann Hosp, Brussels, Belgium; et al)
J Hepatol 53:1117-1122, 2010

Background & Aims.—Severe acute alcoholic hepatitis is associated with a high mortality rate. Oxidative stress is involved in the pathogenesis of acute alcoholic hepatitis. Previous findings had also suggested that enteral nutritional support might increase survival in patients with severe acute alcoholic hepatitis. Therefore, the aim of the present study was to evaluate the efficacy of N-acetylcysteine in combination with adequate nutritional support in patients with severe acute alcoholic hepatitis.

Methods.—Patients with biopsy-proven acute alcoholic hepatitis and mDF ≥32 were randomized to receive N-acetylcysteine intravenously or a placebo perfusion along with adequate nutritional support for 14 days. The primary endpoint was 6-month survival; secondary endpoints were biological parameter evolution and infection rate.

Results.—Fifty-two patients were randomized in the study (28 into the N-acetylcysteine arm, 24 into the control arm), and among them, five were excluded from the analysis for protocol violation. The two groups did not differ in baseline characteristics. Survival rates at 1 and 6 months in N-acetylcysteine and control groups were 70.2 vs. 83.8% ($p = 0.26$) and 62.4 vs. 67.1% ($p = 0.60$), respectively. Early biological changes, documented infection rate at 1 month, and incidence of hepatorenal syndrome did not differ between the two groups.

Conclusions.—In this study, high doses of intravenous N-acetylcysteine therapy for 14 days conferred neither survival benefits nor early biological improvement in severe acute alcoholic hepatitis patients with adequate nutritional support. However, these results must be viewed with caution, since the study suffered from a lack of power.

▶ The authors conducted a single-blind randomized clinical trial evaluating the role of N-acetylcysteine (NAC) combined with enteral nutritional support in the management of patients with acute alcoholic hepatitis. The rationale for the use of NAC is that chronic alcoholism depletes the antioxidants of liver, which could be replaced by infusion of NAC. The authors initially anticipated a 50% reduction of mortality and planned for admittance of 43 patients per group (total = 86) to be an adequate sample size for the study. Instead, they performed an unplanned interim analysis of the data after 52 patients were entered into the trial and 47 patients were eligible for analysis per protocol. No statistical differences were noted between groups. In fact, numerically, 1-month survival was worse in the NAC group ($P = .09$) than in the control group. These data, combined with other studies noted in the authors' article, suggest that administration of NAC to patients with acute alcoholic hepatitis along with enteral nutritional support provides no clinically important outcome value.

J. M. Daly, MD

Physician Attitudes and Practices of Enteral Nutrition as Primary Treatment of Paediatric Crohn Disease in North America
Stewart M, Day AS, Otley A (IWK Health Centre, Halifax, Nova Scotia, Canada; Univ of New South Wales, Australia)
J Pediatr Gastroenterol Nutr 52:38-42, 2011

Background.—The use of exclusive enteral nutrition (EEN) in children with Crohn disease has not been universally adopted by North American paediatric gastroenterologists. This is in stark contrast to their European counterparts. The present study aimed to define attitudes and practice patterns of EEN use by members of the North American Society for Paediatric Gastroenterology, Hepatology, and Nutrition.

Methods.—Members were contacted by e-mail and provided with access to a Web-based survey.

Results.—Surveys were completed by 326 of 1162 (30.7%) eligible North American Society for Paediatric Gastroenterology, Hepatology, and Nutrition members from North America (86% United States, 14% Canada). Thirty-one percent of respondents reported never using EEN, 55% reported sparse use, and 12% reported regular use. Physicians in Canada reported significantly more use than those in United States ($P < 0.001$). Currently working and previously working in a centre where EEN was used were highly correlated with both the perceived appropriateness of EEN and the regularity of its use ($P < 0.01$). More American physicians than Canadian physicians reported that concurrent medical therapy was necessary to induce remission ($P < 0.001$). Canadian respondents were more likely to use maintenance therapy than American respondents ($P = 0.02$). Compliance issues were seen as the main disadvantages of EEN and as the major barrier to increased use by nonregular users.

Conclusions.—There are significant variations in the patterns of use and the acceptance of EEN between Canada and the United States, with Canadian physicians showing a greater use of EEN. The use of EEN appears influenced by the extent to which physicians are exposed to its use both in their training and in their current practice setting.

▶ It is well known that attitudes regarding forms of treatment for chronic disease often vary within and among countries. This interesting study attempted to evaluate the use of exclusive enteral feeding in children with Crohn disease using survey methods of pediatric gastroenterologists in the United States and Canada. The response rate (31%) to the survey was good considering an e-mail method. Physicians in the United States used exclusive enteral feeding less often than their Canadian counterparts. Interestingly, Canadian physicians were more likely to use enteral feeding as maintenance therapy than American physicians. Training and exposure to the use of enteral feeding as a treatment modality were the major factors that influenced its use in patients. It appears that appropriate studies and guidelines are called for to help standardize the use of enteral feeding in these children with Crohn disease.

J. M. Daly, MD

Early Enteral Nutrition in Burns: Compliance With Guidelines and Associated Outcomes in a Multicenter Study
Mosier MJ, Pham TN, Klein MB, et al (Loyola Univ Med Ctr, Maywood, IL; Univ of Washington Burn Ctr, Seattle; et al)
J Burn Care Res 32:104-109, 2011

Early nutritional support is an essential component of burn care to prevent ileus, stress ulceration, and the effects of hypermetabolism. The American Burn Association practice guidelines state that enteral feedings should be initiated as soon as practical. The authors sought to evaluate compliance with early enteral nutrition (EN) guidelines, associated complications, and hospitalization outcomes in a prospective multicenter observational study. They conducted a retrospective review of mechanically ventilated burn patients enrolled in the prospective observational multicenter study "Inflammation and the Host Response to Injury." Timing of initiation of tube feedings was recorded, with early EN defined as being started within 24 hours of admission. Univariate and multivariate analyses were performed to distinguish barriers to initiation of EN and the impact of early feeding on development of multiple organ dysfunction syndrome, infectious complications, days on mechanical ventilation, intensive care unit (ICU) length of stay, and survival. A total of 153 patients met study inclusion criteria. The cohort comprised 73% men, with a mean age of 41 ± 15 years and a mean %TBSA burn of $46 \pm 18\%$. One hundred twenty-three patients (80%) began EN in the first 24 hours and 145 (95%) by 48 hours. Age, sex, inhalation injury, and full-thickness burn size were similar between those fed by 24 hours vs after 24 hours, except for higher mean Acute Physiology and Chronic Health Evaluation II scores (26 vs 23, $P = .03$) and smaller total burn size (44 vs 54% TBSA burn, $P = .01$) in those fed early. There was no significant difference in rates of hyperglycemia, abdominal compartment syndrome, or gastrointestinal bleeding between groups. Patients fed early had shorter ICU length of stay (adjusted hazard ratio 0.57, $P = 0.03$, 95% confidence interval 0.35–0.94) and reduced wound infection risk (adjusted odds ratio 0.28, $P = 0.01$, 95% confidence interval 0.10–0.76). The investigators have found early EN to be safe, with no increase in complications and a lower rate of wound infections and shorter ICU length of stay. Across institutions, there has been high compliance with early EN as part of the standard operating procedure in this prospective multicenter observational trial. The investigators advocate that initiation of EN by 24 hours be used as a formal recommendation in nutrition guidelines for severe burns, and that nutrition guidelines be actively disseminated to individual burn centers to permit a change in practice.

▶ Previously, Alexander et al had shown that patients with substantial burn injury had an improved outcome when enteral feeding was started early. But like so many standards of care, the appropriate utilization of therapeutic interventions is not always carried out.

This prospective observational study evaluated retrospectively the implementation of early enteral feeding guidelines in multiple institutions. As noted, 80% of patients started enteral feeding within 24 hours of injury and 95% within 48 hours. As previously shown, early enteral feeding was associated with significantly decreased rates of wound infections and shorter lengths of stay in intensive care unit. Importantly, the vast majority of patients followed established American Burn Association guidelines to start enteral feeding within 24 hours. Further education of hospital personnel and health care providers is needed to get to 100% compliance in all institutions.

J. M. Daly, MD

A Randomized, Double-Blind, Controlled Trial of the Effect of Prebiotic Oligosaccharides on Enteral Tolerance in Preterm Infants (ISRCTN77444690)
Modi N, Uthaya S, Fell J, et al (Imperial College London, UK)
Pediatr Res 68:440-445, 2010

Breast milk prebiotic oligosaccharides are believed to promote enteral tolerance. Many mothers delivering preterm are unable to provide sufficient milk. We conducted a multicenter, randomized, controlled trial comparing preterm formula containing 0.8 g/100 mL short-chain galacto-oligosaccharides/long-chain fructo-oligosaccharides in a 9:1 ratio and an otherwise identical formula, using formula only to augment insufficient maternal milk volume. Infants were randomized within 24 h of birth. The primary outcome (PO) was time to establish a total milk intake of 150 mL/kg/d PO and the principal secondary outcome (PSO) was proportion of time between birth and 28 d/discharge that a total milk intake of ≥150 mL/kg/d was tolerated. Other secondary outcomes included growth, fecal characteristics, gastrointestinal signs, necrotizing enterocolitis, and bloodstream infection. Outcomes were compared adjusted for prespecified covariates. We recruited 160 infants appropriately grown for GA <33 wk. There were no significant differences in PO or PSOs. After covariate adjustment, we showed significant benefit from trial formula in PSO with increasing infant immaturity (2.9% improved tolerance for a baby born at 28-wk gestation and 9.9% at 26-wk gestation; $p < 0.001$) but decreased or no benefit in babies >31-wk gestation. Prebiotic supplementation appears safe and may benefit enteral tolerance in the most immature infants.

▶ Enteral nutrition management of preterm infants is difficult particularly when mothers are unable to provide sufficient milk. This randomized, controlled, multicenter trial compared prebiotic oligosaccharide—supplemented formula with standard formula augmenting insufficient mother's milk. After reviewing the results in 160 infants, no differences in primary or secondary outcomes were noted between groups. There was a suggestion of greater improvement in the most immature (26 and 28 weeks' gestation) babies using the prebiotic-supplemented formulation. To understand these differences, further studies will be required in these immature preterm infants, evaluating enough infants to determine if these differences are significant and sustained and if clinical outcome differences occur.

J. M. Daly, MD

Lactobacillus GG as Treatment for Diarrhea During Enteral Feeding in Critical Illness: Randomized Controlled Trial
Ferrie S, Daley M (Royal Prince Alfred Hosp, Sydney, Australia)
JPEN J Parenter Enteral Nutr 35:43-49, 2011

Background.—Diarrhea is a common problem in critical illness. The aim of this study was to investigate the effect of probiotic treatment with *Lactobacillus rhamnosus* GG on established diarrhea in critically ill patients.

Methods.—This prospective randomized blinded trial in the adult intensive care unit of a large tertiary referral teaching hospital compared probiotic treatment with placebo. Thirty-six consecutive critically ill enterally fed adults with diarrhea were randomized to receive 2 capsules per day for 7 days of either *Lactobacillus* GG in an inulin base (Culturelle) or inulin alone (placebo). Diarrhea was defined as ≥3 unformed stools or >200 mL stool volume within 24 hours. Prospectively defined primary end point was duration of diarrhea, and secondary end point was mean number of loose stools per day during the 14 days from the first capsule.

Results by Intention-to-Treat Analysis.—No significant difference was observed for any end point. There was a trend toward more diarrhea in the probiotic treatment group. Mean (standard deviation) duration of diarrhea was 3.83 (2.39) days for the probiotic group and 2.56 (1.85) days for the placebo group ($P =.096$). Mean number of loose stools per day during the 14 days from the first capsule was 1.58 (0.88) in the probiotic group and 1.10 (0.79) in the placebo group ($P =.150$).

Conclusions.—This study does not support the use of *Lactobacillus* GG as a treatment for established diarrhea in enterally fed critically ill patients.

▶ Unfortunately, negative studies more often do not get published for a variety of reasons. This prospective, randomized, blinded clinical trial evaluated the use of probiotic therapy with *Lactobacillus* GG in patients in intensive care unit (ICU) who suffered from diarrhea. The end points (duration and volume of loose stools) were measured for the 32 patients who entered the study. The duration of the study was 14 days. No statistical difference was noted between groups. Arithmetically, there were longer duration and volume of diarrhea in the experimental group compared with the control group.

Thus, therapy with *Lactobacillus* GG cannot be recommended as treatment for diarrhea in patients in ICU.

J. M. Daly, MD

Gastric residual volume during enteral nutrition in ICU patients: the REGANE study

Montejo JC, Miñambres E, Bordejé L, et al (Hospital Universitario 12 de Octubre, Madrid, Spain; Hospital Universitario Marqués de Valdecilla, Santander, Spain; Hospital Universitari Germans Trias i Pujol, Badalona, Spain; et al)
Intensive Care Med 36:1386-1393, 2010

Objective.—To compare the effects of increasing the limit for gastric residual volume (GRV) in the adequacy of enteral nutrition. Frequency of gastrointestinal complications and outcome variables were secondary goals.

Design.—An open, prospective, randomized study.

Setting.—Twenty-eight intensive care units in Spain.

Patients.—Three hundred twenty-nine intubated and mechanically ventilated adult patients with enteral nutrition (EN).

Interventions.—EN was administered by nasogastric tube. A protocol for management of EN-related gastrointestinal complications was used.

Patients were randomized to be included in a control (GRV = 200 ml) or in study group (GRV = 500 ml).

Measurements and Results.—Diet volume ratio (diet received/diet prescribed), incidence of gastrointestinal complications, ICU-acquired pneumonia, days on mechanical ventilation and ICU length of stay were the study variables. Gastrointestinal complications were higher in the control group (63.6 vs. 47.8%, $P = 0.004$), but the only difference was in the frequency of high GRV (42.4 vs. 26.8%, $P = 0.003$). The diet volume ratio was higher for the study group only during the 1st week (84.48 vs. 88.20%) ($P = 0.0002$). Volume ratio was similar for both groups in weeks 3 and 4. Duration of mechanical ventilation, ICU length of stay or frequency of pneumonia were similar.

Conclusions.—Diet volume ratio of mechanically ventilated patients treated with enteral nutrition is not affected by increasing the limit in GRV. A limit of 500 ml is not associated with adverse effects in gastrointestinal complications or in outcome variables. A value of 500 ml can be equally recommended as a normal limit for GRV.

▶ It seems intuitive that patients fed enterally who have a high gastric residual volume are more likely to develop complications such as vomiting and aspiration. This open prospective study evaluated 329 patients in numerous Spanish intensive care units (ICUs), evaluating complications associated with gastric residual volumes of 250 and 500 cc. Those studied by protocol had fewer complications compared with the control group. The major significant finding was the diet volume ratio (diet received/diet prescribed). Importantly, even with gastric residual volumes of 500 cc, complications were no more frequent than with volumes of 250 cc. Use of protocol-driven enteral nutrition is important in critically ill patients in the ICU.

J. M. Daly, MD

***Bifidobacterium adolescentis* Supplementation Ameliorates Parenteral Nutrition-Induced Liver Injury in Infant Rabbits**
Wu J, Wang X, Cai W, et al (Shanghai Jiao Tong Univ School of Medicine, China)
Dig Dis Sci 55:2814-2820, 2010

Background.—Parenteral nutrition (PN)-induced liver injury is associated with gut atrophy, and probiotics have demonstrated the ability to stabilize the intestinal microecosystem and offer protection against bacterial translocation from the gut to the liver. Therefore, we hypothesized that enteral *Bifidobacterium* supplements could alleviate PN-associated liver injury.

Methods.—Three-week-old New Zealand rabbits were divided into three groups: control, PN, and PN + Bif group (PN plus enteral feeding 0.5×10^8 *Bifidobacterium adolescentis* per day). After 10 days, serum levels of liver enzyme and endotoxin were measured, and histology of liver and ileum were performed. Blood and homogenized samples of tissue from the mesenteric lymph nodes, lung, and spleen were cultured for detecting bacteria translocation. Intestinal permeability was determined by sugar absorption test.

Results.—Serum levels of total bilirubin and bile acid were found to be lower in the PN + Bif group, with considerably improved ileum and liver histology (vs. the PN group). The bacterial translocation rate (15.6%), serum endotoxin level (0.11 ± 0.03 EU/ml), and lactulose/mannitol ratio (0.02 ± 0.004) in the PN + Bif group were obviously lower than those of PN group (77.5%, 0.60 ± 0.09 EU/ml, and 0.038 ± 0.008, respectively) and similar to those of the control group (2.8%, 0.09 ± 0.03 EU/ml, and 0.019 ± 0.005, respectively).

Conclusions.—Enteral probiotic supplementation could reduce gut permeability, bacterial translocation and endotoxemia, and thus attenuate PN-associated gut and liver injuries in infant rabbits.

▶ The development of hepatic biochemical and steatosis abnormalities in infants, children, and adult patients receiving total parenteral nutrition (TPN) is well known. A variety of causative factors have been described, such as decreased choline levels, increased glucose in excess of metabolic needs, use of lipid emulsions, and potential bacterial translocation across the intestinal tract. These authors studied the use of enteral probiotics in association with TPN in infant rabbits receiving TPN to simulate the problems seen clinically. The experimental group receiving *Bifidobacterium adolescentis* had on average lower translocation rates, lower serum endotoxin levels, and lower lactulose/mannitol ratios (a measure of intestinal permeability) compared with the parenteral nutrition—only group. It would be valuable to determine the bacterial composition of the small and large intestine in these 3 groups and to determine if structural mucosal changes occur in the 3 groups.

J. M. Daly, MD

Glucose and protein kinetics in patients undergoing colorectal surgery: perioperative amino acid versus hypocaloric dextrose infusion
Lugli AK, Schricker T, Wykes L, et al (McGill Univ, Montreal, Canada)
Metabolism 59:1649-1655, 2010

Surgical injury provokes a stress response that leads to a catabolic state and, when prolonged, interferes with the postoperative recovery process. This study tests the impact of 2 nutrition support regimens on protein and glucose metabolism as part of an integrated approach in the perioperative period incorporating epidural analgesia in 18 nondiabetic patients undergoing colorectal surgery. To test the hypothesis that parenteral amino acid infusion (amino acid group, n = 9) maintains glucose homeostasis while maintaining normoglycemia and reduces proteolysis compared with infusion of dextrose alone (DEX group, $n = 9$), glucose and protein kinetics were measured before and on the second day after surgery using a stable isotope tracer technique. Postoperatively, the rate of appearance of glucose was higher ($P < .001$) and blood glucose increased more ($P < .001$) in the DEX group than in the amino acid group. The postoperative increase in the appearance of leucine from protein breakdown tended to be greater ($P = .077$) in the DEX group. We conclude that perioperative infusion of a nutrition support regimen delivering amino acids alone maintains blood glucose homeostasis and normoglycemia and tends to have a suppressive effect on protein breakdown compared with infusion of dextrose alone.

▶ The authors studied 18 patients to determine if the infusion of amino acids postoperatively would maintain glucose homeostasis compared with the infusion of glucose alone. In these patients undergoing colorectal surgery, blood glucose increased more in the dextrose-infused group compared with the amino acid–infused group. Leucine breakdown was also created in the dextrose-infused group compared with the amino acid–infused group. Normoglycemia was maintained in the amino acid–infused group.

Previous studies have shown improved nitrogen balance with the peripheral infusion of amino acids after major elective surgery compared with infusion of glucose alone. Interestingly, patients receiving amino acids alone demonstrate ketosis and blood glucose decreases by the fourth to fifth postoperative day compared with patients receiving glucose alone. Serum uric acid levels also decrease markedly in those receiving amino acids alone.

Despite these changes, the short-term use of amino acids has not been shown to affect patient outcomes.

J. M. Daly, MD

Safety and Efficacy of a Lipid Emulsion Containing a Mixture of Soybean Oil, Medium-chain Triglycerides, Olive Oil, and Fish Oil: A Randomised, Double-blind Clinical Trial in Premature Infants Requiring Parenteral Nutrition

Tomsits E, Pataki M, Tölgyesi A, et al (Semmelweis Univ, Budapest, Hungary)
J Pediatr Gastroenterol Nutr 51:514-521, 2010

Objectives.—Safety, tolerability, and efficacy of a novel lipid emulsion containing a mixture of soybean oil, medium-chain triglycerides, olive oil, and fish oil (SMOFlipid 20%) with reduced n-6 fatty acids (FA), increased monounsaturated and n-3 FA, and enriched in vitamin E were evaluated in premature infants compared with a soybean oil-based emulsion.

Patients and Methods.—Sixty (30/30) premature neonates (age 3—7 days, gestational age ≤34 weeks, birth weights 1000—2500 g) received parenteral nutrition (PN) with either SMOFlipid 20% (study group) or a conventional lipid emulsion (Intralipid 20%, control group) for a minimum of 7 up to

14 days. Lipid supply started at 0.5 g·kg body weight^{-1}·day^{-1} on day 1 and increased stepwise (by 0.5 g) up to 2 g·kg body weight^{-1}·day^{-1} on days 4 to 14. Safety and efficacy parameters were assessed on days 0, 8, and 15 if PN was continued.

Results.—Adverse events, serum triglycerides, vital signs, local tolerance, and clinical laboratory did not show noticeable group differences, confirming the safety of study treatment. At study end, γ-glutamyl transferase was lower in the study versus the control group (107.8 ± 81.7 vs 188.8 ± 176.7 IU/L, $P < 0.05$). The relative increase in body weight (day 8 vs baseline) was 5.0% ± 6.5% versus 5.1% ± 6.6% (study vs control, not significant). In the study group, an increase in n-3 FA in red blood cell phospholipids and n-3:n-6 FA ratio was observed. Plasma α-tocopherol (study vs control) was increased versus baseline on day 8 (26.35 ± 10.03 vs 3.67 ± 8.06 μmol/L, $P < 0.05$) and at study termination (26.97 ± 18.32 vs 8.73 ± 11.41 μmol/L, $P < 0.05$).

Conclusions.—Parenteral infusion of SMOFlipid was safe and well tolerated and showed a potential beneficial influence on cholestasis, n-3 FA, and vitamin E status in premature infants requiring PN.

▶ Lipid emulsions are a very important component of total parenteral nutrition. They provide essential fatty acids that are critical for cellular functions and avoiding complications during long-term parenteral nutrition. This study evaluated the safety, tolerability, and efficacy of a new lipid emulsion that contains soybean oil, medium-chain triglycerides, olive oil, and fish oil. The emulsion also had increased vitamin E levels. This emulsion was compared with a standard soybean oil—based emulsion. Sixty premature neonates received these formulations for a minimum of 7 and up to 14 days. There were no differences noted in adverse events. In neonates who were given the new experimental emulsion formula, serum gamma-glutamyltransferase levels were lower compared with results in the control group. In addition, an increase in ω-3 fatty acids was noted in red blood cell phospholipids. This study is important because neonates receiving standard lipid emulsion formulations with total parenteral nutrition have a higher incidence of fatty liver and biochemical abnormalities, including hyperbilirubinemia. It is well known that hyperbilirubinemia in premature neonates is also associated with increased morbidity and potentially mortality. Thus, the use of new lipid emulsions that can prevent hepatic dysfunction would be very important in the management of premature neonates. Further studies are required to be certain of the safety and efficacy of this new formulation. In addition, it would be valuable to test this formulation in adults who require long-term total parenteral nutrition. Studies on immunologic function would be valuable in addition to studies of serum biochemistry values. Lipid emulsion formulas have been standardized for long periods. It will be valuable to develop new emulsion formulations to improve patient outcomes.

J. M. Daly, MD

Lipid-enriched enteral nutrition controls the inflammatory response in murine Gram-negative sepsis

Lubbers T, De Haan J-J, Hadfoune M, et al (Maastricht Univ Med Centre, The Netherlands; et al)
Crit Care Med 38:1996-2002, 2010

Objectives.—Controlling the inflammatory cascade during sepsis remains a major clinical challenge. Recently, it has become evident that the autonomic nervous system reduces inflammation through the vagus nerve. The current study investigates whether nutritional stimulation of the autonomic nervous system effectively attenuates the inflammatory response in murine Gram-negative sepsis.

Design.—Controlled *in vivo* and *ex vivo* experimental study.

Settings.—Research laboratory of a university hospital.

Subjects.—Male C57bl6 mice.

Interventions.—Mice were intraperitoneally challenged with lipopolysaccharide derived from *Escherichia coli*. Before lipopolysaccharide administration, mice were fasted or enterally fed either lipid-rich nutrition or low-lipid nutrition. Antagonists to cholecystokinin receptors or nicotinic receptors were administered before lipopolysaccharide administration. Blood and tissue samples were collected at 90 mins. Mesenteric afferent discharge was determined in *ex vivo* preparations in response to both nutritional compositions.

Measurements and Main Results.—Both lipid-rich and low-lipid nutrition dose-dependently reduced lipopolysaccharide-induced tumor necrosis factor-α release (high dose: both 1.4 ± 0.4 ng/mL) compared with fasted mice (3.7 ± 0.8 ng/mL; $p < .01$). The anti-inflammatory effect of both nutritional compositions was mediated through cholecystokinin receptors ($p < .01$), activation of mesenteric vagal afferents ($p < .05$), and peripheral nicotinic receptors ($p < .05$). Lipid-rich nutrition attenuated the inflammatory response at lower dosages than low-lipid nutrition, indicating that enrichment of enteral nutrition with lipid augments the anti-inflammatory potential. Administration of lipid-rich nutrition prevented endotoxin-induced small intestinal epithelium damage and reduced inflammation in the liver and spleen compared with fasted (all $p < .01$) and low-lipid nutrition controls (all $p < .05$).

Conclusions.—The current study demonstrates that lipid-rich nutrition attenuates intestinal damage and systemic as well as organ-specific inflammation in murine Gram-negative sepsis through the nutritional vagal anti-inflammatory pathway. These findings implicate enteral administration of lipid-enriched nutrition as a promising intervention to modulate the inflammatory response during septic conditions.

▶ Interruption or diminishment of the cytokine and inflammatory cellular response to sepsis would be of major benefit for critically ill patients. Specific antibodies and pharmacologic agents such as steroids have been used with little or minimal effectiveness. It has been previously shown that lipid emulsions can alter the local cellular and systemic effects of endotoxin.

This animal study evaluated the effects of lipid-rich or low-lipid enteral formulas compared with that in fasted controls that received intraperitoneal endotoxin (lipopolysaccharide [LPS]). The high-lipid enteral formula was of greatest benefit. The authors suggested that the mechanism was because of stimulation of the autonomic nervous system (vagus nerve).

This interesting study raises questions as to the mechanisms involved. Because lipid emulsions bind endotoxin, it is possible that intraperitoneal LPS, which is absorbed into mesenteric lymphatics and the bloodstream, was bound by the lipid emulsion, resulting in less stimulation of the sympathetic nervous system. However, the studies evaluating nicotinic and cholecystokinin receptors do suggest a vagal mechanism of action.

J. M. Daly, MD

Long-term follow-up of patients on home parenteral nutrition in Europe: implications for intestinal transplantation
Pironi L, Home Artificial Nutrition & Chronic Intestinal Failure Working Group of the European Society for Clinical Nutrition and Metabolism (ESPEN) (Univ of Bologna, Italy; et al)
Gut 60:17-25, 2011

Background.—The indications for intestinal transplantation (ITx) are still debated. Knowing survival rates and causes of death on home parenteral nutrition (HPN) will improve decisions.

Methods.—A prospective 5-year study compared 389 non-candidates (no indication, no contraindication) and 156 candidates (indication, no contraindication) for ITx. Indications were: HPN failure (liver failure; multiple episodes of catheter-related venous thrombosis or sepsis; severe dehydration), high-risk underlying disease (intra-abdominal desmoids; congenital mucosal disorders; ultra-short bowel), high morbidity intestinal failure. Causes of death were defined as: HPN-related, underlying disease, or other cause.

Results.—The survival rate was 87% in non-candidates, 73% in candidates with HPN failure, 84% in those with high-risk underlying disease, 100% in those with high morbidity intestinal failure, and 54% in ITx recipients (one non-candidate and 21 candidates) (p<0.001). The primary cause of death on HPN was underlying disease-related in patients with HPN duration ≤2 years, and HPN-related in those on HPN duration >2 years (p=0.006). In candidates, the death HRs were increased in those with desmoids (7.1; 95% CI 2.5 to 20.5; p=0.003) or liver failure (3.4; 95% CI 1.6 to 7.3; p=0.002) compared to non-candidates. In deceased candidates, the indications for ITx were the causes of death in 92% of those with desmoids or liver failure, and in 38% of those with other indications (p=0.041). In candidates with catheter-related complications or ultra-short bowel, the survival rate was 83% in those who remained on HPN and 78% after ITx (p=0.767).

Conclusions.—HPN is confirmed as the primary treatment for intestinal failure. Desmoids and HPN-related liver failure constitute indications for life-saving ITx. Catheter-related complications and ultra-short bowel might be indications for pre-emptive/rehabilitative ITx. In the early years after commencing HPN a life-saving ITx could be required for some patients at higher risk of death from their underlying disease.

▶ It is difficult to determine definitively when a patient should undergo intestinal transplantation because of the morbidity and short- and long-term mortality.

This very interesting prospective study followed over 500 patients who were either candidates or noncandidates for intestinal transplantation. In those deemed to be noncandidates for transplantation, the survival rate was 87% compared with only 73% in those with liver failure, multiple episodes of catheter-related sepsis and venous thrombosis, and severe dehydration and 54% in those with intestinal transplant. In those on home parenteral nutrition (HPN) for more than 2 years, the primary cause of death was complications related to parenteral nutrition itself. Interestingly, in those on HPN with catheter-related complications or ultrashort bowel, survival rates were similar in those with and without intestinal transplantation.

One must recognize that the decision for intestinal transplantation is not taken lightly, and there may be a multitude of factors that were not identified in this study, which may affect the conclusions. Only a true randomized trial regarding transplantation in patients with short bowel will answer these outcome questions.

J. M. Daly, MD

Intravenous arginine and human skin graft donor site healing: A randomized controlled trial

Debats IBJG, Koeneman MM, Booi DI, et al (Univ Hosp Maastricht, The Netherlands)

Burns 37:420-426, 2011

Background and Aims.—Studies evaluating the effect of arginine supplementation in human wound healing are inhomogeneous with conflicting results. This study aims to clarify the role of arginine supplementation in the healing of human skin graft donor sites.

Methods.—35 subjects undergoing skin autografting were randomly assigned to receive intravenous arginine ($n = 16$) or placebo ($n = 19$) for 5 days in a dose of 30 g of arginine or an isovolumetric amount of placebo (25.2 g of alanine). Wound healing was evaluated at the donor sites by objectifying angiogenesis, reepithelialization and neutrophil influx. Plasma amino acid concentrations were measured to evaluate our intervention.

Results.—The two groups were comparable in age, morbidity and nutritional, metabolic and inflammatory state. Plasma arginine and alanine levels increased significantly upon supplementation in the two groups, respectively. No differences were found between the arginine supplementation group and the placebo group in the studied parameters. Placebo vs. arginine; mean ± SD: neutrophil influx on day 2: 6.67 ± 3.0 vs. 6.57 ± 3.3, $p = 0.66$; angiogenesis on day 10: 8.0 ± 2.8 vs. 8.9 ± 3.1; reepithelialization in % on day 10: 81 ± 8.5 vs. 85 ± 7.1.

Conclusion.—Intravenous arginine supplementation does not improve angiogenesis, reepithelialization or neutrophil influx in healing of human skin graft donor sites.

▶ It has been shown previously that collagen formation in different volunteer populations can be improved when 30 g of arginine is administered. These studies were carried out using subcutaneously implanted synthetic tubes. In this article, the authors sought to determine if the use of arginine would improve angiogenesis, reepithelialization, and neutrophil influx following human skin graft donation. A randomized prospective study was carried out. The control group received nitrogen in the form of amino acids, while the experimental group received only arginine. No differences in the measured parameters were observed except for the expected increase in plasma arginine levels in the experimental group.

Former studies measured collagen formation while different end points were measured in this trial. Thus, arginine may have very specific roles in wound healing that are not generally applicable to all wounds.

J. M. Daly, MD

Addition of Polydextrose and Galactooligosaccharide to Formula Does Not Affect Bacterial Translocation in the Neonatal Piglet

Monaco MH, Kashtanov DO, Wang M, et al (Univ of Illinois, Urbana; et al)
J Pediatr Gastroenterol Nutr 52:210-216, 2011

Objectives.—The aim of the study was to determine the effect of polydextrose (PDX) and galactooligosaccharide (GOS) on bacterial translocation (BT) in neonatal piglets.

Materials and Methods.—Piglets (n = 36) were randomized 12 hours after birth to receive total enteral nutrition (TEN) as formula; TEN + GOS (4 g/L), TEN + PDX (4 g/L), or TEN + GOS + PDX (2 g/L each) for 7 days or were supported by total parenteral nutrition (TPN) as a positive control for BT (n = 8). Blood, spleen, liver, and mesenteric lymph node (MLN) samples were cultured for aerobic and anaerobic bacteria. Colon microbiota 16S rDNA was measured by polymerase chain reaction. Myeloperoxidase activity and tumor necrosis factor-α expression were measured in ileum and ascending colon.

Results.—Among the enterally fed groups, no difference was seen in the *Lactobacillus* and *Bacteroides* 16S rDNA copies per gram of colonic contents, yet total bacterial levels were lower (*P* < 0.05) in the TEN + GOS group compared with TEN alone. Bacteria were detected in the blood, liver spleen, and MLN of TPN piglets. In contrast, bacterial counts were predominantly detected in the MLN of TEN piglets, at much lower levels than in TPN, and levels were not affected by GOS and PDX addition. TPN piglets had elevated (*P* < 0.05) ileal myeloperoxidase activity and a trend in elevated ascending colon tumor necrosis factor-α expression (*P* = 0.1).

Conclusions.—PDX and GOS added to formula do not induce BT in healthy piglets. Low levels of bacteria in MLN of healthy neonatal piglets may reflect mucosal sampling rather than pathological BT.

▶ It has been suggested that the use of prebiotics may offer benefit in infants and others. Polydextrose (PDX), a randomly bonded combination of dextrose, sorbitol, and citric acid, and galactooligosaccharide (GOS) have been suggested to increase bacterial translocation from the intestine, which may be harmful in certain circumstances. It is well known that the total enteral nutrition decreases bacterial translocation in animal models compared with total parenteral nutrition. When PDX or GOS was added to total enteral nutrition either alone or together and given to newborn piglets, there was no indication of increased bacterial translocation.

Thus, results from these animal studies suggest that these substances may be of benefit when given to infants as prebiotic therapy.

J. M. Daly, MD

Parenteral Fish Oil as Monotherapy Improves Lipid Profiles in Children With Parenteral Nutrition—Associated Liver Disease
Le HD, de Meijer VE, Zurakowski D, et al (Children's Hosp Boston, MA)
JPEN J Parenter Enteral Nutr 34:477-484, 2010

Background.—Parenteral nutrition (PN) is a life-saving therapy but has been associated with dyslipidemia. Because fish oil has been shown to have positive effects on lipid profiles, the authors hypothesize that a parenteral fish oil lipid emulsion will improve lipid profiles in children who are PN dependent.

Methods.—The authors examined the lipid profiles of a unique cohort of 10 children who were exclusively administered a fish oil—based lipid emulsion while on PN for a median duration of 14 weeks. Longitudinal data analysis with a generalized estimating equations approach was used to determine the sterol and bilirubin levels based on duration of the fish oil—based lipid emulsion.

Results.—After 14 weeks of fish oil monotherapy, children had a 24% increase in high-density lipoprotein. Compared to baseline, serum low-density lipoprotein, very low-density lipoprotein, total cholesterol, and triglyceride levels all significantly decreased by 22%, 41%, 17%, and 46%, respectively. Eight children had their bilirubin improved with a decreased direct bilirubin from 6.9 mg/dL (range, 4.4-10.7) at baseline to 2.3 mg/dL (range, 1.3-4.0) after 14 weeks, and a decrease in total bilirubin from 8.7 mg/dL (range, 5.5-13.7) to 3.8 mg/dL (range, 2.2-6.5).

Conclusion.—A fish oil–based lipid emulsion used as monotherapy in children who exclusively depended on PN for survival was associated with significant improvement in all major lipid panels as well as improvement of hyperbilirubinemia. Parenteral fish oil may be the preferred lipid source in children with dyslipidemia.

▶ Previous studies have evaluated the use of parenteral fish oil emulsions as part of the caloric sources in children undergoing total parenteral nutrition (TPN). The hypothesis is that these emulsions will result in less hyperbilirubinemia associated with fatty liver in these individuals. This is particularly important in those who are dependent for a long term on parenteral nutrition.

In this longitudinal study, 10 children were followed up for 14 weeks and were exclusively administered a fish oil–based lipid emulsion while on parenteral nutrition. Importantly, serum low-density lipoprotein, total cholesterol, and triglyceride levels decreased substantially, and 8 of 10 children showed improvement in their serum bilirubin (total and direct) levels. Studies such as these are very important, as it has been shown that the chronic increases in bilirubin levels seen in children on long-term TPN are extremely deleterious. There are known complications of chronic administration of fish oil emulsions, and the ultimate therapy for children on long-term TPN may be the alternation of various emulsions over time to improve outcomes.

J. M. Daly, MD

Computer-Assisted Glucose Regulation During Rapid Step-Wise Increases of Parenteral Nutrition in Critically Ill Patients: A Proof of Concept Study
Hoekstra M, Schoorl MA, van der Horst ICC, et al (Univ of Groningen, the Netherlands)
JPEN J Parenter Enteral Nutr 34:549-553, 2010

Background.—Early delivery of calories is important in critically ill patients, and the administration of parenteral nutrition (PN) is sometimes required to achieve this goal. However, PN can induce acute hyperglycemia, which is associated with adverse outcome. We hypothesized that initiation of PN using a rapid "step-up" approach, coupled with a computerized insulin-dosing protocol, would result in a desirable caloric intake within 24 hours without causing hyperglycemia.

Methods.—In our surgical intensive care unit (ICU), glucose is regulated by a nurse-centered computerized glucose regulation program. When adequate enteral feeding was not possible, PN was initiated according to a simple step-up rule at an infusion rate of 10 mL/h (approximately 10 kcal/h) and subsequently increased by steps of 10 mL/h every 4 hours, provided glucose was <10 mmol/L, until the target caloric intake

(1 kcal/kg/h) was reached. All glucose levels and insulin doses were collected during the step-up period and for 24 hours after achieving target feeding.

Results.—In all 23 consecutive patients requiring PN, mean intake was 1 kcal/kg/h within 24 hours. Of the 280 glucose samples during the 48-hour study period, mean ± standard deviation glucose level was 7.4 ± 1.4 mmol/L. Only 4.5% of glucose measurements during the step-up period were transiently ≥10 mmol/L. After initiating PN, the insulin requirement rose from 1.1 ± 1.5 units/h to 2.9 ± 2.5 units/h ($P < .001$).

Conclusions.—This proof of concept study shows that rapid initiation of PN using a step-up approach coupled with computerized glucose control resulted in adequate caloric intake within 24 hours while maintaining adequate glycemic control.

▶ The use of total parenteral nutrition (TPN) is common in intensive care settings, but its use is often complicated by the development of hyperglycemia. A prospective randomized trial suggested that hyperglycemia in critically ill patients in the intensive care setting increases the risk of morbidity and mortality. Although controversial at the present time, most intensive care units continue to advocate for precise control of blood glucose levels, despite the risk and morbidity of hypoglycemia. This proof of concept study establishes that progressive increases in the rate of TPN administration can be done safely in patients in the intensive care unit using computerized glucose control models. Obviously, this model requires testing in larger numbers of patients outside of a single institution to be certain that it can be applied safely. However, this first step is an important one.

J. M. Daly, MD

The Impact of Glutamine Dipeptide—Supplemented Parenteral Nutrition on Outcomes of Surgical Patients: A Meta-Analysis of Randomized Clinical Trials

Wang Y, Jiang Z-M, Nolan MT, et al (Peking Union Med College Hosp, Beijing, China; The Johns Hopkins Univ, Baltimore, MD; et al)
JPEN J Parenter Enteral Nutr 34:521-529, 2010

Objective.—To evaluate the impact of glutamine dipeptide—supplemented parenteral nutrition (GLN-PN) on clinical outcomes in surgical patients.

Methods.—MEDLINE, EMBASE, Web of Science, and the Cochrane Controlled Clinical Trials Register were searched to retrieve the eligible studies. The studies were included if they were randomized controlled trials that evaluated the effect of GLN-PN and standard PN on clinical outcomes of surgical patients. Clinical outcomes of interest were postoperative morbidity of infectious complication, mortality, length of hospital stay, and cost. Statistical analysis was conducted by RevMan 4.2 software from the Cochrane Collaboration.

Results.—Fourteen randomized controlled trials (RCTs) (N = 587) were included in this meta-analysis. The results showed that glutamine dipeptide significantly reduced the length of hospital stay by around 4 days in the form of alanyl-glutamine (weighted mean difference [WMD] = −3.84; 95% confidence interval [CI] −5.40, −2.28; z = 4.82; P < .001) and about 5 days in the form of glycyl-glutamine (WMD = −5.40; 95% CI −8.46, −2.33; z = 3.45; P < .001). The overall effect indicated a significant decrease in the infectious complication rates of surgical patients receiving GLN-PN (risk ratio = 0.69; 95% CI 0.50, 0.95; z = 2.26; P = .02).

Conclusion.—GLN-PN was beneficial to postoperative patients by shortening the length of hospital stay and reducing the morbidity of post-operative infectious complications.

▶ The authors performed a meta-analysis of randomized clinical trials to evaluate the impact of glutamine dipeptide—supplemented parenteral nutrition on clinical outcomes in surgical patients. Fourteen randomized controlled trials consisting of 587 patients were included in the analysis to determine the effect of glutamine dipeptide—supplemented parenteral nutrition compared with standard parenteral nutrition. Use of parenteral nutrition supplemented with glutamine dipeptide significantly reduced the average length of hospital stay and resulted in a significant decrease in infectious complication rates. Previous studies have shown that glutamine improves muscle amino acid metabolism while also preserving the gastrointestinal mucosa. Preservation of muscle mass and reduction of gastrointestinal bacterial translocation are important. The results of this meta-analysis of randomized clinical trials strongly suggest that parenteral nutrition with glutamine dipeptide may have important benefits in clinical outcomes of surgical patients.

J. M. Daly, MD

A New Intravenous Fat Emulsion Containing Soybean Oil, Medium-Chain Triglycerides, Olive Oil, and Fish Oil: A Single-Center, Double-Blind Randomized Study on Efficacy and Safety in Pediatric Patients Receiving Home Parenteral Nutrition
Goulet O, Antébi H, Wolf C, et al (Univ of Paris, France; Faculté de Médecine Paris Ouest, France; Hôpital Saint Antoine, Paris, France)
JPEN J Parenter Enteral Nutr 34:485-495, 2010

Background.—SMOFlipid 20% is an intravenous lipid emulsion (ILE) containing soybean oil, medium-chain triglycerides, olive oil, and fish oil developed to provide energy, essential fatty acids (FAs), and long-chain ω-3 FAs as a mixed emulsion containing α-tocopherol. The aim was to assess the efficacy and safety of this new ILE in pediatric patients receiving home parenteral nutrition (HPN) compared with soybean oil emulsion (SOE).

Methods.—This single-center, randomized, double-blind study included 28 children on HPN allocated to receive either SMOFlipid 20% (n = 15) or a standard SOE (Intralipid 20%, n = 13). ILE was administered 4 to 5 times per week (goal dose, 2.0 g/kg/d) within a parenteral nutrition regimen. Assessments, including safety and efficacy parameters, were performed on day 0 and after the last study infusion (day 29). Lipid peroxidation was determined by measurement of thiobarbituric acid reactive substances (TBARS).

Results.—There were no significant differences in laboratory safety parameters, including liver enzymes, between the groups on day 29. The mean ± standard deviation changes in the total bilirubin concentration between the initial and final values (day 29 to day 0) were significantly different between groups: SMOFlipid group −1.5 ± 2.4 µmol/L vs SOE group 2.3 ± 3.5 µmol/L, P < .01; 95% confidence interval [CI], −6.2 to −1.4). In plasma and red blood cell (RBC) phospholipids, the ω-3 FAs C20:5ω-3 (eicosapentaenoic acid) and + C22:6ω-3 (docosahexaenoic acid) increased significantly in the SMOFlipid group on day 29. The ω-3:ω-6 FA ratio was significantly elevated with SMOFlipid 20% compared with SOE group (plasma, day 29: 0.15 ± 0.06 vs 0.07 ± 0.02, P < .01, 95% CI, 0.04−0.11; and RBC, day 29: 0.23 ± 0.07 vs 0.14 ± 0.04, P < .01, 95% CI, 0.04−0.13). Plasma α-tocopherol concentration increased significantly more with SMOFlipid 20% (15.7 ± 15.9 vs 5.4 ± 15.2 µmol/L, P < .05; 95% CI, −2.1 to 22.6). The low-density lipoprotein−TBARS concentrations were not significantly different between both groups, indicating that lipid peroxidation did not differ between groups.

Conclusions.—SMOFlipid 20%, which contains 15% fish oil, was safe and well tolerated, decreased plasma bilirubin, and increased ω-3 FA and α-tocopherol status without changing lipid peroxidation.

▶ Intravenous lipid emulsions are critical to provide essential fatty acids for patients unable to eat adequately. For patients on long-term home parenteral nutrition, they are essential. In the past, studies have shown that standard soybean oil emulsions do not provide enough omega-3 fatty acids and may be harmful because of immunosuppression. Thus, it is important to develop new lipid emulsion formulations to provide these critical nutrients. This study is important because it was randomized and double blind. It showed a lowering of serum bilirubin levels versus an increase with the control formulation with no evidence of increased lipid peroxidation.

The formulation also included alpha-tocopherol and medium-chain triglycerides, giving more easily utilizable energy sources. Importantly, no differences in liver functions were noted between the control and experimental groups. Thus, this new lipid formulation passed the first safety test for 28-day use. It will be valuable as testing continues to evaluate other energy, biochemical, and immunological parameters for use in children and adults.

J. M. Daly, MD

The Inflammatory Modulation Effect of Glutamine-Enriched Total Parenteral Nutrition in Postoperative Gastrointestinal Cancer Patients

Lu C-Y, Shih Y-L, Sun L-C, et al (Kaohsiung Med Univ Hosp, Taiwan)
Am Surg 77:59-64, 2011

The objective of this study is to explore the inflammatory modulation effect of glutamine-enriched total parenteral nutrition (TPN) by investigating the alterations of inflammation-related cytokines in gastrointestinal (GI) cancer patients postoperatively. Fifty GI cancer patients received postoperative 7 days of isocaloric and isonitrogenous TPN after operation. They were randomly divided to receive either glutamine-enriched TPN or standard TPN. The inflammation-related cytokines including interleukin-6, interleukin-10, and tumor necrosis factor-α were also determined. Records of nutritional assessments, inflammatory status, and postoperative complications were compared between the two groups. Of 50 enrolled patients, 25 patients were classified as the intervention group, and the control group also comprised 25 patients. The differences of gender, age, primary GI malignancies, and hematological and biochemical data between the two compared groups were not statistically significant (all $P > 0.05$). Compared with standard TPN, a higher serum prealbumin level and better nitrogen balance were observed in glutamine-enriched TPN ($P = 0.039$ and 0.048 respectively). A significantly lower serum interleukin-6 level was found in comparing glutamine-enriched with standard TPN ($P = 0.01$), but not in interleukin-10 ($P = 0.374$) and tumor necrosis factor-α levels ($P = 0.653$). Moreover, a significant lower serum C-reactive protein level was detected in glutamine-enriched TPN compared with standard TPN ($P = 0.013$). Indeed, four cases of postoperative infectious complications were noted in the control group, but no postoperative infectious complications were observed in the interventional group ($P = 0.037$). Our present study shows that glutamine-enriched TPN may be beneficial in improving the inflammatory status and decreasing the infectious morbidity in postoperative GI cancer patients.

▶ Many studies have been carried out in perioperative patients to determine if the use of nutritional supplementation either enterally or parenterally may be beneficial. In various meta-analysis reports, the use of immunologic-modulated total parenteral nutrition (TPN) appeared to be beneficial in postoperative patients. However, in critically ill septic patients in the intensive care unit, it may be harmful. This small study evaluated 50 patients undergoing resection for colon cancer. Demographics between groups were similar. The group given glutamine-supplemented TPN showed improved prealbumin levels and nitrogen balance.

Mean serum interleukin 6 and C-reactive protein levels were significantly lower in the glutamine-supplemented group compared with results in controls given standard TPN. The authors noted 2 cases of postoperative pneumonia and 2 cases of central venous catheter infections in the standard group compared with the supplemented group.

Clearly, postoperative morbidity was not a primary end point of this study; serum cytokines, etc, were the end points. Patients with colon cancer undergoing surgery are not usually malnourished, so the explanation for these results is unclear. Further studies should be undertaken to determine if patient outcome is truly improved with glutamine-supplemented TPN.

J. M. Daly, MD

Assessing Appropriate Parenteral Nutrition Ordering Practices in Tertiary Care Medical Centers

Martin K, DeLegge M, Nichols M, et al (Med Univ of South Carolina, Charleston; Univ of South Carolina, Columbia)
JPEN J Parenter Enteral Nutr 35:122-130, 2011

Background.—Parenteral nutrition (PN) is an essential feeding route for specific patient populations. Despite its utility, PN is invasive, costly, and associated with clinical complications. In most U.S. hospitals, PN is over-prescribed. This study measured rates of inappropriate PN use in hospitalized adults, as determined by the 2002 American Society for Parenteral and Enteral Nutrition guidelines, at 4 tertiary care South Carolina hospitals (facilities A—D). Secondary aims were to identify indicators of inappropriate use and estimated preventable costs.

Methods.—Over a 3-month period, trained registered dietitians at each site collected data retrospectively and prospectively to determine PN appropriateness and indicators of use in 278 randomly selected PN cases.

Results.—PN therapy was inappropriately prescribed in 32% of cases, resulting in approximately 552 days and $138,000 in preventable hospital costs. Thirteen percent of patients who were prescribed inappropriate PN were discharged on home PN. Mean duration of PN therapy was higher in inappropriate cases vs appropriate cases (6 ± 7 days [range, 1—78 days] vs 10 ± 10.6 days [range, 1—51 days]; $P < .004$). Facility B had lower rates of inappropriately prescribed PN (23%) compared with facilities A (33%), C (35%), and D (38%). Dietitians recommended against PN in >70% of all inappropriate cases at facilities A and D compared with <45% at facilities B and D ($P < .001$). Facility B employed more certified nutrition support dietitians (68% of staff) and was among the 2 hospitals using a nutrition support team (NST).

Conclusion.—This study was novel by comparing PN practices in state-wide hospitals. Results indicate that NSTs and certified nutrition support clinicians can curtail preventable spending from inappropriate PN use. Future studies should identify barriers in implementing evidence-based practice.

▶ In the past, nutrition support teams were the major providers of total parenteral nutrition (TPN) in hospitals. As hospital budgets became tight, these teams were often dispersed. At the same time, all physicians were able to order TPN for their patients using a formulaic approach that reduced metabolic complications. However, the appropriate use of TPN in the hospitalized setting is unclear.

This study investigated the use of TPN in 4 South Carolina hospitals, evaluating the appropriateness of TPN in a particular patient setting. Nearly 300 patients were studied. In one-third of patients, the use of TPN was inappropriate as deemed by expert nutritionists. The cost savings to the hospitals would have amounted to nearly $140 000. The cost may have been even higher if they took into account complications of therapy.

It is incumbent on hospital administrators to understand the need for expert nutritionists to help guide the appropriate use of TPN to improve patient care and reduce costs.

J. M. Daly, MD

Local Administration of Antibiotics by Gentamicin–Collagen Sponge does not Improve Wound Healing or Reduce Recurrence Rate After Pilonidal Excision with Primary Suture: A Prospective Randomized Controlled Trial
Andersson RE, Lukas G, Skullman S, et al (Länssjukhuset Ryhov, Jönköping, Sweden; Kärnsjukhuset, Skövde, Sweden)
World J Surg 34:3042-3046, 2010

Background.—Excision and primary suture for pilonidal disease is associated with a high rate of wound infection and recurrences. This randomized, controlled study was designed to analyze the effect of local application of a gentamicin-containing collagen sponge (Collatamp®) in reducing the wound infection rate and recurrences after excision of pilonidal sinus and wound closure with primary midline suture.

Methods.—From March 2003 to November 2005, 161 patients with symptomatic pilonidal disease were operated on at 11 hospitals with traditional wide excision of the sinus and all of its tracts. The patients were randomized to filling of the cavity with a gentamicin-containing collagen sponge (Collatamp®) before wound closure or to closure with no additional treatment. Information about the treatment allocation was hidden until the end of the study. Information about wound healing was noted at follow-up at the outpatient department after 2–4 days, 2 weeks, 3 months, and 1 year.

Results.—No statistically significant differences were observed between the groups during follow-up. Patients who received prophylaxis with Collatamp® had slightly fewer wounds with exudate at 2–4 days and 2 weeks of follow-up (2% vs. 10%, $p = 0.051$ and 57% vs. 65%, $p = 0.325$, respectively), a slightly larger proportion of healed wounds at 3 months follow-up (77% vs. 66%, $p = 0.138$) but not at 1 year (85% vs. 90%, $p = 0.42$, respectively), and slightly more reoperations (10% vs. 4%, $p = 0.213$).

Conclusions.—This randomized, controlled study showed no significant differences in the rates of wound infection, wound healing, and recurrences when a gentamicin–collagen sponge was added to the surgical treatment of pilonidal disease with excision and primary midline suture. This does not support the use of gentamicin—collagen sponge for the surgical treatment of pilonidal disease.

▶ As the authors have described, excision and primary closure of pilonidal cysts often result in infection and wound breakdown. The authors performed a prospective randomized trial, whereby they studied 161 patients in 11 institutions. Ultimately, there were no differences between the control group and the group which had the gentamicin-impregnated sponge placed in the wound prior to closure. This could be for several reasons, such as the overall low rate of infection, the increased rate of reoperations in the sponge group, or the lack of effectiveness of the sponge.

This study is important for its straightforward results in a large multi-institutional trial.

J. M. Daly, MD

Influence of Glycemic Control on Tympanic Membrane Healing in Diabetic Rats
Kaftan H, Reuther L, Miehe B, et al (Ernst Moritz Arndt Univ, Greifswald, Germany)
Laryngoscope 121:823-827, 2011

Objectives/Hypothesis.—It is generally assumed that glycemic control in diabetic patients is important in optimizing wound healing. The goal of this study was to examine tympanic membrane (TM) wound healing in spontaneously diabetic rats depending on the diabetic metabolic state compared to nondiabetic control animals.

Study Design.—Prospective controlled study in experimental animals.

Methods.—Right-sided myringotomy was performed in 20 normoglycemic rats, 17 well-compensated, and 23 poorly compensated diabetic rats. TMs were observed for a total of 3 weeks. Effect of diabetic metabolic state on the healing of the TMs was evaluated by closure rates and histology.

Results.—Diabetic rats showed a significant delay in TM wound healing compared to the control group, but there were no significant differences between both diabetes groups.

Conclusions.—Glycemic control does not influence TM wound repair in an animal model of type 1 diabetes.

▶ This interesting animal study evaluated a model of tympanic membrane healing to assess the effects of glycemic control in diabetic animals. It is well known that wound healing is impaired in diabetic animals and patients. It has been suggested that tight glycemic control for patients in the intensive care unit setting reduces infectious complications so commonplace in these hospital areas. In this study, the presence of experimental type I diabetes in rats led to impaired tympanic healing. However, glycemic control did not lead to improvements in these diabetic animals.

Further work clearly needs to be done in animal models such as these to understand the mechanisms whereby specific areas of healing remain impaired despite treatment of hyperglycemia.

J. M. Daly, MD

9 Wound Healing

Timing of Administration of Bevacizumab Chemotherapy Affects Wound Healing After Chest Wall Port Placement

Erinjeri JP, Fong AJ, Kemeny NE, et al (Memorial Sloan-Kettering Cancer Ctr, NY)

Cancer 117:1296-1301, 2011

Background.—The authors investigated how the timing of administration of bevacizumab, a targeted vascular endothelial growth factor-inhibiting chemotherapeutic agent, affected the risk of wound healing in patients undergoing chest wall port placement.

Methods.—The authors performed a retrospective search of an institutional review board approved, Health Insurance Portability and Accountability Act compliant database between 2002 and 2008, identifying 1108 port placements in patients who were treated with bevacizumab. One hundred twenty of these ports eventually required explant. Data analyzed included patient demographics, indication for port removal, and schedule of bevacizumab therapy.

Results.—Wound healing complications requiring port explant were seen in 0.9% of placements (10/1108). When bevacizumab was given within 1 day of port placement, the absolute risk (AR) of port removal for wound dehiscence was 2.4% (2/82), compared with 0.3% (3/1021) when 2 or more days had passed between port placement and bevacizumab administration, yielding a statistically significant relative risk (RR) of 8.1 ($P < .02$). Similarly, when bevacizumab was administered within 7 days of port insertion, there was a significant RR of dehiscence-related port explant (AR 1.4% vs 0.1%, RR 11.5, $P < .028$). However, no significant RR for dehiscence-related port removal was observed when bevacizumab was administered within 14 days (AR 0.9% vs 0.2%, RR 6.2, $P < .09$) or 30 days (AR 0.7% vs 0.2%, RR 3.7, $P < .23$) of port placement.

Conclusions.—The risk of a wound dehiscence requiring chest wall port explant in patients treated with bevacizumab was inversely proportional to the interval between bevacizumab administration and port placement, with significantly higher risk seen when the interval is less than 14 days.

▶ It has been well known that administration of chemotherapy prior to or immediately after wounding inhibits the ultimate healing. It is less clear regarding the timing of administration of specific biologics such as bevacizumab, a vascular endothelial growth factor—inhibiting agent, may affect wound healing. In this large but retrospective study, port placement was chosen as the wound to examine. When the agent was administered within 14 days and certainly within 2 days, the port had to be removed much more frequently than if a longer duration had occurred between administration and port placement.

Studies such as these are important to demonstrate in a very practical way the importance of timing of drug administration with the planned elective surgical procedure.

J. M. Daly, MD

Human Cadaveric Dermal Matrix for Management of Challenging Surgical Defects on the Scalp
Stebbins WG, Hanke CW, Petersen J (Laser and Skin Surgery Ctr of Indiana, Carmel)
Dermatol Surg 37:301-310, 2011

Background.—Biologic scaffolds have shown promise in patients unable to tolerate prolonged surgical closure or extensive wound care, but there has been little research in the field of Mohs micrographic surgery (MMS) on human cadaveric dermis in this capacity.

Objective.—To evaluate the utility of human cadaveric dermis as a means of decreasing operative time, minimizing postoperative wound care, and improving aesthetic outcomes in selected patients with deep surgical defects, including those with exposed bone.

Methods.—Fourteen patients (8 men, 6 women) with deep postoperative defects after MMS were treated with a cadaveric dermal allograft as part or all of their postoperative wound management.

Results.—Allograft placement was well tolerated, with high satisfaction levels relating to minimal postoperative wound care and aesthetic outcome. Significantly shorter operative times were noted in all patients than with primary closure or grafting.

Conclusion.—In patients with significant comorbidities, inability to tolerate extended surgical repairs, or inability to perform extensive wound care, human cadaveric dermal allografts can decrease operative time and minimize wound care complexity while providing an excellent aesthetic outcome in many cases. Shorter healing times than expected were also noted in a number of patients.

▶ It is important to use all possible means to improve wound closure and maximize cosmetic appearances after major Mohs surgery. This study was undertaken to evaluate human cadaveric dermis in this setting. This small prospective clinical study evaluated 14 patients who underwent deep Mohs excision. Operative times were less, and cosmetic appearances were deemed quite good from a subjective review of results.

Clearly, this form of therapy needs further rigorous evaluation, but this small study suggests benefit in a defined population.

J. M. Daly, MD

A review of topical negative pressure therapy in wound healing: sufficient evidence?
Mouës CM, Heule F, Hovius SER (Erasmus Univ Med Ctr, Rotterdam, The Netherlands)
Am J Surg 201:544-556, 2011

Background.—Topical negative pressure (TNP) therapy has become a useful adjunct in the management of various types of wounds. However, the TNP system still has characteristics of a "black box" with uncertain efficacy for many users. We extensively examined the effectiveness of TNP therapy reported in research studies.

Data Sources.—A database search was undertaken, and over 400 peer-reviewed articles related to the use of TNP therapy (animal, human, and in vitro studies) were identified.

Conclusions.—Almost all encountered studies were related to the use of the commercial VAC device (KCI Medical, United States). Mechanisms of action that can be attributed to TNP therapy are an increase in blood flow, the promotion of angiogenesis, a reduction of wound surface area in certain types of wounds, a modulation of the inhibitory contents in wound fluid, and the induction of cell proliferation. Edema reduction and bacterial clearance, mechanisms that were attributed to TNP therapy, were not proven in basic research.

▶ Topical negative pressure is a major therapeutic tool in the management of difficult wounds. While often bulky and noisy machines are used in the hospital setting, portable equipment is available for the patients who are ambulatory and discharged to the home setting. The use of this therapy developed out of relatively simple concepts. This review article summarizes very nicely the current status of this treatment for large acute and chronic wounds. Physiologically, the wound area demonstrates promotion of angiogenesis, which leads to increased cell proliferation. Wound contraction appears to occur faster than with other treatments leading to a decrease in the size of the wound surface area. Topical negative pressure applied to difficult wounds has made an enormous difference in surgical patient care.

J. M. Daly, MD

Is There a Benefit to Drains With a Kocher-Langenbeck Approach? A Prospective Randomized Pilot Study
Hsu JR, Stinner DJ, Rosenzweig SD, et al (Brooke Army Med Ctr, Fort Sam Houston, TX; Director of Sports Medicine, North Lewis New Iberia, LA; et al)
J Trauma 69:1222-1225, 2010

Background.—Closed suction drainage is a routine part of wound management for patients undergoing surgical treatment of acetabulum fractures. This pilot study seeks to determine if there is a difference in wound healing for a Kocher-Langenbeck approach with and without the use of drains.

Methods.—We conducted a prospective, randomized study including 39 patients with acetabulum fractures treated through a Kocher-Langenbeck approach. During wound closure, patients were randomized into two groups: 20 patients (group I) received drains and 19 (group II) were closed without drains. All were followed up for drain output, quality and quantity of drainage, signs of infection, and duration of drainage. Patients were then evaluated at 2 weeks and 8 weeks for wound healing and any signs of infection.

Results.—By the 8-week follow-up, all wounds healed without any signs of infection. There was no difference in the average number of days of drainage between groups: 7.45 days and 7.95 days for group I and group II, respectively ($p = 0.37$). There were two wound complications (5.13%), with one in each group. Both complications consisted of cellulitis without signs of deep infection and had complete resolution with intravenous antibiotics. A post hoc power analysis determined that a test population of 1,264 patients would be needed to show a reduction in wound drainage time by 1 day.

Conclusion.—With the numbers available in this pilot study, we showed no benefit to the use of drains for acetabular surgery performed through a Kocher-Langenbeck approach.

▶ Many studies have evaluated the use of drains in wounds of postoperative patients. For example, it was common to place drains after cholecystectomy, appendectomy, liver resection, etc. Prospective randomized trials have been conducted that have not demonstrated any benefit with the use of drains after many individual abdominal procedures as well as soft-tissue procedures in terms of infection and wound healing.

This randomized prospective trial also demonstrated no benefit to the use of drains after treatment of acetabular fractures. Measured healing parameters and infectious complications were similar in the drained versus nondrained groups. One could argue that the study was underpowered with only 39 patients entered in the trial. However, as the authors note, over 1000 patients would need to be studied to determine if a meaningful difference could be found. It certainly appears that these results, coupled with many previous trials, recommend against the routine use of drains after many surgical procedures.

J. M. Daly, MD

Biomechanical Properties of a New Multilocking Loop Peripheral Suture Technique for the Repair of Flexor Tendons: A Comparative Experimental Study
Turk YC, Guney A, Oner M, et al (Erciyes Univ Med Faculty, Kayseri, Turkey)
Ann Plast Surg 65:425-429, 2010

We aimed to evaluate the biomechanical properties of a new multilocking loop peripheral suture technique. For this aim, 40-deep digital flexor tendons of adult male sheep front limb were divided and then repaired using one of the following methods: simple peripheral suture plus 2- or 4-strand Kessler core suture or a new multilocking loop peripheral suture combined with either 2- or 4-strand Kessler core suture. Intact tendons were used as controls. The following biomechanical parameters were tested: ultimate tensile strength, energy to failure, 2-mm gap formation force, stiffness, and mechanism of failure. Regardless of the number of core suture strands, the new technique resulted in greater ultimate tensile strength, energy to failure, 2-mm gap formation force, and stiffness values, compared with simple running peripheral suture. In conclusion, the new multilocking loop peripheral suture technique represents a biomechanically strong and technically suitable method for flexor tendon repair.

▶ Issues of flexor tendon repair methods are extremely important. After repair, it is important to begin some motion to decrease the potential for adhesion formation. Because of this, the type of suture material and method of suturing the tendons together are critical to maximize the opportunity for healing. Commonly, the core and peripheral suture technique is used. The authors used the same material in a sheep tendon model and demonstrated that the use of an interlocking suture technique along with either 2 or 4 core sutures maximized the strength of the tendons' healing. This technique needs to be studied in a prospective randomized trial, preferably a multi-institutional clinical trial. End point markers of healing should then be studied to determine strength of healing, adhesion formation, and clinical outcome measures.

J. M. Daly, MD

Management of Split-Thickness Donor Sites With Synthetic Wound Dressings: Results of a Comparative Clinical Study

Markl P, Prantl L, Schreml S, et al (Univ Hosp Regensburg, Germany)
Ann Plast Surg 65:490-496, 2010

This prospective, randomized, single-blinded, clinical study aimed at evaluating 3 different synthetic wound dressings for treating split-thickness skin graft donor sites. Seventy-seven patients were randomly assigned to 3 study groups: Suprathel, Biatain-Ibu, Mepitel. Wounds were inspected daily until complete reepithelization. Ease of care, treatment costs, and scar development after a 6 months follow-up were evaluated. Suprathel showed significant ($P \leq 0.001$) pain reduction after 24 hours but increasing pain scores on the 5th day of treatment. Biatain-Ibu showed significant pain relief immediately after application and during the entire treatment period ($P < 0.05$). Mepitel did not show any significant pain reduction. No differences were seen with regard to healing time, quality of reepithelization, and scar development. Biatain-Ibu had the lowest overall treatment costs ($P \leq 0.001$). The investigated materials did not differ with regard to quality and acceleration of the healing process, but Biatain-Ibu seems to be the most appropriate dressing material in terms of cost-effectiveness.

▶ Coverage methods for those receiving split-thickness skin grafts vary greatly. The ultimate outcome measure is complete healing of the graft. This randomized, prospective, clinical trial in 77 patients evaluated 3 different wound dressings after split-thickness skin grafts. Biatain-Ibu, a nonadhesive foam dressing containing ibuprofen, clearly reduced pain at the site of the skin graft and was the least expensive method of skin graft coverage chosen for study in this clinical trial. There were no differences in the mean times to reepithelialization among the 3 groups nor in the ultimate cosmetic outcome; however, use of Biatain-Ibu did require lengthier and more complex dressing changes.

Studies such as these are important to better define the least expensive yet best type of wound dressings, not only for skin grafts but also for all types of wounds.

J. M. Daly, MD

Continuous Subcutaneous Instillation of Bupivacaine Compared to Saline Reduces Interleukin 10 and Increases Substance P in Surgical Wounds After Cesarean Delivery

Carvalho B, Clark DJ, Yeomans DC, et al (Stanford Univ School of Medicine, CA)
Anesth Analg 111:1452-1459, 2010

Background.—Recent evidence suggests that locally delivered local anesthetics may exert tissue-damaging effects such as chondrolysis after intraarticular injection. Alteration of the inflammatory response is a potential mechanism for local anesthetic-induced tissue toxicity. In this study, we tested the effects of continuous local anesthetic infiltration on the release of inflammatory and nociceptive mediators in skin wounds after cesarean delivery.

Methods.—Thirty-eight healthy women undergoing cesarean delivery with spinal anesthesia were enrolled in this study, and were randomized to receive subcutaneous surgical wound infiltration with bupivacaine 5 mg/mL or saline at 2 mL/h for 24 hours after cesarean delivery. Wound exudate was sampled at 1, 3, 5, 7, and 24 hours after cesarean delivery using a subcutaneous wound drain technique. Cytokines, chemokines, substance P, prostaglandin E_2, and nerve growth factor were assayed using multiplex Bio-Plex® (Bio-Rad, Hercules, CA) and enzyme-linked immunosorbent assays.

Results.—Bupivacaine wound infusion resulted in a significant decrease of interleukin 10 and increase of substance P in wounds compared with saline infusion (area under the 24-hour concentration-time curve; $P < 0.001$). No statistically significant differences were detected for other cytokines, nerve growth factor, and prostaglandin E_2.

Conclusions.—This study demonstrates that the continuous administration of clinically used doses of bupivacaine into wounds affects the local composition of wound mediators. Observed changes in interleukin 10 are compatible with a disruption of antiinflammatory mechanisms. Whether such modulation combined with the release of the proinflammatory mediator substance P results in an overall proinflammatory wound response will require future studies of wound healing.

▶ Postoperative pain control is critical in the management of surgical patients. Use of epidural analgesia and patient-controlled analgesia is a common method for achieving better control of pain in postoperative patients. Subcutaneous instillation of bupivacaine has also been used in this setting to specifically reduce incisional pain. This randomized clinical study by Carvalho et al demonstrates that infusion of bupivacaine compared with saline alone significantly reduced wound levels of interleukin 10 and increased levels of substance P. Importantly, there was no evidence of wound problems with the bupivacaine infusions. As a follow-up study, the authors should evaluate the relationship, if any, of interleukin 10 and substance P to wound healing, rates of infection, and incisional pain control in a larger patient population.

J. M. Daly, MD

Use of Acellular Dermal Replacement in Reconstruction of Nonhealing Lower Extremity Wounds

Kahn SA, Beers RJ, Lentz CW (Univ of Rochester Med Ctr, NY; Univ of New Mexico Health Sciences Ctr, Albuquerque)
J Burn Care Res 32:124-128, 2011

Dermal templates are well established in the treatment of burn wounds and acute nonburn wounds. However, the literature regarding their use for reconstruction of chronic, nonhealing wounds is limited. This study describes a series of patients with chronic wounds reconstructed with a commercially available bilayer, acellular dermal replacement (ADR) containing a collagen-glycosaminoglycan dermal template and a silicone outer layer. A retrospective review was performed of 10 patients treated for chronic wounds with ADR and negative pressure dressing followed by split-thickness skin graft between July 2006 and January 2009. Data collected included age, gender, comorbidities, medications, wound type or location, wound size, the number of applications of ADR, the amount of ADR applied (in square centimeter), the amount of time between ADR placement and grafting, complications, need for reoperation, and percentage of graft take after 5 and 14 days. The mean age of study subjects was 44 years. All patients in the study had comorbidities that interfere with wound healing and were treated for lower extremity wounds (four to legs, five to ankles, and one to foot). The wounds had a variety of causative factors including venostasis ulcers (6, 60%), trauma in diabetic patients (2, 20%), brown recluse bite (1, 10%), and a wound caused from purpura fulminans (1, 10%). The average wound size and amount of ADR applied was 162 ± 182 cm^2. Each patient required only one application of ADR. The average time between ADR placement and skin grafting was 36.5 days. The mean percentage of graft take at 5 days was 89.55%, 14 days was 90%, and 21 days was 87.3%. Only two patients required regrafting, and one of these grafts was lost because of patient noncompliance. ADR can be used successfully in the treatment of chronic wounds. ADR provides direct wound coverage and can conform to a variety of anatomical sites. This study demonstrates that the use of ADR in treating chronic wounds results in high rates of skin graft take. Favorable results were obtained despite the majority of patients having comorbidities that would normally interfere with wound healing.

▶ Patients with nonhealing chronic wounds present difficult situations. A variety of methods have been tried in the past, including various growth factors as well as mechanical means, to improve wound healing. This study used dermal templates as part of the reconstruction process in patients with chronic nonhealing wounds. Acellular dermal replacement (ADR), a commercially available bilayer, was applied to the wounds of 10 patients along with negative pressure dressings followed by split-thickness skin grafts. In this retrospective review, each patient only required one application of ADR. The mean percentage of split-thickness wound varied from 87% to 90% over 21 days after application of the graft.

Clearly the use of ADR appeared to improve the wound setting, making it more receptive to the graft when it was applied.

J. M. Daly, MD

Randomized clinical trial of mesh *versus* sutured wound closure after open abdominal aortic aneurysm surgery
Bevis PM, Windhaber RAJ, Lear PA, et al (Cheltenham General Hosp, UK; Univ of Bristol, UK; Southmead Hosp, Bristol, UK; et al)
Br J Surg 97:1497-1502, 2010

Background.—Incisional herniation is a common complication of abdominal aortic aneurysm (AAA) repair. This study investigated whether prophylactic mesh placement could reduce the rate of postoperative incisional hernia after open repair of AAA.

Methods.—This randomized clinical trial was undertaken in three hospitals. Patients undergoing elective open AAA repair were randomized to routine abdominal mass closure after AAA repair or to prophylactic placement of polypropylene mesh in the preperitoneal plane.

Results.—Eighty-five patients with a mean age of 73 (range 59–89) years were recruited, 77 (91 per cent) of whom were men. There were five perioperative deaths (6 per cent), two in the control group and three in the mesh group ($P = 0 \cdot 663$), none related to the mesh. Sixteen patients in the control group and five in the mesh group developed a postoperative incisional hernia (hazard ratio $4 \cdot 10$, 95 per cent confidence interval $1 \cdot 72$ to $9 \cdot 82$; $P = 0 \cdot 002$). Hernias developed between 170 and 585 days after surgery in the control group, and between 336 and 1122 days in the mesh group. Four patients in the control group and one in the mesh group underwent incisional hernia repair ($P = 0 \cdot 375$). No mesh became infected, but one was subsequently removed owing to seroma formation during laparotomy for small bowel obstruction.

Conclusion.—Mesh placement significantly reduced the rate of postoperative incisional hernia after open AAA repair without increasing the rate of complications. Registration number: ISRCTN28485581 (http://www.controlled-trials.com).

▶ The development of incisional hernias after major abdominal surgery is a significant problem. However, the prophylactic use of nonabsorbable mesh also poses problems, specifically wound infections and chronic reactions to the mesh. In this prospective randomized trial, 85 patients were randomized to either receive or not receive a preperitoneal placement of polypropylene mesh after abdominal aortic aneurysm (AAA) repair. Three important points were made as a result of this study. First, no increase in immediate wound complications occurred because of the mesh. Second, there was a significant decrease in the later development of incisional hernias in the group that underwent closure with the mesh versus controls. Third, the development of incisional hernias occurred late in the patient's courses. However, they occurred earlier in the control group (170-585 days postoperatively) versus 336 to 1122 days in the mesh-treated group. These results, if replicated in further trials, suggest that a standard of care may include the use of mesh for abdominal wound closure after AAA repair.

J. M. Daly, MD

Evaluation of Chronic Wound Treatment with the SNaP Wound Care System versus Modern Dressing Protocols

Lerman B, Oldenbrook L, Eichstadt SL, et al (O'Connor Hosp, San Jose, CA; Stanford Univ, CA; Spiracur, Inc, Sunnyvale, CA)
Plast Reconstr Surg 126:1253-1261, 2010

Background.—Traditional negative-pressure wound therapy systems use an electrically powered pump to generate negative pressure at the wound bed. The SNaP Wound Care System is a novel, ultraportable device that delivers negative-pressure wound therapy without the use of an electrically powered pump.

Methods.—At an outpatient wound care clinic, 21 subjects with difficult-to-treat lower extremity ulcers received treatment with the SNaP System and were evaluated for wound healing for up to 4 months.

Outcomes were then compared with 42 patient-matched controls treated at the same center with modern wound care protocols that included the use of Apligraf, Regranex, and skin grafting.

Results.—In the SNaP-treated group, 100 percent of subjects demonstrated improvement in wound size and 86 percent (18 of 21) exhibited a statistically significant healing trend ($p < 0.05$). Using Kaplan-Meier estimates of wound healing, SNaP-treated subjects healed in an average of 74.25 ± 20.1 days from the start of SNaP treatment and the matched controls healed in an average of 148.73 ± 63.1 days from the start of conventional treatment. This significantly faster healing time represents a 50 percent absolute reduction in time to healing ($p < 0.0001$) for subjects treated with the SNaP device.

Conclusions.—The findings reported here for the SNaP Wound Care System are similar to published reports for powered negative-pressure wound therapy devices for the treatment of highly challenging lower extremity wounds. This study suggests that the SNaP Wound Care System may be a useful addition to the techniques available to the wound care clinician.

▶ The authors reviewed 21 patients treated with negative-pressure wound care using a new portable device (Smart Negative Pressure [SNaP]) and compared the wound healing results with 42 patient-matched controls treated with other protocols. The results suggested marked improvement in healing (74 days) compared with controls (149 days) treated by conventional means.

The study is confounded by the use of patient-matched controls rather than a prospective randomized trial being conducted. This can result in bias, for example, by more frequent observations of the patients and more frequent dressing changes. The authors also note that Apligraf was often used in combination with negative pressure delivered by SNaP. However, despite these shortcomings, patients did heal well, which is the critical end point. The device appears simple and is quiet. Clearly, a prospective randomized trial is indicated.

J. M. Daly, MD

Randomized clinical trial of Chinese herbal medications to reduce wound complications after mastectomy for breast carcinoma
Chen J, Lv Q, Yu M, et al (Sichuan Univ, China; et al)
Br J Surg 97:1798-1804, 2010

Background.—Ischaemia and necrosis of skin flaps is a common complication after mastectomy. This study evaluated the influence of anisodamine and *Salvia miltiorrhiza* on wound complications after mastectomy for breast cancer.

Methods.—Ninety patients undergoing mastectomy for breast carcinoma were divided into three groups. Group 1 received routine wound care, group 2 received intravenous *Salvia miltiorrhiza* after surgery for 3 days and group 3 similarly received intravenous anisodamine. Skin flaps were observed on postoperative days 4 and 8; areas of wound ischaemia and necrosis were graded and adverse events recorded.

Results.—There was no difference in demographic characteristics between the groups. At 4 days after surgery the rate of ischaemia and necrosis in groups 2 and 3 was significantly reduced compared with that in control group 1 (median wound score $6 \cdot 80$ *versus* $23 \cdot 38$, $P = 0 \cdot 002$, and $3 \cdot 76$ *versus* $23 \cdot 38$, $P < 0 \cdot 001$, respectively). This improvement in groups 2 and 3 continued to postoperative day 8 (both $P < 0 \cdot 001$), but wound scores at this stage were better in group 3 than in group 2 ($1 \cdot 82$ *versus* $6 \cdot 92$ respectively; $P = 0 \cdot 022$). The volume of wound drainage was lower in group 3 than in group 1 ($P = 0 \cdot 004$). The incidence of adverse effects was highest in group 3, and two patients in this group discontinued treatment. No significant complications were noted in group 2.

Conclusion.—Anisodamine and *S. miltiorrhiza* were both effective in reducing skin flap ischaemia and necrosis after mastectomy, although anisodamine was associated with a higher rate of adverse effects.

▶ Skin flap necrosis after performing a mastectomy is a major complication resulting in difficult cosmesis and potentially infected prosthesis problems. Previous studies have evaluated vasodilator creams placed on flaps to improve wound healing. This prospective randomized trial studied the effects of anisodamine and *Salvia miltiorrhiza* on skin flap necrosis in patients undergoing mastectomies. Anisodamine is a belladonna alkaloid that blocks the M acetylcholine receptor, thereby reducing vessel spasm and improving microcirculation. *S miltiorrhiza*, also known as red sage, also has been suggested to improve microcirculation. At day 4, both experimental groups showed significant improvement in wound healing without necrosis compared with the control group, which became more significant in group 3 at day 8, although the anisodamine group had more adverse complications. Studies such as these evaluating both Eastern and Western medicines for common surgical problems are important as we seek the best quality care for our patients.

J. M. Daly, MD

Acceleration of wound healing by growth hormone-releasing hormone and its agonists

Dioufa N, Schally AV, Chatzistamou I, et al (Univ of Athens Med School, Greece; Veterans Affairs Med Ctr and South Florida Veterans Affairs Foundation for Res and Education, Miami, FL; Univ of Athens, Greece; et al)
Proc Natl Acad Sci U S A 107:18611-18615, 2010

Despite the well-documented action of growth hormone-releasing hormone (GHRH) on the stimulation of production and release of growth hormone (GH), the effects of GHRH in peripheral tissues are incompletely explored. In this study, we show that GHRH plays a role in wound healing and tissue repair by acting primarily on wound-associated fibroblasts. Mouse embryonic fibroblasts (MEFs) in culture and wound-associated fibroblasts in mice expressed a splice variant of the receptors for GHRH (SV1). Exposure of MEFs to 100 nM and 500 nM GHRH or the GHRH agonist JI-38 stimulated the expression of α-smooth muscle actin (αSMA) based on immunoblot analyses as well as the expression of an αSMA-β-galactosidase reporter transgene in primary cultures of fibroblasts isolated from transgenic mice. Consistent with this induction of αSMA expression, results of transwell-based migration assays and in vitro wound healing (scratch) assays showed that both GHRH and GHRH agonist JI-38 stimulated the migration of MEFs in vitro. In vivo, local application of GHRH or JI-38 accelerated healing in skin wounds of mice. Histological evaluation of skin biopsies showed that wounds treated with GHRH and JI-38 were both characterized by increased abundance of fibroblasts during the early stages of wound healing and accelerated reformation of the covering epithelium at later stages. These results identify another function of GHRH in promoting skin tissue wound healing and repair. Our findings suggest that GHRH may have clinical utility for augmenting healing of skin wounds resulting from trauma, surgery, or disease.

▶ Growth factors such as vascular endothelial growth factor, growth hormone, and others have been studied as a way to enhance the healing of wounds. This is particularly important in circumstances in which wound healing is impaired. While growth hormone has been shown to improve anabolic processes when administered systemically and wound healing when administered locally and systemically, growth hormone—releasing hormone (GHRH) has not been studied for these effects. GHRH has been shown to increase fibroblast proliferation, which is one of many critical processes in the maturation of the wound healing process leading to improved collagen deposition. This study identified the GHRH agonist JI-38 as effective as well regarding both fibroblast proliferation and epithelial coverage of the wound.

Studies such as these are very important, as they will eventually lead to combinations that improve the closure, contracture, and epithelialization of wounds. It will be important to test these substances for efficacy in models of impaired wound healing.

J. M. Daly, MD

The Effect of Percutaneous Intervention on Wound Healing in Patients With Mixed Arterial Venous Disease

Lantis JC II, Boone D, Lee L, et al (Columbia Univ, NY)
Ann Vasc Surg 25:79-86, 2011

Background.—Open venous ulcers in patients with combined arterial and venous insufficiency are notoriously hard to treat. Patients with an ankle—brachial index (ABI) of 0.5-0.8 have been shown to heal poorly. Because adequate compression therapy is contraindicated in patients with an ABI of <0.7, we decided to undertake an aggressive approach of percutaneous revascularization for these patients.

Methods.—A total of 27 patients with clinical and duplex scan evidence of chronic venous insufficiency, active leg ulcers, and impaired arterial perfusion (ABI: <0.7) were treated using a protocol that required performing percutaneous revascularization before ambulatory compression therapy. The patients were followed at 2-week intervals (average) before and after revascularization. Wound measurements and time to complete closure were also recorded.

Results.—The results of the patients were compared with their own previous wound healing trajectories. Additionally, their healing rate was compared with previously published rates of impaired arterial perfusion venous wound closure; 25% closure at 10 weeks, 50% at 19 weeks. At enrollment, the average ABI and wound sizes were 0.56 and 12 cm^2, respectively. On average, the wounds had remained open for 17 weeks. After the intervention, the average ABI was 0.97, average time taken to complete closure was 10 weeks, closure rate at 10 weeks was 75%, and absolute closure rate was 100%.

Conclusion.—Although previous studies have shown that closure of mixed arterial venous ulcers occur without arterial intervention, attaining a near normal ABI allows for timelier wound closure. Therefore, we advocate an aggressive approach of percutaneous revascularization in this population.

▶ This observational interventional study evaluated a series of 27 patients with very difficult extremity ulcer healing problems. Lower extremity ulcers associated with mixed arterial-venous insufficiency have a very poor healing rate, despite multiple different management approaches. The conservative approach does not appear beneficial when the insufficiency is severe. These authors were aggressive in their percutaneous revascularization attempts. However, they were able to improve mean ankle-brachial index scores and then apply ambulatory compression therapy. Compared with historical controls, they achieved markedly improved healing for ulcers that were 12 cm^2 in size at enrollment.

This report shows the importance of being safe, yet aggressive, in the management of these patients. Percutaneous revascularization provides an approach with less of an insult to the patient and should clearly be tried wherever possible.

J. M. Daly, MD

Tendon Healing In Vivo and In Vitro: Neutralizing Antibody to TGF-β Improves Range of Motion After Flexor Tendon Repair
Xia C, Yang X, Wang Y-Z, et al (Qingdao Univ, China)
Orthopedics 33:809, 2010

Adhesion formation between the flexor tendon and its surrounding fibro-osseous sheath results in a decreased postoperative range of motion (ROM) in the hand. Transforming growth factor-beta (TGF-β) is a key cytokine in the pathogenesis of tissue fibrosis. In this study, the effects of TGF-β1 neutralizing antibody were investigated in vitro and in vivo.

In the in vitro investigation, primary cell cultures from rabbit flexor tendon sheath, epitenon, and endotenon were established and each was supplemented with TGF-β along with increasing doses of TGF-β1 neutralizing antibody. Collagen I production was measured with enzyme-linked immunosorbent assay. In the in vivo study, rabbit zone-II flexor tendons were transected and then immediately repaired. Transforming growth factor-β1 neutralizing antibody or phosphate-buffered saline solution (control) was added to the repair sites, and the forepaws were tested for ROM and repair strength at 8 weeks postoperatively.

Transforming growth factor-β1 neutralizing antibody reduced TGF-β upregulated collagen production. Intraoperative application of TGF-β1 neutralizing antibody significantly improved the ROM of the operatively treated digits. The effect on breaking strength of the tendon repair was inconclusive.

▶ Tendon repair in the hand can be fraught with difficulties. It is critical to have a strong bond between the 2 tendon ends while at the same time minimizing the adhesion formation to adjacent tissues. It is well known that transforming growth factor β (TGF-β) is associated with scar formation. In this interesting study, the authors measured in vitro collagen formation with TGF-β added to cell cultures. The increase in collagen I formation seen in control cultures was diminished when TGF-β antibody was added to the culture in increasing amounts. Using a rabbit tendon healing model in vivo, the authors noted that addition of TGF-β1 neutralizing antibody improved the sliding score (range of motion) while not decreasing the breaking strength of the repaired tendons.

Studies such as these are important because they define mechanisms and test hypotheses that can lead to clinical trials. Further work is needed, but this is an interesting approach to the problem of maintaining strength of the repaired tendons while minimizing adhesion formation at the repair site.

J. M. Daly, MD

Wound Macrophages as Key Regulators of Repair: *Origin, Phenotype, and Function*
Brancato SK, Albina JE (Alpert Med School of Brown Univ, Providence, RI)
Am J Pathol 178:19-25, 2011

Recent results call for the reexamination of the phenotype of wound macrophages and their role in tissue repair. These results include the characterization of distinct circulating monocyte populations with temporally restricted capacities to migrate into wounds and the observation that the phenotype of macrophages isolated from murine wounds partially reflects those of their precursor monocytes, changes with time, and does not conform to current macrophage classifications. Moreover, findings in genetically modified mice lacking macrophages have confirmed that these cells are essential to normal wound healing because their depletion results in retarded and abnormal repair. This mini-review focuses on current knowledge of the phenotype of wound macrophages, their origin and fate, and the specific macrophage functions that underlie their reparative role in injured tissues, including the regulation of the cellular infiltration of the wound and the production of transforming growth factor-β and vascular endothelial growth factor.

▶ Macrophages are critical to the wound healing process because of the many roles they serve, such as the local production of cytokines and other biochemical substances, their scavenging role relative to debris and bacteria, and the cell-cell interactive roles they play to encourage other cells to migrate into the wounded area. This article critically reviews the literature as to the phenotypes of wound macrophages and the roles they play in the wound healing process. The review provides insight as to potential mechanisms for improving wound healing in difficult situations. As such, it is important reading.

J. M. Daly, MD

Wound Complications in Thyroxine-Supplemented Patients Following Foot and Ankle Surgery
Grunfeld R, Kunselman A, Bustillo J, et al (Penn State Milton S. Hershey Med Ctr, PA)
Foot Ankle Int 32:38-46, 2011

Background.—Our hypothesis was that thyroxine supplementation in patients undergoing foot and ankle surgery would be associated with increased postoperative wound complications and wound dehiscence compared to patients without thyroxine supplementation.

Materials and Methods.—A retrospective review of 48 patients supplemented with thyroxine that underwent foot and ankle surgery was conducted and analyzed for wound complications. All patients were non-diabetic. A total of 94 historical controls were used to compare the incidence of wound complications to the thyroxine sample. Patient demographics, medical comorbidities, principal diagnosis and procedure performed were recorded. The presence or absence of wound dehiscence, infection or other wound complications was recorded for all patients based on the followup clinical notes in the electronic record.

Results.—In the thyroxine group, the most common diagnosis was degenerative arthritis (31%, $n = 15$), which also occurred in 28.7% of control patients ($n = 27$). Wound dehiscence was reported in 36.2% ($n = 17$) of thyroxine-supplemented patients compared to 10.8% of control patients ($n = 10$). After adjusting for age, gender, hypertension diagnosis, and vascular disease diagnosis, the odds for wound dehiscence remained significantly greater for the thyroxine group compared to control patients (adjusted OR = 3.7; 95% CI: (1.3, 11.4); $p = 0.01$).

Conclusion.—Overall, our results suggest increased wound dehiscence complications in the postoperative period for thyroxine-supplemented patients compared to control patients. This finding remained even after adjusting for the associated cardiovascular comorbidities seen in thyroxine-supplemented patients.

▶ In this study, the authors hypothesized that administration of thyroxine to patients with presumable previous hypothyroidism would be associated with increased postoperative complications. Using historical controls, the authors noted that increased infections and wound complications occurred in the thyroxine-supplemented group compared with historical controls. The authors discussed hypothyroidism and its effects on wound healing, which has previously been noted in the literature. This article points out several issues. First, the use of historical controls truly does not provide good scientific evidence for comparison. Medical records are notoriously inaccurate and omit many findings. Second, no measurements of thyroid or thyroid-stimulating hormone levels were undertaken, so there is no true understanding of the endocrine status of these patients. Finally, historical controls almost always show worse results than contemporaneous patients.

The authors will be commended if they begin a prospective database of patients undergoing foot and ankle surgery evaluating the patient's endocrine status as well as other factors know to be important to postoperative morbidity after such surgery.

J. M. Daly, MD

Blockade of Transforming Growth Factor-β1 Accelerates Lymphatic Regeneration During Wound Repair

Avraham T, Daluvoy S, Zampell J, et al (Memorial Sloan-Kettering Cancer Ctr, NY; et al)
Am J Pathol 177:3202-3214, 2010

Lymphedema is a complication of cancer treatment occurring in approximately 50% of patients who undergo lymph node resection. Despite its prevalence, the etiology of this disorder remains unknown. In this study, we determined the effect of soft tissue fibrosis on lymphatic function and the role of transforming growth factor (TGF)-β1 in the regulation of this response. We determined TGF-β expression patterns in matched biopsy specimens collected from lymphedematous and normal limbs of patients with secondary lymphedema. To determine the role of TGF-β in regulating tissue fibrosis, we used a mouse model of lymphedema and inhibited TGF-β function either systemically with a monoclonal antibody or locally by using a soluble, defective TGF-β receptor. Lymphedematous tissue demonstrated a nearly threefold increase in the number of cells that stained for TGF-β1. TGF-β inhibition markedly decreased tissue fibrosis, increased lymphangiogenesis, and improved lymphatic function compared with controls. In addition, inhibition of TGF-β not only decreased TGF-β expression in lymphedematous tissues, but also diminished inflammation, migration of T-helper type 2 (Th2) cells, and expression of profibrotic Th2 cytokines. Similarly, systemic depletion of T-cells markedly decreased TGF-β expression in tail tissues. Inhibition of TGF-β function promoted lymphatic regeneration, decreased tissue fibrosis, decreased chronic inflammation and Th2 cell migration, and improved lymphatic function. The use of these strategies may represent a novel means of preventing lymphedema after lymph node resection.

▶ Performance of complete axillary or groin dissections can lead to limb lymphedema, which can be quite disabling to patients. Disruption of lymphatic channels is thought to be the major cause of peripheral limb edema. Whenever radiation therapy is given to the lymphatic drainage area after surgical therapy, lymphedema is almost assured. This suggests that fibrosis coupled with lymphatic channel disruption is the major cause of lymphedema.

The authors thought to evaluate intracellular mechanisms with a focus on transforming growth factor (TGF)-β expression in lymphedematous tissues. Interestingly, they found increased expression of TGF-β in lymphedematous tissues, and inhibition of TGF-β decreased inflammation and fibrosis. This is an interesting approach to reduce the potential for development of lymphedema clinically. However, the effects of TGF-β inhibition on overall wound healing and the strength of healing wounds would have to be examined.

J. M. Daly, MD

Safety and efficacy of patient specific intramuscular injection of HGF plasmid gene therapy on limb perfusion and wound healing in patients with ischemic lower extremity ulceration: Results of the HGF-0205 trial

Powell RJ, for the HGF-0205 Trial Investigators (Dartmouth Hitchcock Med Ctr, Lebanon, NH; et al)

J Vasc Surg 52:1525-1530, 2010

Objectives.—We have previously reported the results of a dose-finding phase II trial showing that HGF angiogenic gene therapy can increase TcPO2 compared with placebo in patients with critical limb ischemia (CLI). The purpose of this randomized placebo controlled multi-center trial was to further assess the safety and clinical efficacy of a modified HGF gene delivery technique in patients with CLI and no revascularization options.

Methods.—Patients with lower extremity ischemic tissue loss (Rutherford 5 and 6) received three sets of eight intramuscular injections every 2 weeks of HGF plasmid under duplex ultrasound guidance. Injection locations were individualized for each patient based on arteriographically defined vascular anatomy. Primary safety end point was incidence of adverse events (AE) or serious adverse events (SAE). Clinical end points included change from baseline in toe brachial index (TBI), rest pain assessment by a 10 cm visual analogue scale (VAS) as well as wound healing, amputation, and survival at 3 and 6 months.

Results.—Randomization ratio was 3:1 HGF (n = 21) vs placebo (n = 6). Mean age was 76 ± 2 years, with 56% male and 59% diabetic. There was no difference in demographics between groups. There was no difference in AEs or SAEs, which consisted mostly of transient injection site discomfort, worsening of CLI, and intercurrent illnesses. Change in TBI significantly improved from baseline at 6 months in the HGF-treated group compared with placebo (0.05 ± 0.05 vs −0.17 ± 0.04; P =.047). Change in VAS from baseline at 6 months was also significantly improved in the HGF-treated group compared with placebo (−1.9 ± 1.3 vs +0.06 ± 0.2; P =.04). Complete ulcer healing at 12 months occurred in 31% of the HGF group and 0% of the placebo (P =.28) There was no difference in major amputation of the treated limb (HGF 29% vs placebo 33%) or mortality at 12 months (HGF 19% vs placebo 17%) between groups.

Conclusion.—HGF gene therapy using a patient vascular anatomy specific delivery technique appears safe, maintained limb perfusion, and decreased rest pain in patients with CLI compared with placebo. A larger study to assess the efficacy of this therapy on more clinically relevant end points is warranted.

▶ This randomized prospective clinical trial was carried out in 8 major medical centers to evaluate the safety and efficacy of patient-specific intramuscular injection of hepatocyte growth factor (HGF) plasmid gene therapy on limb perfusion and wound healing in patients with ischemic lower extremity ulceration. As this was a phase 2 safety trial, the primary end points were adverse effects due to therapy. Other outcome measures determined potential improvement in blood flow to the extremities, improvement in healing of vascular ulcers, avoidance of amputation, and overall vascular outcomes at various time points after therapy. Either placebo or HGF was injected intramuscularly at specific points in the limb determined by vascular studies. The authors noted significant improvement in toe brachial index and visual analog scale at 6 months after initiating therapy with HGF compared with placebo. Unfortunately, the amputation rate was similar between both groups of patients. Nevertheless, this is an important study in humans evaluating the effects of growth factors on improving the vascular supply in patients with ischemic lower extremity ulcerations.

J. M. Daly, MD

Manganese superoxide dismutase expression in endothelial progenitor cells accelerates wound healing in diabetic mice
Marrotte EJ, Chen D-D, Hakim JS, et al (Univ of Pittsburgh School of Medicine, PA)
J Clin Invest 120:4207-4219, 2010

Amputation as a result of impaired wound healing is a serious complication of diabetes. Inadequate angiogenesis contributes to poor wound healing in diabetic patients. Endothelial progenitor cells (EPCs) normally augment angiogenesis and wound repair but are functionally impaired in diabetics. Here we report that decreased expression of manganese superoxide dismutase (MnSOD) in EPCs contributes to impaired would healing in a mouse model of type 2 diabetes. A decreased frequency of circulating EPCs was detected in type 2 diabetic (*db/db*) mice, and when isolated, these cells exhibited decreased expression and activity of MnSOD. Wound healing and angiogenesis were markedly delayed in diabetic mice compared with normal controls. For cell therapy, topical transplantation of EPCs onto excisional wounds in diabetic mice demonstrated that diabetic EPCs were less effective than normal EPCs at accelerating wound closure. Transplantation of diabetic EPCs after *MnSOD* gene therapy restored their ability to mediate angiogenesis and wound repair. Conversely, siRNA-mediated knockdown of MnSOD in normal EPCs reduced their activity in diabetic wound healing assays. Increasing the number of transplanted diabetic EPCs also improved the rate of wound closure. Our findings demonstrate that cell therapy using diabetic EPCs after ex vivo MnSOD gene transfer accelerates their ability to heal wounds in a mouse model of type 2 diabetes.

▶ It is well known that diabetic patients have poor wound healing capabilities. This can often result in loss of skin flaps, chronically infected wounds, and potential loss of limbs. Multiple methods have been suggested to improve diabetic wound healing, including local application of growth factors, angiogenic factors, and pharmacologic agents. In this animal study in diabetic (*db/db*) mice, cellular therapy was applied based on the knowledge that endothelial progenitor cells (EPCs) have decreased expression of manganese superoxide dismutase (MnSOD) in the diabetic *db/db* animal model. The proof of concept is that gene therapy directed at correcting this deficiency improved wound healing and angiogenesis in this model. In addition, inhibition of EPC cellular MnSOD using small interfering RNA techniques resulted in impaired wound healing and angiogenesis in normal animals.

This concept of EPC cellular deficiency of MnSOD in diabetic animals and its repair using gene therapy techniques may have applicability in diabetic humans if circulating epithelial progenitor cells can be multiplied and transfected to increase MnSOD activity.

J. M. Daly, MD

Improved diabetic wound healing through topical silencing of p53 is associated with augmented vasculogenic mediators
Nguyen PD, Tutela JP, Thanik VD, et al (New York Univ Langone Med Ctr)
Wound Repair Regen 18:553-559, 2010

Diabetes is characterized by several poorly understood phenomena including dysfunctional wound healing and impaired vasculogenesis.

p53, a master cell cycle regulator, is upregulated in diabetic wounds and has recently been shown to play a regulatory role in vasculogenic pathways. We have previously described a novel method to topically silence target genes in a wound bed with small interfering (si)RNA. We hypothesized that silencing p53 results in improved diabetic wound healing and augmentation of vasculogenic mediators. Paired 4-mm stented wounds were created on diabetic db/db mice. Topically applied p53 siRNA, evenly distributed in an agarose matrix, was applied to wounds at postwound day 1 and 7 (matrix alone and nonsense siRNA served as controls). Animals were sacrificed at postwound days 10 and 24. Wound time to closure was photometrically assessed, and wounds were harvested for histology, immunohistochemistry, and immunofluorescence. Vasculogenic cytokine expression was evaluated via Western blot, reverse transcription-polymerase chain reaction, and enzyme-linked immunosorbent assay. The ANOVA/t-test was used to determine significance ($p \leq 0.05$). Local p53 silencing resulted in faster wound healing with wound closure at 18 ± 1.3 d in the treated group vs. 28 ± 1.0 d in controls. The treated group demonstrated improved wound architecture at each time point while demonstrating near-complete local p53 knockdown. Moreover, treated wounds showed a 1.92-fold increase in CD31 endothelial cell staining over controls. Western blot analysis confirmed near-complete p53 knockdown in treated wounds. At day 10, VEGF secretion (enzyme-linked immunosorbent assay) was significantly increased in treated wounds (109.3 ± 13.9 pg/mL) vs. controls (33.0 ± 3.8 pg/mL) while reverse transcription-polymerase chain reaction demonstrated a 1.86-fold increase in SDF-1 expression in treated wounds vs. controls. This profile was reversed after the treated wounds healed and before closure of controls (day 24). Augmented vasculogenic cytokine profile and endothelial cell markers are associated with improved diabetic wound healing in topical gene therapy with p53 siRNA.

▶ It is well known that impaired wound healing occurs in diabetic subjects. All the mechanisms involved in this delay process have not been identified. However, p53 is a major cell regulator that has been shown to be upregulated in wounds of diabetic patients. The authors used a novel technique to inhibit/silence p53 locally using small interfering RNA (siRNA) in an agarose matrix gel. Significantly less time to closure was noted in those wounds treated with p53 siRNA matrix than control wounds and showed near complete silencing of p53 in the local wound area. They also noted improved vasculogenesis with increased CD31 endothelial cell staining compared with results in controls. Increased stromal cell–derived factor 1 expression also occurred in treated wounds compared with controls.

This is a novel method to silence genes in vivo to accomplish improvement in healing the wounds of diabetic mice. If safety is proven, then this methodology should be attempted in diabetic patients who have difficult wound healing problems.

J. M. Daly, MD

Limitations of the *db/db* mouse in translational wound healing research: Is the NONcNZO10 polygenic mouse model superior?

Fang RC, Kryger ZB, Buck DW II, et al (Northwestern Univ Feinberg School of Medicine, Chicago, IL)

Wound Repair Regen 18:605-613, 2010

Murine models have provided valuable insights into the pathogenesis of both diabetes and chronic wounds. However, only a few published reports to date have investigated wound healing differences among the differing diabetic mouse models. The goal of the present study was to further define the wound healing deficiency phenotypes of streptozotocin-induced (STZ-induced), *Akita*, and *db/db* diabetic mice in comparison with a promising new polygenic strain of Type 2 diabetes (NONcNZO10) by using three specific wound models that targeted different critical processes in the pathogenesis of chronic wounds. Incisional, excisional, and ischemia/ reperfusion wound models were established on mice of each strain. Wound healing parameters including tensile strength, epithelial gap, and wound necrosis were evaluated. In contrast to the other diabetic mice, the NONcNZO10 strain was found to have significant wound healing impairments in all wound healing models. Not only do the NONcNZO10 mice appear to better model human Type 2 diabetes, these provocative findings suggest that the mice may show more clinically relevant wound healing deficiencies than previous diabetic mouse models.

▶ The search for clinically relevant animals for research is never-ending. It is well known that diabetic patients have impaired wound healing. Previously, streptozotocin-induced or *db/db* diabetic mice were commonly used to measure the effectiveness of pharmacologic or biologic agents on various types of wounds. Often, the authors would then surmise effectiveness in diabetic patients.

This interesting study presents a different genetic (NONcNZO10) model of diabetes in mice. The results show a consistent negative effect on wound healing in these genetically modified animals using incisional, excisional, and ischemia/ reperfusion models compared with the other 2 types of diabetic animal models. It will be interesting in studies going forward to compare biologic, pharmacologic, and other means of improving healing of wounds in these NONcNZO10 mice.

J. M. Daly, MD

Accelerated wound healing mediated by activation of Toll-like receptor 9

Sato T, Yamamoto M, Shimosato T, et al (Natl Cancer Inst, Frederick, MD)

Wound Repair Regen 18:586-593, 2010

Wound healing is mediated through complex interactions between circulating immune cells and local epithelial and endothelial cells. Elements of the innate immune system are triggered when Toll-like receptors (TLR) are stimulated by their cognate ligands, and previous studies suggest that such interactions can accelerate wound healing. This work examines the effect of treating excisional skin biopsies with immunostimulatory CpG oligodeoxynucleotides (ODN) that trigger via TLR9. Results indicate that CpG (but not control) ODN accelerate wound closure and reduce the total wound area exposed over time by >40% ($p < 0.01$). TLR9 knockout mice, a strain unresponsive to the immunomodulatory effects of CpG stimulation, are unresponsive to ODN treatment and exhibit a general delay in healing when compared with wild-type mice. CpG ODN administration promoted the influx of macrophages to the wound site and increased the production of vascular endothelial growth factor, expediting neovascularization of the wound bed ($p < 0.01$ for both parameters). Stimulation via TLR9 thus represents a novel strategy to accelerate wound healing.

▶ The ability to accelerate wound healing has been the holy grail sought by many investigators. Physical environment changes (mild stress), chemical (increased oxygenation), and growth factor administration locally have all been tested in efforts to improve the healing of wounds. Animal models of diabetes, radiation, chemotherapy, and malnutrition have been studied.

In this study, local administration of CpG oligodeoxynucleotides (ODN) markedly reduced the wound area after skin excision in animal models compared with controls. The authors studied toll-like receptor 9 (TLR9) knockout mice showing that administration of ODN had no effect, thus demonstrating that TLR9 pathways are critical to this stimulus. It will be important for the authors to study models of impaired wound healing to determine if stimulation of these pathways can return the healing process to normal.

J. M. Daly, MD

Mechanisms of improved wound healing in Murphy Roths Large (MRL) mice after skin transplantation

Tolba RH, Schildberg FA, Decker D, et al (Univ of Bonn, Germany)
Wound Rep Reg 18:662-670, 2010

Scars arise in the late phase of wound healing and are characterized by fibroplasia. Previous controversial studies have discussed the regenerative wound healing capacity of Murphy Roths Large (MRL) mice. The aim of this study was to investigate the mechanisms of improved wound healing in a skin transplantation model. Skin grafts from MRL and haplotypically identical B10.BR mice were cross-transplanted. At day 10, B10.BR and MRL grafts on B10.BR recipients deposited collagen and showed severe apoptosis. Grafts of MRL recipients were not affected by such alterations and showed an enhanced healing progress. They were characterized by higher partial pressure of tissue oxygen, increased microcirculation, exceptionally intense neovascularization, and a blunted inflammatory response.

This phenotype was accompanied by increased vascular endothelial growth factor expression, augmented by enhanced signal transducer and activator of transcription 3 (STAT3) phosphorylation. These effects were combined with a decreased STAT1 expression and phosphorylation. STAT1 pattern variation was associated with decreased Smad7 levels. Furthermore, MRL recipients showed improved stem cell recruitment to the wound area. The basic accelerated wound healing mechanism in MRL mice found in this skin transplantation model is improved engraftment; this is based on enhanced neovascularization and reduced inflammation. These effects are most likely due to higher vascular endothelial growth factor levels and changes in the STAT/Smad signal pathway, which may enhance transforming growth factor-β signaling, reducing proinflammatory responses.

▶ Many animal models of wound healing exist in an effort try to either replicate the healing of wounds in humans or isolate specific mechanisms of the healing process that can be inhibited or enhanced to improve the healing process.

This animal study used Murphy Roths Large (MRL) mice to investigate the mechanisms of wound healing in a skin transplantation model. The results showed enhanced healing in the MRL mice associated with improved stem cell recruitment to the wound area along with improved oxygen levels in the wound area. This was associated with reduced inflammation and higher vascular endothelial growth factor levels. Possible mechanisms included an increase in the signal transducer and activator of transcription 3 (STAT3) along with decreased STAT1 expression.

These studies are very important as they attempt to isolate specific mechanisms of the wound healing processes with the ultimate goal of improving the human condition.

J. M. Daly, MD

Effects of Human Cord Blood Mesenchymal Stem Cells on Cutaneous Wound Healing in Lepr^{db} Mice

Tark K-C, Hong J-W, Kim Y-S, et al (Yonsei Univ College of Medicine, Seoul, Korea; BONA Plastic Surgery Clinic, Seoul, Korea)
Ann Plast Surg 65:565-572, 2010

Purpose.—In the present study, we used the diabetic mouse as a model of delayed wound healing to investigate the effects of human cord blood mesenchymal stem cells (CB-MSC) on wound healing.

Methods.—A delayed wound healing model was used by *db/db* mice. Study models were divided by an injection of human CB-MSC with phosphate buffered solution (PBS) by a different method. One was a locally topical injection, the other was a systemic injection via the end tail vein. Both models were treated with 2.0×10^6 CB-MSC after an 8-mm full thickness defect was made by a skin punch biopsy on the back. We evaluated the wound size, transforming growth factor (TGF)-β, and vascular endothelial growth factor histologic evaluation, and vessel counts. Engraft of CB-MSC was detected by an antihuman antibody.

Result.—Wound healing was accelerated in the experimental group in the topical injection model with statistical significance on the 6th, 9th, and 12th day ($P < 0.05$). In the systemic injection model, wound healing was completed from the 9th day, but there was no statistical significance. TGF-β increased in the first week and decreased in the third week in the experimental groups of both models. But there were opposite results in the control groups of both models. The statistical differences were found in first and third week in topical injection and in the third week in systemic injection ($P < 0.05$). Vascular endothelial growth factor increased in all groups and in all models as the wound healing. But statistical significance did not show between all experimental and control groups. Anti-human antibody immunochemical staining was positive in the wound.

Conclusion.—We concluded that CB-MSC had a positive effect on wound healing. Statistically significant results were noted in the topical injection model. We also reported good effects on the systemic injection model, although we did not find any statistical significance. CB-MSC may influence wound healing by TGF-β.

▶ It is critical to define mechanisms to improve the healing of difficult wounds. Growth factors, drugs, and cellular injection techniques continue to be investigated. This study used *db/db* diabetic mice as a model of impaired wound healing and investigated the use of human cord blood mesenchymal stem cells (CB-MSC) in a skin excision model. The authors noted that local injection of CB-MSC accelerated wound healing within the first 12 days compared with that in controls. Interestingly, wound transforming growth factor-β increased in the local injection group, opposite to the results found in controls. The mechanisms whereby mesenchymal stem cells improve healing can be both direct by having these stem cells differentiate into fibroblasts and other inflammatory cells or indirect via secretion of growth factors affecting the behavior and multiplication of cells in the local wound area. While the exact mechanism is unclear from this study, the positive beneficial effect of local wound injection of CB-MSC is clear.

J. M. Daly, MD

Systemic Transplantation of Progenitor Cells Accelerates Wound Epithelialization and Neovascularization in the Hairless Mouse Ear Wound Model

Sander AL, Jakob H, Henrich D, et al (Hosp of the Johann Wolfgang Goethe-Univ, Frankfurt am Main, Germany; et al)
J Surg Res 165:165-170, 2011

Background.—Impaired wound healing due to local injury, infection, or systemic diseases, such as diabetes, is a major clinical problem. Recent studies have shown that endothelial progenitor cells (EPC) isolated from peripheral blood, bone marrow, as well as the spleen accumulate in granulation tissue at the site of neovascularization, causing secretion of growth factors and cytokines and thus accelerating wound healing.

Materials and Methods.—In the present study, we transplanted systemic EPC and then measured epithelialization and neovascularization in the hairless mouse ear wound model.

Results.—Systemic EPC transplantation significantly accelerated epithelialization and neovascularization compared with control wounds receiving phosphate-buffered saline without calcium and magnesium (PBS). The EPC group had significantly higher vascular density than did the PBS-treated group as determined by immunohistochemistry for CD31 and CD90. Fluorescence microscopy revealed accumulation "homing" of the transplanted EPC at the sites of neovascularization in the granulation tissue throughout healing. Furthermore, transplantation of EPC also increased the expression of the angiogenic cytokine stromal cell-derived factor 1α (SDF1α).

Conclusions.—This appears to be the first demonstration of EPC recruitment to the site of wound neovascularization throughout the healing process. These findings demonstrate that transplanting systemic EPC into "normal" healing wounds promotes epithelialization and neovascularization and thus could be a useful method for accelerating wound healing.

▶ The ability to improve wound healing remains the Holy Grail of scientists working in this area of research. Multiple types of interventions continue to be investigated. Unfortunately, many seem to be beneficial in animal studies only to be found ineffective in humans. This study used endothelial progenitor cells (EPCs) isolated from peripheral blood, bone marrow, and spleen. After systemic injection, they appeared to localize in the area of the wound. In this report, transplantation of EPCs improved epithelialization and neovascularization in an ear wound model. It will be very interesting to determine whether these cells traffic specifically to a wound or whether they become trapped in the lung, liver, or elsewhere. The dose-response of these cells should also be determined. It will also be important to evaluate the many other parameters of wound healing, such as tensile strength, deposition of collagen, wound contracture, etc. Finally, any adverse effects should be noted, particularly in the dose-response experiments.

This is an interesting approach to improving the healing process in wounds and needs further study.

J. M. Daly, MD

Stem cells and bronchial stump healing

Gomez-de-Antonio D, Zurita M, Santos M, et al (Hospital Universitario Puerta de Hierro, Majadahonda, Madrid, Spain)
J Thorac Cardiovasc Surg 140:1397-1401, 2010

Objective.—Bronchial stump dehiscence is still the most feared complication for the thoracic surgeon, with mortality rates ranging from 25% to 75%. This study reports the histologic effect of adult stem cells in the healing process of the bronchial stump after lung resection.

Methods.—A left pneumonectomy was performed in 36 Wistar rats. Half of them received previously labeled bone marrow-derived stem cells applied to the bronchial stump. In each group, 7 rats were sacrificed on day 7 and 11 rats were sacrificed on day 21. Macroscopic variables and histopathologic features were analyzed.

Results.—On days 7 and 21, there were fewer adhesions in the stem cell group ($P = .042$ and $.031$, respectively). Bronchial stump *restitutio ad integrum* on day 21 was found predominantly in rats from the stem cell group ($P = .012$). At that time, the same group showed significantly less inflammation in every layer of the stump ($P < .050$).

Conclusions.—Bone marrow-derived stem cells administered topically on a bronchial stump are able to migrate, reach the bronchial wall, and participate in the healing process. This induces fewer adhesions, less inflammatory response, and better regeneration of the tissue.

▶ This experiment in animals demonstrated that bone marrow—derived stem cells could be applied topically to the bronchial stump of mice that had undergone pneumonectomy. Importantly, the authors demonstrated that these stem cells would migrate to the area of the bronchial stump and they would participate in the healing process. The authors noted that there was improved healing with less complications from adhesions and a more solid bronchial stump when measured histologically at varying times after the transection of the bronchus. This study has important implications for wound healing in humans who have undergone lung resection. It would have been interesting if the authors had actually measured the tensile strength of the bronchial stump to determine whether collagen synthesis and tensile strength is improved in this model of wound healing.

J. M. Daly, MD

10 Gastrointestinal

Utility of Removable Esophageal Covered Self-Expanding Metal Stents for Leak and Fistula Management

Blackmon SH, Santora R, Schwarz P, et al (The Methodist Hosp, Houston, TX)
Ann Thorac Surg 89:931-937, 2010

Background.—Esophageal or gastric leakage from anastomotic wound dehiscence, perforation, staple line dehiscence, or trauma can be a devastating event. Traditional therapy has often consisted of either surgical repair for rapidly diagnosed leaks or diversion for more complicated cases, commonly associated with a delayed diagnosis. This study summarizes our experience treating leaks or fistulas with novel, covered self-expanding metal stents (cSEMS). The primary objective of this study was to determine the efficacy and safety of covered self-expanding metal stents when used to treat complicated leaks and fistulas.

Methods.—Over 15 months, 25 patients with esophageal or gastric leaks were evaluated for stenting as primary treatment. A prospective database was used to collect data. Stents were placed endoscopically, with contrast evaluation used for leak evaluation. Patients who did not improve clinically after stenting or whose leak could not be sealed underwent operative management.

Results.—During a mean follow-up of 15 months, 23 of the 25 patients with esophageal or gastric leaks during a 15-month period were managed with endoscopic stenting as primary treatment. Healing occurred in patients who were stented for anastomotic leakage after gastric bypass or sleeve gastrectomy (n = 10). One patient with three esophageal iatrogenic perforations healed with stenting. Eight patients successfully avoided esophageal diversion and healed with stenting and adjunctive therapy. Two of the 4 patients with tracheoesophageal fistulas sealed with the assistance of a new pexy technique to prevent stent migration; 1 additional patient had this same technique used to successfully heal an upper esophageal perforation.

Conclusions.—Esophageal leaks and fistulas can be effectively managed with cSEMS as a primary modality. The potential benefits of esophageal stenting are healing without diversion or reconstruction and early return to an oral diet.

▶ Gastroesophageal leaks and fistulae were nearly uniformly fatal only 15 to 20 years ago. For example, patients with barotrauma to the esophagus with rupture into the chest most often had delayed diagnosis with subsequent open thoracic surgery for drainage, debridement, and/or diversion. However, the outcome was frequently death or a prolonged recovery from sepsis that was followed by further major surgery for esophageal reconstruction. Blackmon et al offer the intriguing alternative of esophageal stenting with drainage and demonstrate promising results. Although this approach was used in only 23 patients, it is remarkable to note that most patients were successfully treated by stent management and, in fact, the patients returned to oral intake in a short period of time, despite having a delayed presentation to the treating institution. Furthermore, it is important to note that these patients were treated in a multidisciplinary fashion with gastroenterologists and surgeons participating in the decision making and care. This study is a superb example of the best that an academic medical center can offer in terms of patient care. These complex patients received innovative, multidisciplinary care that provided high-quality results. Although these results are encouraging, they are preliminary and the product of a relatively small number of patients. Further studies that provide criteria for stent therapy will be required and likely these studies will come along rather slowly because of the low number of patients afflicted by esophageal perforation. This patient population provides an excellent study group for a multi-institutional investigation.

K. E. Behrns, MD

Surgical gastrojejunostomy or endoscopic stent placement for the palliation of malignant gastric outlet obstruction (SUSTENT study): a multicenter randomized trial
Jeurnink SM, for the Dutch SUSTENT Study Group (Erasmus MC-Univ Med Ctr Rotterdam, The Netherlands; et al)
Gastrointest Endosc 71:490-499, 2010

Background.—Both gastrojejunostomy (GJJ) and stent placement are commonly used palliative treatments of obstructive symptoms caused by malignant gastric outlet obstruction (GOO).
Objective.—Compare GJJ and stent placement.
Design.—Multicenter, randomized trial.
Setting.—Twenty-one centers in The Netherlands.
Patients.—Patients with GOO.
Interventions.—GJJ and stent placement.
Main Outcome Measurements.—Outcomes were medical effects, quality of life, and costs. Analysis was by intent to treat.
Results.—Eighteen patients were randomized to GJJ and 21 to stent placement. Food intake improved more rapidly after stent placement than after GJJ (GOO Scoring System score ≥2: median 5 vs 8 days, respectively; $P < .01$) but long-term relief was better after GJJ, with more patients living more days with a GOO Scoring System score of 2 or more than after stent placement (72 vs 50 days, respectively; $P = .05$). More major complications (stent: 6 in 4 patients vs GJJ: 0; $P = .02$), recurrent obstructive

symptoms (stent: 8 in 5 patients vs GJJ: 1 in 1 patient; $P = .02$), and rein-terventions (stent: 10 in 7 patients vs GJJ: 2 in 2 patients; $P < .01$) were observed after stent placement compared with GJJ. When stent obstruction was not regarded as a major complication, no differences in complications were found ($P = .4$). There were also no differences in median survival (stent: 56 days vs GJJ: 78 days) and quality of life. Mean total costs of GJJ were higher compared with stent placement ($16,535 vs $11,720, respectively; $P = .049$ [comparing medians]). Because of the small study population, only initial hospital costs would have been statistically significant if the Bonferroni correction for multiple testing had been applied.

Limitations.—Relatively small patient population.

Conclusions.—Despite slow initial symptom improvement, GJJ was associated with better long-term results and is therefore the treatment of choice in patients with a life expectancy of 2 months or longer. Because stent placement was associated with better short-term outcomes, this treatment is preferable for patients expected to live less than 2 months. (Clinical trial registration number: ISRCTN 06702358).

▶ Surgical palliation for advanced malignant disease is often complicated by long hospital stays and poor patient outcomes; therefore, alternatives to the treatment of conditions such as gastric outlet obstruction are welcome. In this randomized trial by Jeurnink et al, malignant gastric outlet obstruction was treated by either endoscopic stent placement or by surgical gastrojejunostomy. Importantly, we learned that if the patients will live less than 2 months then a stent is likely the treatment of choice, whereas anticipated survival longer than 2 months is best treated by gastrojejunostomy. A second important lesson is that biliary obstruction should be anticipated before the treatment for gastric outlet obstruction and addressed either by endoscopic or percutaneous stenting or by surgical palliation. It should not be surprising that stents have a functional lifespan of about 2 months, a time when significant tumor in-growth may occur. We know from surgical bypasses in which the decompressive loop may traverse nearby the tumor that this type of palliation will have a limited lifespan. Though stent placement is a good alternative, the surgical patients in this study appeared to have an excessive length of stay, which not only may have been related to delayed gastric emptying but also may be decreased by minimally invasive approaches to these surgical procedures. Nonetheless, we must continue to develop less invasive methods to relieve these desperate patient symptoms and return them to their home environment in the shortest, most humane manner.

K. E. Behrns, MD

Endoscopic, endoluminal fundoplication for gastroesophageal reflux disease: Initial experience and lessons learned
Velanovich V (Henry Ford Hosp, Detroit, MI)
Surgery 148:646-653, 2010

Background.—Several devices have been developed to create an antire-flux barrier endoscopically for the treatment of gastroesophageal reflux disease. All have failed to provide long-term symptom relief, were associated with clinically important complications, or were otherwise removed from the market. A new device, the Esophyx (Endogastric Solutions, Redmond, WA), provides the closest approximation experimentally to a standard Belsy fundoplication. This report describes an initial experience with this device.

Methods.—Patients considered candidates for endoscopic fundoplication include those with symptomatic gastroesophageal reflux disease, a small (<2 cm) hiatal hernia, objective pathologic evidence of gastroesophageal reflux disease, and an absence of other esophageal motility disorders. The procedure was conducted under general anesthesia with a surgeon operating the device and an endoscopist operating the gastroscope. H-fasteners were placed from the esophagus to the gastric cardia with the goal of creating an approximately 270–300° fundoplication approximately 3–4 cm in length. Symptom severity was measured with the GERD-HRQL instrument (best possible score 0, worst possible score 50). The patients were followed-up for complications and symptom improvement.

Results.—In all, 26 patients underwent an attempted endoscopic fundo-plication. Two patients could not be completed because of the inability to pass the device. Of the 24 patients who underwent endoscopic fundoplica-tion, 20 had the typical symptoms of gastroesophageal reflux disease, 4 had symptoms of laryngopharyngeal reflux, and 4 had recurrent symp-toms after a Nissen fundoplication. There was 1 major complication of a gastric mucosal tear that led to bleeding and the need for a blood trans-fusion. Nineteen (79%) patients reported satisfaction with their symptom relief. Of those dissatisfied, 2 had symptoms of laryngopharyngeal reflux, 1 had functional heartburn, 1 had associated gastroparesis, and 1 had clear failure with gastroesophageal reflux disease. The median GERD-HRQL score improved from 25 (interquartile range, 19.5–28.5) to 5 (interquar-tile range, 3–9; $P = .0004$).

Conclusion.—Endoscopic fundoplication with the Esophyx device is feasible with satisfactory initial results. Endoscopic fundoplication seems to be best suited for patients with small hiatal hernias and mild-to-moderate typical symptoms; however, subsequent trials are needed to assess the long-term effectiveness of the technique (Fig 4).

▶ Endoscopic approaches to the treatment of gastroesophageal reflux disease have been a topic of considerable interest for 2 decades or more. However, the success rate of fundoplication with these devices has been disappointing, and the number of patients harmed has not been insignificant. In our institution,

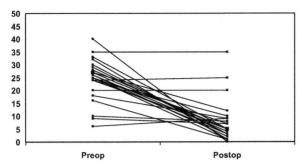

FIGURE 4.—Individual changes in preoperative and postoperative total GERD-HRQL scores. (Reprinted from Velanovich V. Endoscopic, endoluminal fundoplication for gastroesophageal reflux disease: initial experience and lessons learned. *Surgery*. 2010;148:646-653. Copyright 2010, with permission from Mosby, Inc.)

we have had 2 patients referred for major esophageal perforations using the described device. Therefore, safety is a major consideration. In addition, effectiveness of the fundoplication should be measured by relief of clinical symptoms and proof that esophageal acid exposure is decreased. Velanovich demonstrates that the procedure can be safely performed. However, effectiveness is not convincingly shown since the follow-up is short and 6 patients or 23% of the group (Fig 4) had little symptomatic relief. Furthermore, the absence of 24-hour esophageal pH monitoring following treatment is worrisome since this objective measure would significantly augment clinical findings and may explain failure of symptomatic relief in some patients. This single-investigator study is a reasonable start to examining the utility of this endoscopic device, but further studies examining the effectiveness are warranted and randomized controlled trials comparing the outcomes with this device to laparoscopic fundoplication and/or best medical therapy are needed.

K. E. Behrns, MD

Laparoscopic Surgery for Gastric Cancer: A Collective Review with Meta-Analysis of Randomized Trials

Kodera Y, Fujiwara M, Ohashi N, et al (Nagoya Univ Graduate School of Medicine, Aichi, Japan; et al)
J Am Coll Surg 211:677-686, 2010

Background.—Laparoscopy has been successfully used to treat cholelithiasis and stage abdominal tumors but is only gradually being introduced to treat gastric cancers. Within the last 10 years laparoscopic resection for colon cancer has produced oncologic outcomes comparable to those with open resection and involve less pain and a shorter hospital stay. However, the laparoscopic approach to gastric cancer surgery is seldom used in Western medicine because resectable disease is rarely encountered. In Eastern countries such as Japan and Korea, early-stage disease is commonly handled surgically, but laparoscopy-assisted gastrectomy is indicated only for stage IA and IB cancers. The current status of laparoscopic surgery for gastric cancer was summarized, noting controversies among Asian surgeons that could alter the standard of care.

Nodal Dissection.—Both the East and West support extended lymph node dissection. D2 dissection that involves en bloc or anatomical dissection of retroperitoneal lymph nodes has been the standard of care in Japan since the 1960s and still achieves superior stage-by-stage survival rates compared to not using D2 dissection. A high proportion of patients who have confirmed retroperitoneal node metastases, which can only be addressed by D2 dissection, are alive 5 years postoperatively. Patients with confirmed N2-stage disease survive only when D2 dissection is performed. D2 lowers the risk for cancer-related death long term. The Japanese Gastric Cancer Guidelines defines D2 as a standard procedure for T2-stage cancer or higher but also permits its use for T1-stage cancer with extensive invasion of the submucosa, when about 20% of patients harbor nodal metastasis. Cancer relapse is rare but possible with suboptimal dissection.

Surgical Training.—In the beginning, laparoscopic surgeons were generally already experts in performing open surgery. They then faced the challenge of using long straight devices with a limited range of motion while dealing with insufficient psychomotor skills and a two-dimensional field of view. Assisted by innovations in surgical instruments such as staplers and vessel sealing systems, the surgeons' determination finally produced surgical quality comparable to that of contemporary open surgery. Lymph node retrieval via laparoscopic approach has consistently equaled that of open surgery. However, the learning curve needed to perform laparoscopic surgery well is considerable.

Outcomes.—Short-term outcomes after laparoscopic gastrectomy demonstrate less blood loss, longer operating time, and no marked increase in morbidity or mortality compared to open surgical outcomes. Fewer surgical complications attend laparoscopic versus open approaches. Looking at long-term data, laparoscopic gastrectomy has achieved excellent results, especially using the modified D2 dissection in patients with mucosal or smaller submucosal cancer. The 5-year disease-free survival rates are 99.8% for stage IA, 98.7% for stage IB, and 85.7% for stage II. These excellent results prompted experienced investigators in Japan and Korea to extend the indications to more advanced cancers. The result was longer operating time, less blood loss, and faster recovery, with lymph node retrieval and short-term survival equal to those with open surgery. Peculiar port-site recurrences have complicated the use of the laparoscopic approach, however.

Controversies.—Port-site recurrence is a troubling complication even though most oncologic outcomes after laparoscopic surgery are comparable to or better than those after open surgery. Patients report less pain, which means better preservation of lung function and physical well-being with the laparoscopic approach. This permits an earlier and/or more intensive use of adjuvant therapies because the patient is stronger.

Research into expanding the indications for laparoscopic gastrectomy is principally conducted in Eastern nations, where earlier-stage cancers are more common. Studies are hampered by comorbidity of patients, lack of experience for the surgeon, small available patient samples, philosophical differences in treatment objectives, and the current wide use of laparoscopy for gastric cancer in Japan that has not waited for evidence-based confirmation. Total gastrectomy is still challenging under laparoscopic guidance with no standardized technique. In Korea gastric cancer surgery is only available in high-volume hospitals by a few highly trained surgeons. Having evidentiary support for the technique would be readily accepted there.

Conclusions.—Eastern nations are currently at the forefront in investigating the use of the laparoscopic approach to treat early-stage gastric cancer. Because this entity is rarely seen in Western nations, the results may not be widely applicable in Western settings. Support for extending the laparoscopic approach to more advanced cancer does not currently exist but a randomized trial is under way. New techniques are more readily applied when the incidence of gastric cancer is lower and more procedures are done by a few experts located in high-volume hospitals. A program of training is needed to prepare new graduates who have little experience in the open surgical technique.

▶ The collective review by Kodera et al is focused on the laparoscopic treatment of gastric cancer, a relatively rare malignancy in the United States. This article has several pertinent lessons that address not only gastric cancer but also surgical training and the conduct of trials. First, this work demonstrates that laparoscopic resection for gastric cancer is safe, effective, and compares favorably with open gastric resection for early gastric cancer. The collective review shows that lymph node harvest, blood loss, morbidity, and mortality for laparoscopic surgery are comparable with open gastric surgery. The laparoscopic approach, however, is more time consuming. The operative approach for advanced gastric cancers, however, is not settled because of the risk of port-site recurrence. Several studies in Japan and Korea are ongoing. Importantly, in the conduct of these trials, it is evident that the training of surgeons from Asia must change if high-quality operative care is to be delivered to all patients with gastric cancer. This emphasis on training is refreshing because the Japanese and Korean surgeons have strict guidelines for the care of patients with gastric cancer, and these guidelines must be met to perform gastric resections for gastric cancer. This has led to uniformity in care and standardization of process, operational issues with which most medical centers in the United States are grappling. Finally, many of the clinical trials that are ongoing in the east arise from surgical societies, an approach that infrequently occurs in the United States. The origination of clinical trials from surgical societies is an attractive concept that should be examined in the United States.

K. E. Behrns, MD

Proximal Esophageal pH Monitoring: Improved Definition of Normal Values and Determination of a Composite pH Score

Ayazi S, Hagen JA, Zehetner J, et al (Univ of Southern California, Los Angeles, CA)
J Am Coll Surg 210:345-350, 2010

Background.—Patients with respiratory and laryngeal symptoms are commonly referred for evaluation of reflux disease as a potential cause. Dual-probe pH monitoring is often performed, although data on normal acid exposure in the proximal esophagus are limited because of the small number of normal subjects and inconsistent placement of the proximal pH sensor in relation to the upper esophageal sphincter. We measured proximal esophageal acid exposure using dual-probe pH and calculated a composite pH score in a large number of asymptomatic volunteers to better define normal values.

Study Design.—Eighty-one normal subjects free of reflux, laryngeal, or respiratory symptoms were recruited. All had video esophagraphy to exclude hiatal hernia. Esophageal pH monitoring was performed using 1 of 3 different dual-probe catheters with sensors spaced 10, 15, or 18 cm apart. The standard components of esophageal acid exposure were measured, excluding meal periods. A composite pH score for the proximal esophagus was calculated using these components.

Results.—The final study population consisted of 59 (49% male) subjects, with a median age of 27 years. All had normal distal esophageal acid exposure and no hiatal hernia. The 95th percentile values for the percent time the pH was < 4 for the total, upright, and supine periods were 0.9%, 1.2%, and 0.4%, respectively. The 95th percentile for the number of reflux episodes was 24 and for the calculated proximal esophageal composite pH score was 16.4.

Conclusions.—In a large population of normal subjects, we have defined the normal values and calculated a composite pH score for proximal esophageal acid exposure. The total percent time pH < 4 was similar to previously published normal values, but the number of reflux episodes was greater.

▶ Gastroesophageal reflux as a cause of pulmonary or upper respiratory symptoms is a difficult diagnosis that too frequently is based on nonspecific symptoms or unreliable tests. Antireflux procedures performed for these symptoms often result in either a homerun in that the patient is markedly improved or a strikeout with the patient undergoing a significant operation for little or no improvement. Ayazi et al in their report advance our understanding of basic esophageal function by using appropriately sized pH catheters to measure reflux episodes as close as possible to the upper esophageal sphincter (UES). Their data show that with exclusion of meal-induced reflux episodes, the number of reflux episodes and the acid exposure at the UES can be carefully quantified to produce a reliable composite reflux score. Presumably, this will aid in the diagnosis of patients with true gastric content reflux to the respiratory tract.

However, a few caveats should be noted. First, the study population was nearly ideal, but as noted by the authors, the age was younger than the typical patient population. In addition, the body mass index was ideal, not a typical finding in the patient population with upper esophageal reflux. In addition the size of the catheter was determined by the findings on manometry. Therefore, all patients must undergo manometry as a prerequisite to a pH study. Some may argue that this is required in this patient population, but it would be nice to know that acid reflux is the cause of respiratory symptoms prior to mandating manometry. Finally, although these data are encouraging, this study did not test symptomatic patients, and the follow-up study will set the standard. The real question will be answered by the study that correlates patient's symptoms, pH score, and outcome over time.

K. E. Behrns, MD

Necessity for improvement in endoscopy training during surgical residency

Subhas G, Gupta A, Mittal VK (Providence Hosp and Med Ctrs, Southfield, MI)
Am J Surg 199:331-335, 2010

Background.—The Residency Review Committee for Surgery has recently increased the required number of cases needed to achieve competency in endoscopy training.

Methods.—A 10-question survey was sent to program directors for general surgery residencies. Endoscopic training patterns, facilities, perspectives, and residents' performance were examined.

Results.—Seventy-one surgery programs (30%) responded to the survey. Of these, 42% (n = 30) had a program size of 3 to 4 residents. Ten percent (n = 7) of all programs could not fulfill the minimum Accreditation Council for Graduate Medical Education (ACGME) requirements. Only 55% (n = 39) of programs had a dedicated rotation in endoscopy and an endoscopic skills training laboratory in their program. Few programs had their residents performing more than 100 cases of gastroscopy (18%) and colonoscopy (21%).

Conclusions.—Future endoscopy training for surgical residents needs to be improved to comply with the new requirements. This would include provision of an endoscopic skills laboratory, dedicated endoscopic rotations, and increasing the number of staff surgeons who perform endoscopic procedures.

▶ The field of gastrointestinal surgery has continued to evolve since the introduction of laparoscopy, and recent emphasis has been placed on general surgery trainees receiving adequate endoscopic training. As defined by the Residency Review Committee for Surgery, adequate training would include 50 colonoscopies and 35 esophagogastroduodenoscopies. The obvious question is "Does achievement of these numeric milestones represent adequate training?" The obvious answer is no since competency is not defined by numbers alone but by achievements in knowledge, patient evaluation, technical skills, and postprocedure management. This is true not only for endoscopy but also for all areas of surgical expertise; however, endoscopy training, I suspect, falls short in delivering competency, and the article by Subhas et al highlights the shortcomings. First, we are not training complete endoscopists because most of our trainees are comfortable with diagnostic but not therapeutic endoscopy. In addition, we delegate a significant amount of endoscopic training to our medical colleagues who are superb teachers but have a different perspective and commitment to our trainees. As noted in this article, only 55% of programs had adequate structural organization and laboratory facilities to provide a satisfactory experience for our residents. Furthermore, the number of competent surgeons who can serve as instructors of endoscopy is limited. As gastrointestinal surgeons strive to improve patient care, advancement of endoscopic teaching and surgical endoscopy must move to the forefront of our training programs. No longer can a rotation in endoscopy suffice as our teaching unit. We should look for opportunities to integrate endoscopy in our practices, and, yes, that means that some of us will need to retrain.

K. E. Behrns, MD

Genetic Variations in Angiogenesis Pathway Genes Predict Tumor Recurrence in Localized Adenocarcinoma of the Esophagus
Lurje G, Leers JM, Pohl A, et al (Univ of Southern California/Norris Comprehensive Cancer Ctr, Los Angeles)
Ann Surg 251:857-864, 2010

Objective.—The aim of this study was to determine whether the risk of systemic disease after esophagectomy could be predicted by angiogenesis-related gene polymorphisms.

Summary Background Data.—Systemic tumor recurrence after curative resection continues to impose a significant problem in the management of patients with localized esophageal adenocarcinoma (EA). The identification of molecular markers of prognosis will help to better define tumor stage, indicate disease progression, identify novel therapeutic targets, and monitor response to therapy. Proteinase-activated-receptor 1 (PAR-1) and epidermal growth factor (EGF) have been shown to mediate the regulation of local and early-onset angiogenesis, and in turn may impact the process of tumor growth and disease progression.

Methods.—We investigated tissue samples from 239 patients with localized EA treated with surgery alone. DNA was isolated from formalin-fixed paraffin-embedded normal esophageal tissue samples and polymorphisms were analyzed using polymerase chain reaction-restriction fragment length polymorphism and 5'-end [γ-^{33}P] ATP-labeled polymerase chain reaction methods.

Results.—PAR-1 −506 ins/del (adjusted P value = 0.011) and EGF +61 A>G (adjusted P value = 0.035) showed to be adverse prognostic markers, in both univariate and multivariable analyses. In combined analysis, grouping alleles into favorable versus nonfavorable alleles, high expression variants of *PAR-1* −506 ins/del (any insertion allele) and *EGF* +61 A>G (A/A) were associated with a higher likelihood of developing tumor recurrence (adjusted *P* value < 0.001).

Conclusion.—This study supports the role of functional *PAR-1* and *EGF* polymorphisms as independent prognostic markers in localized EA and may therefore help to identify patient subgroups at high risk for tumor recurrence.

▶ Sequencing of the human genome represented a tremendous scientific accomplishment that ultimately should lead to improved understanding of the pathobiology of many diseases. In this article, Lurje et al perform a thoughtful genetic assessment of polymorphisms of genes that are involved in the angiogenic processes in human esophageal adenocarcinoma. They examined 7 genes for variants that may be associated with tumor recurrence or overall survival from adenocarcinoma. To study these genes the authors used a highly select group of patients with esophageal adenocarcinoma: patients with localized disease who underwent surgery only without neoadjuvant or adjuvant therapy. Furthermore, they examined a single biologic process, angiogenesis, that is known to be involved in tumor development and recurrence. Angiogenesis is regulated by multiple genes, of which 7 were selected for genetic variations. Each of these genes may have multiple polymorphisms that may be associated with altered protein expression, the ultimate regulatory molecule from altered gene expression. In addition, expression of each of the genes studied may be influenced by a vast array of signal transduction pathways. The network of interacting genes and proteins is obviously voluminous and complicated. This well-designed study is a good example of our current understanding of the involvement of genetic alterations in malignant disease, but as one can see, the process is complicated and highly select patient populations currently serve as the models of investigation. Are the combinations of pathobiologic processes, gene expression, and protein expression networks so complex that the promise of personalized medicine is empty? Likely not, but it will take time, energy, and resources to fulfill the vision of personalized medicine.

K. E. Behrns, MD

Self-expanding metal stents as an alternative to surgical bypass for malignant gastric outlet obstruction
Shaw JM, Bornman PC, Krige JEJ, et al (Univ of Cape Town Health Sciences Faculty, South Africa)
Br J Surg 97:872-876, 2010

Background.—Gastroduodenal obstruction due to malignancy can be difficult to palliate. Self-expanding metal stents (SEMS) are gaining acceptance as an effective alternative to surgical bypass.

Methods.—Patients not suitable for surgical bypass, with complete gastric outlet obstruction as a result of malignancy, were offered palliation with SEMS from November 2004 to December 2008. The procedure was performed under fluoroscopic guidance and conscious sedation. Data were collected prospectively.

Results.—Seventy patients underwent SEMS placement (hepatobiliary and pancreatic malignancy, 44; antral gastric carcinoma, 19; other, seven). Follow-up was complete in 69 patients (99 per cent). Technical and clinical success rates were 93 and 95 per cent respectively. Median hospital stay was 2 (range 1—18) days, median survival was $1 \cdot 8$ $(0 \cdot 1 - 19 \cdot 0)$ months, and 87 per cent had improved intake after SEMS placement, as determined by Gastric Outlet Obstruction Severity Score before and after stenting $(P < 0 \cdot 001)$. Complications included two episodes of minor bleeding.

Conclusion.—The use of SEMS to alleviate complete malignant gastric outlet obstruction in patients with limited life expectancy is successful in re-establishing enteral intake in most patients, with minimal morbidity, no mortality and a short hospital stay.

▶ Obstruction of the stomach from regionally advanced carcinoma is a difficult decision-making process because many patients with this condition are in poor clinical condition and have a severely limited lifespan. To further complicate the decision-making process, many of these patients have biliary obstruction that must also be addressed, but, as this article shows, jaundice most often requires palliation before gastric outlet obstruction. In addition, a prospective randomized trial has demonstrated that 17% of patients who have a surgical biliary bypass without enteric bypass will subsequently have a need for intervention of the obstructed stomach. In these patients, either open or laparoscopic palliation late in the course of disease leads to prolonged hospitalization and often no meaningful recovery from surgery. Surgical gastroenterostomy is too often complicated by delayed gastric emptying and a lengthy hospital stay in patients with precious little time to spare. Shaw et al present excellent results on the use of endoscopically placed self-expanding metal stents for gastric outlet obstruction. Nearly 90% of the patients had improved intake following the procedure. This work brings clarity to the management of patients with gastric outlet obstruction due to advanced malignancy. First, the success of this procedure should be the death knell for double bypass surgery. This is a significant operation in very ill patients and should be abandoned. This commentator has not performed this procedure for years. Second, though it is laudable that the authors proved beyond doubt that these patients had significant obstruction, why wait until they are nearly completely obstructed when the diagnosis is evident previously? We should offer the earliest and best palliation available for the comfort of these patients.

K. E. Behrns, MD

Endoscopic Treatment of Zenker Diverticulum: Results of a 7-Year Experience

Al-Kadi AS, Maghrabi AA, Thomson D, et al (Peter-Lougheed Ctr, Calgary, Alberta, Canada; Univ of Manitoba, Winnipeg, Canada; Brandon Regional Health Centre, Manitoba, Canada)
J Am Coll Surg 211:239-243, 2010

Background.—Zenker diverticulum (ZD) is a rare disease usually seen in elderly patients who present with symptoms of worsening dysphagia and regurgitation. Although open surgical approach is still the standard management for symptomatic patients, the endoscopic technique has evolved as an alternative approach, especially for highly morbid patients. We are reporting our experience for treating ZD using endoscopic needle-knife papillotome.

Study Design.—A total of 18 patients with a mean age of 80 years (range 68 to 91 years) were included in our prospective cohort study. All patients underwent endoscopic cricopharyngeal myotomy for symptomatic ZD using needle-knife papillotome at Brandon Regional Health Centre during a 7-year period. Mean follow-up was 27.5 months. A dysphagia score system from 0 (no dysphagia) to 4 (severe dysphagia) was used. All patients' baseline characteristics, pre- and postoperative symptoms, operative time, time to oral intake, length of hospital stay, recurrence of symptoms, and complications were analyzed.

Results.—Dysphagia score and regurgitation symptoms improved substantially after treatment. Mean operative time was 28.4 minutes. Oral intake was resumed within 24 hours in all but 1 patient. Hospital stay for the majority was 24 to 48 hours. Only 1 patient had a micro-perforation treated conservatively and 2 patients had re-do procedures for persistence of dysphagia.

Conclusions.—Endoscopic cricopharyngeal myotomy using needle-knife papillotome is an effective approach to manage ZD for highly morbid patients. It is minimally invasive, decreases anesthetic time, shortens hospital stay, and has a low complication rate.

▶ Zenker diverticulum is an uncommon affliction that is most frequently seen in the elderly. The presentation of these patients results in 2 immediate issues. First, as the authors point out, the aged population with this diverticulum often has significant comorbidities and are not suitable candidates for a major operation. The second concern is related to the rarity of the condition; many surgeons have little experience with the treatment of this disease. Thus, the management should be straightforward and carry little risk. Al-Kadi et al present a simple, relatively low-risk endoscopic procedure that can be completed in one or more stages. Importantly, the procedure duration was under 30 minutes and the complication rate was low. Therefore, this treatment may be a suitable replacement for open surgery or more complicated endoscopic surgery requiring stapling devices. However, we still must address the dilemma of few surgeons having experience treating the disease, and in fact, most surgeons have little upper endoscopic experience. In recent years, the number of cases of upper and lower endoscopy for general surgery trainees has increased and most residency programs have adapted. Yet surgeon experience with therapeutic endoscopy is limited. As we continue to look for minimally invasive approaches to gastrointestinal diseases and identify opportunities as described in this article, we must take the extra step in identifying how surgeons of the future will be trained to competently conduct endoscopic procedures. Minimally invasive operations including endoscopic procedures continue to evolve at a rapid pace, and we must adapt our training to meet these needs.

K. E. Behrns, MD

Impact of symptom–reflux association analysis on long-term outcome after Nissen fundoplication
Broeders JA, Draaisma WA, Bredenoord AJ, et al (Gastrointestinal Res Unit of the Univ Med Ctr Utrecht, The Netherlands; et al)
Br J Surg 98:247-254, 2011

Background.—A positive symptom association probability (SAP) is regarded as an important selection criterion for antireflux surgery by many physicians. However, no data corroborate the relationship between symptom–reflux association and outcome, nor is it clear what impact a negative SAP has on the outcome of antireflux surgery in patients with abnormal oesophageal acid exposure. This study compared long-term outcomes of Nissen fundoplication in patients with a negative *versus* positive SAP.

Methods.—Five-year outcome of Nissen fundoplication in patients with proton-pump inhibitor (PPI)-refractory reflux and pathological acid exposure was compared between those with (SAP+, 109) and without (SAP−, 29 patients) a positive symptom association. Symptoms, quality of life (QoL), PPI use, endoscopic findings, manometry and acid exposure were evaluated.

Results.—At 5 years' follow-up, relief of reflux symptoms (95 *versus* 87 per cent), reduction in PPI use (80 to 25 per cent *versus* 85 to 14 per cent; $P < 0.050$) and improvement in QoL were similar in the SAP− and SAP+ groups. Reduction in acid exposure time (13·4 to 1·6 per cent *versus* 11·1 to 0·2 per cent of total time; $P < 0.010$), improvement in oesophagitis (44 to 6 per cent *versus* 61 to 13 per cent; $P < 0.050$) and increase in lower oesophageal sphincter pressure were also comparable.

Conclusion.—The subjective and objective outcomes of fundoplication in patients with pathological acid exposure are comparable among those with a positive and negative SAP. Patients with pathological acid exposure and a negative SAP can also benefit from antireflux surgery (Fig 1).

▶ Laparoscopic Nissen fundoplication is an operation designed to improve the functional performance of the gastroesophageal junction. However, like all

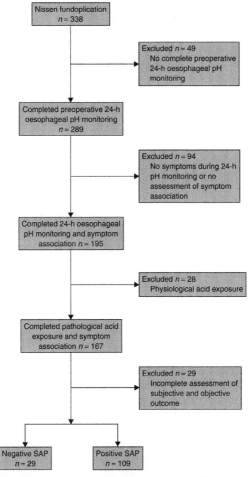

FIGURE 1.—Study profile. (Reprinted from Broeders JA, Draaisma WA, Bredenoord AJ, et al. Impact of symptom—reflux association analysis on long-term outcome after Nissen fundoplication. *Br J Surg.* 2011;98:247-254. Copyright ©, British Journal of Surgery Society Ltd. Reproduced with permission. Permission is granted by John Wiley & Sons Ltd on behalf of the BJSS Ltd).

functional gastrointestinal surgeries, the outcomes of this nonextirpative operation can be variable and, thus, proper selection of patients is of paramount importance. Broeders et al performed an excellent study to examine the association of symptoms with pathological reflux documented by 24-hour pH probe assessment. This nicely designed trial compared the short- and long-term outcome of patients with documented pathological reflux demonstrated via pH probe results and the association of symptoms by a validated symptom-associated probability. The results demonstrated that the outcomes were similar in patients who had pathologic reflux whether symptom association was present or absent. These findings are important since many patients with pathologic reflux, but without associated symptoms, are denied surgical treatment for fear of long-term failure of a functional operation. These results show that the failure rate is similar, albeit high, in patients with pathologic reflux. Importantly, this study originated in a surgical unit focused on the outcome study of patients with reflux, yet as Fig 1 demonstrates and the authors acknowledge, the number of patients who underwent complete evaluation was limited. Clearly this study shows the value of rigid adherence to a complete evaluation in patients with reflux disease, and this type of preoperative evaluation should be the standard for all patients potentially undergoing reflux surgery.

K. E. Behrns, MD

A Multicenter Study of Survival After Neoadjuvant Radiotherapy/ Chemotherapy and Esophagectomy for ypT0N0M0R0 Esophageal Cancer

Vallböhmer D, Hölscher AH, DeMeester S, et al (Univ of Cologne, Germany; Univ of Southern California, Los Angeles, CA; et al)
Ann Surg 252:744-749, 2010

Objective.—To evaluate 5-year survival of patients with locally advanced esophageal cancer (LAEC) who have undergone multimodality treatment with complete histopathologic response.

Background.—Patients with LAEC may obtain excellent local-regional response to multimodality therapy. The overall benefit of a complete histopathologic response, when no viable tumor is present in the surgical specimen, is incompletely understood and existing data are limited to single-center studies with relatively few patients. The aim of this multi-center study was to define the outcome of patients with complete histopathologic response after multimodality therapy for LAEC.

Methods.—The study population included 299 patients (229 male, 70 female; median age: 60 years) with LAEC (cT2N1M0, T3-4N0-1M0; 181 adenocarcinomas, 118 squamous carcinomas) who underwent either neoadjuvant radiochemotherapy (n = 284) or chemotherapy (n = 15) followed by esophagectomy at 6 specialized centers: Europe (3) and United States (3). All patients in the study had stage ypT0N0M0R0 after resection.

Results.—Esophagectomy with thoracotomy (n = 255) was more frequent than with a transhiatal approach (n = 44). The median number of analyzed lymph nodes in the surgical specimens was 20 (minimum-maximum: 1−77). Thirty-day mortality rate was 2.4% and 90-day mortality rate was 5.7%. Overall 5-year survival rate was 55%. The disease-specific 5-year survival rate was 68%, with a recurrence rate of 23.4% (n = 70; local vs distant recurrence: 3.3% vs 20.1%). Cox regression analysis identified age as the only independent predictor of survival, whereas gender, histology, type of esophagectomy, type of neoadjuvant therapy, and the number of resected lymph nodes had no prognostic impact.

Conclusion.—Patients with histopathologic complete response at the time of resection of LAEC achieve excellent survival.

▶ The use of neoadjuvant therapy for esophageal cancer has been under scrutiny for a decade or more. The effect of radiochemotherapy on esophageal cancer survival has been debated, and this article addresses a small subset of patients undergoing neoadjuvant therapy. Vallböhmer et al gathered data from 6 international centers to test the hypothesis that neoadjuvant therapy that resulted in a complete pathologic response was associated with improved survival. The data are convincing in that the disease-specific 5-year survival was 68%, while the overall survival was 55%. Notable, however, was the 23% recurrence rate indicating that complete pathologic response is not synonymous with freedom from disease. Although these data were collected from highly specialized centers over a long period, the results are important from a proof of concept standpoint; that is, patients with esophageal cancer can potentially be cured by the use of neoadjuvant therapy. Although the authors adamantly defend the necessity of surgery following neoadjuvant therapy, colorectal surgeons previously espoused a similar response regarding neoadjuvant therapy for rectal cancer. However, subsequent studies have suggested that surgery may not be necessary following complete clinical response from radiochemotherapy for rectal cancer. Generally speaking, the surgical community purports the need for resection following neoadjuvant therapy, and this may be the correct response, but perhaps surgery could be viewed as a salvage therapy in patients with local recurrence and surgery may truly be unnecessary in some patients and futile in patients with systemic disease. Answers to these complex questions will require well-constructed, multi-institutional, randomized trials, which will require substantial effort and funding. However, these questions are perfect for comparative effectiveness research.

K. E. Behrns, MD

A Multicenter, Randomized Efficacy Study of the EndoBarrier Gastrointestinal Liner for Presurgical Weight Loss Prior to Bariatric Surgery

Schouten R, Rijs CS, Bouvy ND, et al (Atrium Med Centre Parkstad, Heerlen, The Netherlands; Rijnstate Hosp, Arnhem, The Netherlands; Maastricht Univ Med Centre, The Netherlands)
Ann Surg 251:236-243, 2010

Background.—The endoscopically placed duodenal-jejunal bypass sleeve or EndoBarrier Gastrointestinal Liner has been designed to achieve weight loss in morbidly obese patients. We report on the first European experience with this device.

Methods.—A multicenter, randomized clinical trial was performed. Forty-one patients were included and 30 underwent sleeve implantation. Eleven patients served as a diet control group. All patients followed the same low-calorie diet during the study period. The purpose of the study was to determine the safety and efficacy of the device.

Results.—Twenty-six devices were successfully implanted. In 4 patients, implantation could not be achieved. Four devices were explanted prior to the initial protocol end point because of migration (1), dislocation of the anchor (1), sleeve obstruction (1), and continuous epigastric pain (1). The remaining patients all completed the study. Mean procedure time was 35 minutes (range: 12−102 minutes) for a successful implantation and 17 minutes (range: 5−99 minutes) for explantation. There were no procedure related adverse events. During the study period the 26 duodenal-jejunal bypass sleeve patients (100%) had at least one adverse event, mainly abdominal pain and nausea during the first week after implantation. Initial mean body mass index (BMI, kg/m^2) was 48.9 and 47.4 kg/m^2 for the device and control patients, respectively. Mean excess weight loss after 3 months was 19.0% for device patients versus 6.9% for control patients ($P < 0.002$). Absolute change in BMI at 3 months was 5.5 and 1.9 kg/m^2, respectively. Type 2 diabetes mellitus was present at baseline in 8 patients of the device group and improved in 7 patients during the study period (lower glucose levels, HbA1c, and medication requirements).

Conclusion.—The EndoBarrier Gastrointestinal Liner is a feasible and safe noninvasive device with excellent short-term weight loss results. The device also has a significant positive effect on type 2 diabetes mellitus. Long-term randomized and sham studies for weight loss and treatment of diabetes are necessary to determine the role of the device in the treatment of morbid obesity.

This study was registered at www.clinicaltrials.gov (registration number: NCT00830440).

▶ The optimal treatment for morbid obesity has been elusive for several decades because behavioral therapy and pharmacologic therapy have essentially failed to produce lasting results, and invasive therapies are all associated with complications, albeit the rate of these complications has improved over time and the weight loss after invasive therapies is markedly better than noninvasive therapies. In an attempt to make operative approaches to the treatment of obesity safer, presurgical weight loss has been proposed. The study by Shouten et al provides an example of a barrier device that when implanted prior to definitive operative therapy would, in theory, decrease operative complications. Though the authors tout this device as noninvasive and deem it a success, careful inspection of the data reveal that only 10% of the patients completed the 24-week study and 100% of the patients in the device arm of the trial had adverse events. Weight loss was modest. Furthermore, even though the barrier device would purportedly be used prior to definitive operative therapy for obesity, the trial did not study this hypothesis. The control group was a diet-only group without surgical intervention; thus, the hypothesis that the barrier device would lead to presurgical weight loss and decrease the risk of definitive operative therapy was not tested. Given these results, it is difficult to know where this device fits in the treatment algorithm of morbid obesity, and, perhaps, given these results it should not be used. The zeal for less invasive treatments for obesity should not result in procedures that are universally associated with adverse events for minimal results.

K. E. Behrns, MD

Overall Mortality, Incremental Life Expectancy, and Cause of Death at 25 Years in the Program on the Surgical Control of the Hyperlipidemias

Buchwald H, Rudser KD, Williams SE, et al (Univ of Minnesota, Minneapolis)
Ann Surg 251:1034-1040, 2010

Objective.—To present the longest follow-up report of any lipid-atherosclerosis intervention trial.

Summary of Background Data.—The Program on the Surgical Control of the Hyperlipidemias (POSCH), a secondary, clinical/arteriographic, randomized controlled trial, was the first lipid-atherosclerosis trial to demonstrate unequivocally that low density lipoprotein cholesterol reduction reduced the incidence of coronary heart disease death and myocardial infarction.

Methods.—We report POSCH 25 years follow-up for overall mortality, specific cause of death, and certain subgroup analyses, as well as a prediction for increase in life expectancy derived from the POSCH database, supplemented by the 2006 National Death Index, 1989—2006.

Results.—There were 838 patients randomized in POSCH (421 surgery, 417 control). At 25 years follow-up, the difference in the restricted mean survival and the logrank (Mantel-Haenszel) statistic was statistically significant, with survival probabilities of 0.57 (surgery) and 0.51 (controls). Cause of death data indicated a significant increase in cardiovascular deaths in the control group; cancer deaths were also greater in the control group but this was not significant. The most compelling subgroup analysis was a significant increase in survival, starting at 5 years after randomization, in the surgery group for patients with an ejection fraction ≥50%, with relative probabilities of 0.61 (surgery) and 0.51 (control). The estimated incremental increase in life expectancy over more than 25 years of follow-up was 1.0 year overall and 1.7 years in the cohort with an ejection fraction ≥50%.

Conclusions.—A 25-year mortality follow-up in POSCH shows statistically significant gains in overall survival, cardiovascular disease-free survival, and life expectancy in the surgery group compared with the control group.

▶ Frequently, gastrointestinal surgery results in surgical anatomy that may cause metabolic disturbances. However, surgery is rarely viewed as a viable therapeutic approach to metabolic diseases. The Program on the Surgical Control of the Hyperlipidemias (POSCH), however, is an outstanding example—and one of the few examples—of a well-conceived surgical approach to a metabolic disease such as hyperlipidemia. Although results from POSCH have been published previously, this article clearly highlights the benefits of long-term (25 years) follow-up. Dr Buchwald and colleagues have conducted a model clinical trial that continues to show benefits long after patient enrollment and initial data analysis. This study is remarkable for several features, but 2 findings deserve special attention. First, the momentum and perseverance required to follow patients enrolled in a clinical trial for 25 years is enormous and is a testament to the study team and principal investigator. Almost never do we see such a commitment. Second, as mentioned previously, surgical investigators too infrequently consider a surgical approach to metabolic diseases. This study is an excellent example of work that is based on the sound principles of gastrointestinal physiology that led to a well-designed clinical trial. The era of comparative effectiveness trials is emerging, and we should not assume that drug discovery is the lone approach to the treatment of metabolic diseases. We should consider surgical approaches to metabolic diseases and begin basic science in vivo investigations that will lead to clinical trials of comparative effectiveness. Comparative effectiveness trials should become a large component of surgical research.

K. E. Behrns, MD

Medical and Surgical Treatments for Obesity Have Opposite Effects on Peptide YY and Appetite: A Prospective Study Controlled for Weight Loss
Valderas JP, Irribarra V, Boza C, et al (Pontificia Universidad Católica de Chile, Santiago, Chile)
J Clin Endocrinol Metab 95:1069-1075, 2010

Context.—The effects of medical and surgical treatments for obesity on peptide YY (PYY) levels, in patients with similar weight loss, remain unclear.

Objective.—The objective of the study was to assess PYY and appetite before and after Roux-en-Y gastric bypass (RYGB), sleeve gastrectomy (SG), and medical treatment (MED).

Design.—This was a prospective, controlled, nonrandomized study.

Setting.—The study was conducted at the Departments of Nutrition and Digestive Surgery at a university hospital.

Participants.—Participants included three groups of eight patients with similar body mass indexes (RYGB 37.8 ± 0.8, SG 35.3 ± 0.7, and MED 39.1 ± 1.7 kg/m², $P = $ NS) and eight lean controls (body mass index 21.7 ± 0.7 kg/m²).

Main Outcome Measures.—Total plasma PYY, hunger, and satiety visual analog scales in fasting and after ingestion of a standard test meal were measured.

Results.—At baseline there were no differences in the area under the curve (AUC) of PYY, hunger, or satiety in obese groups. Two months after the interventions, RYGB, SG, and MED groups achieved similar weight loss (17.7 ± 3, 14.9 ± 2.4, 16.6 ± 4%, respectively, $P = $ NS).

PYY AUC increased in RYGB (*P* < 0.001) and SG (*P* < 0.05) and did not change in MED. PYY levels decreased at fasting, 30 min, and 180 min after a standard test meal in MED (*P* < 0.05). Hunger AUC decreased in RYGB (*P* < 0.05). Satiety AUC increased in RYGB (*P* < 0.05) and SG (*P* < 0.05). Appetite did not change in MED. PYY AUC correlated with satiety AUC (r = 0.35, *P* < 0.05).

Conclusion.—RYGB and SG increased PYY and reduced appetite. MED failed to produce changes. Different effects occur despite similar weight loss. This suggests that the weight-loss effects of these procedures are enhanced by an increase in PYY and satiety.

▶ Valderas et al designed a simple, yet elegant, study of the effects of various weight loss methods on peptide YY concentrations in the serum of obese patients or controls. Four groups of patients were evaluated: lean controls, medically treated obese patients, and obese patients treated with either Roux-en-Y gastric bypass or sleeve gastrectomy. Peptide YY was studied at various time points following a meal, and hunger and appetite were appropriately assessed. Peptide YY is secreted from the intestine by L-secreting cells that are located predominantly in the distal small bowel. This peptide provides feedback to the upper gut to slow gastric emptying and secretion and to decrease food intake. At times, this peptide has been deemed responsible for the ileal brake phenomenon in which distal small bowel enteric contents induce feedback to the proximal bowel to slow down. However, if this were the sole mechanism, then decreased delivery of caloric content or other nutrient constituents by decreased intake from medical treatment or surgical treatment would result in changes in peptide YY. However, this was not the case, and, therefore, alternative mechanisms must be in play. Could changes in ghrelin concentrations after surgical treatment be responsible for altered peptide YY concentrations? This important question will no doubt be addressed soon. This article represents a throwback study in which important gastrointestinal physiology questions were addressed because of the importance in creating a physiologically sound surgical approach. Although funding agencies have not supported this type of work recently, it is obvious that we still do not have a sound physiologic basis for some of our surgical treatments and that many of these questions remain unanswered.

K. E. Behrns, MD

---

15 Years of Litigation Following Laparoscopic Cholecystectomy in England
Alkhaffaf B, Decadt B (Stockport NHS Foundation Trust, Manchester, UK)
Ann Surg 251:682-685, 2010

Objective.—We aimed to analyze trends in litigation following laparoscopic cholecystectomy (LC) in England and compare our findings with data from the United States.

Background.—Several studies from the United States have highlighted the medico-legal repercussions of complications following LC. In

2007–2008, litigation claims cost the National Health Service in England over 660 million Great British Pounds (GBP) (1.1 billion USD). Despite this, there has been little examination of litigation following LC in England.

Methods.—Data from the National Health Service Litigation Authority on clinical negligence claims between 1995 and 2009 following LC were obtained and analyzed.

Results.—Four hundred eighteen claims were made of which 303 were settled. One hundred ninety-eight (65%) were found to be in the claimants favor for a total cost of 20.4 million GBP (33.4 million USD). Litigation claims have leveled since 2001. Operator error was the most likely cause to result in a claim and the only cause associated with a successful claim ($P = 0.023$). A delay in the recognition of complications was the second most common reason for initiation of a claim. Bile duct injury was the most frequent injury resulting in litigation and the most likely injury associated with a successful claim ($P < 0.001$). The average payout for a successful claim was 102,827 GBP/168,337 USD. Findings from US studies were similar, although the magnitude of payouts was 4 times higher.

Conclusion.—Strategies that minimize bile duct injury and speed up recognition of injuries should be adopted to reduce the litigation burden and improve patient care.

▶ Since the introduction of laparoscopic cholecystectomy, bile duct injury has been the most feared complication because of potential loss of life and long-term consequences such as chronic liver injury. Not surprisingly, this complication is often viewed as resulting in litigation, and in the United States several studies have demonstrated the association between bile duct injury and financial compensation. This study by Alkhaffaf and Decadt shows the results of litigation for bile duct injury in the National Health System in England. The causes for legal claims in the United Kingdom are similar to that in the United States, with bile duct injury being the most common cause for litigation and associated with the highest likelihood of success. Overall, 65% of claims were successful and resulted in over $33 million dollar (USD) payout. However, there ends the similarity between legal claims following laparoscopic cholecystectomy in the United States and United Kingdom since the individual award in the United States was about 4 times higher than in the United Kingdom. This study is important for several reasons. First, intraoperative error was the most common cause of injury and, therefore, securing the critical view of safety of the triangle of Calot remains an important operative principle. Second, early recognition of a complication can reduce the chance of lawsuit and award. Finally, the discrepancy in financial remuneration between the United States and United Kingdom has little justification. This surely speaks to the need for liability reform as an integral component of improving our health care system.

K. E. Behrns, MD

Evolution of a Reliable Biliary Reconstructive Technique in 400 Consecutive Living Donor Liver Transplants

Soin AS, Kumaran V, Rastogi AN, et al (Sir Ganga Ram Hosp, New Delhi, India)
J Am Coll Surg 211:24-32, 2010

Background.—Biliary complications (BCs) are a major cause of morbidity and mortality after living donor liver transplantation (LDLT). They occur because the graft hepatic ducts are often small, thin walled, multiple, and may become ischemic during transection.

Study Design.—Of the 460 LDLTs done at our center before November 2009, the first 402 partial liver grafts had at least 3 months of follow-up. In the first 158, conventional hepatic duct isolation was used in the donor (group C). In the last 244 cases, the complete hilar plate and Glissonian sheath approach (HPGS) was used (group H). We compared the incidence and outcomes of BCs in the 2 groups.

Results.—The rate of BC was significantly lower in group H (5.3%) than in group C (15.8%, p = 0.000). The incidence of early (within 3 months of transplant) BCs was similarly significantly lower in group H (3.3%) than in group C (13.2%, P = 0.000). The incidence of late BCs in the 145 patients in group H who had completed at least 12 months of follow-up was 2.8%. The proportion of BCs needing surgical correction was much higher in group C (44%) than in group H (7.7%, p = 0.022).

Conclusions.—By providing a graft with a well-vascularized hepatic duct or ducts with a sheath of supporting tissue that holds sutures well, the HPGS approach minimizes the incidence and severity of BCs in LDLT (Table 4).

▶ Biliary complications following liver transplantation, especially living donor liver transplantation, have been problematic and can be difficult complications that may result in graft loss. Many alternative techniques and the use of

TABLE 4.—Analysis of Demographic Data and Other Possible Associations with Biliary Complications

Parameter	Group C (n = 158)	Group H (n = 244)	p Value
Recipient age, y, mean ± SD (range)	43.64 ± 15.87; (1−69)	45.02 ± 15.32; (0.6−69)	0.438
Recipient gender (M/F), n	123/35	198/46	0.421
Roux anastomosis, n (%)	22 (13.9)	31 (12.7)	0.725
Use of cystic duct, n (%)	6 (3.8)	11 (4.5)	0.729
Arterial complications, n (%)	0 (0)	4 (1.6)	0.106
CMV episodes, n (%)	4 (2.5)	12 (4.9)	0.232
Acute rejection episodes, n (%)	26 (16.5)	37 (15.2)	0.728
Cold ischemia time, min	89.97 ± 43.64	93.04 ± 34.12	0.052
Type of graft-right/left lobe, n	128/30	218/26	0.026
Warm ischemia time, min	53.43 ± 14.46	48.88 ± 13.92	0.001
Multiple ducts, n (%)	30 (18.9)	103 (42.2)	0.000

Group C, conventional; Group H, hilar plate−Glissonian sheath.

duct-to-duct anastomosis versus Roux-en-Y hepaticojejunostomy have been hotly debated. Fortunately, Soin et al describe a new approach that appears to have a sound physiologic basis: preservation of hepatic duct blood supply. Most biliary complications are believed to result from ischemic complications and, therefore, a technique that permits adequate perfusion is attractive. These authors describe a hilar plate and Glissonian sheath approach in which the thick surrounding tissue of the donor hepatic duct is left intact and multiple ducts remain as individual orifices rather than disruption of surrounding tissue for a ductoplasty. The early outcomes using this approach were markedly improved compared with the traditional technique used by this group. Surprisingly, whether this technique was used in a duct-to-duct approach or in combination with a Roux-en-Y limb, did not make a significant difference (Table 4). A limitation of this study is the lack of information about donor outcome, but presumably the outcome was good or the authors would not have perpetuated the use of it in more than 400 patients. Importantly, this technique may be applicable to hepatic resection aside from donor transplantation and in cases of biliary reconstruction. Preservation of arterial inflow tissue surrounding the hepatic ducts should be appropriately considered in any operation that involves biliary reconstruction.

K. E. Behrns, MD

Is There a Role for Endoscopic Therapy as a Definitive Treatment for Post-Laparoscopic Bile Duct Injuries?
Fatima J, Barton JG, Grotz TE, et al (Mayo Clinic, Rochester, MN)
J Am Coll Surg 211:495-502, 2010

Background.—Excellent results of surgical reconstruction of major bile duct injuries (BDIs) have been well-documented. Reports of successful definitive management of central bile duct leakage and stenoses have been reported infrequently. The aim of this study was to assess treatment and outcomes for operative and endoscopic treatment of BDI after laparoscopic cholecystectomy (LC) and define the role of endoscopy in management.

Study Design.—All patients undergoing treatment for post-laparoscopic BDI from 1998 to 2007 at Mayo Clinic, Rochester, Minnesota were reviewed. Outcomes of surgical and endoscopic intervention were analyzed.

Results.—BDI was identified in 159 patients (mean age 51 years). Injury was recognized intraoperatively in 39 (25%) patients. Primary intervention was surgical in 59 (37%) and endoscopic in 100 (63%) patients. Class A BDIs (n = 77) were successfully treated endoscopically in 76 (99%) patients. Seven had class D BDIs; 4 were managed surgically, and 3 endoscopically. Of 66 patients with E1 to E4 BDI, 44 (67%) were initially managed surgically and 22 (33%) endoscopically. Thirteen of the latter 22 underwent sustained endoscopic therapy (median stent time 7 months), which was successful in 10 (77%). Four patients with E5 were managed surgically. Median follow-up was 45 months. Sixty-three patients underwent Roux-en-Y hepaticojejunostomy reconstruction at

Mayo; 3 (5%) failed and required stenting. None required operative revision.

Conclusions.—Endoscopic management of class A BDI has excellent outcomes. Although surgical management remains the preferred therapy, short-term endoscopic treatment for class E1 to E4 can optimize the patient and operative field for reconstruction. Prolonged stenting in select patients with E1 to E4 characterized by stenosis is successful in the majority.

▶ Surprisingly, the number of bile duct injuries sustained during the performance of laparoscopic cholecystectomy has changed considerably in recent years. Fortunately, many of these injuries are bile leaks from the cystic duct remnant or small transected ducts in the bed of the gallbladder. These injuries are successfully treated by endoscopic stenting. However, central biliary system injuries with leaks, stenoses, or occlusions represent difficult management problems that require multidisciplinary approaches to achieve successful resolution. Fatima et al report their experience with all bile duct leaks treated endoscopically or surgically. Special attention should be paid to those patients with central biliary system injuries. Eleven of 66 patients had attempted definitive therapy by endoscopic means and 8 of the 11 were treated successfully. Therefore, there certainly is a role for endoscopic therapy; however, this comes at a cost of multiple endoscopic sessions, and over half of the patients had stents in place for more than 3 months. These results should be compared with surgical treatment that resulted in a 92% stricture-free rate at 5 years. Thus, the surgical gold standard sets a high bar. No doubt, endoscopic and percutaneous approaches are invaluable in the treatment of central biliary strictures, but the data are irrefutable that the best long-term outcome is achieved with surgical care. Importantly, as we strive to limit the cycle of care for a specific diagnosis like bile duct injury, we must keep in mind the safest and most direct route to long-term resolution. In the case of central bile duct injury, this would appear to be surgical repair.

K. E. Behrns, MD

Management of Giant Hemangioma of the Liver: Resection versus Observation

Schnelldorfer T, Ware AL, Smoot R, et al (Mayo Clinic, Rochester, MN)
J Am Coll Surg 211:724-730, 2010

Background.—Management of patients with giant hemangiomas of the liver encounters persistent controversy. Although recent case series suggest a low complication rate with nonoperative management, the classic paradigm of preventive operative resection remains.

Study Design.—A retrospective cohort study was conducted of 492 patients with giant hepatic hemangioma (>4 cm in size) diagnosed between 1985 and 2005 at Mayo Clinic Rochester. Long-term outcomes were assessed by patient survey, with a follow-up of 11 ± 6.4 years.

Results.—Of 492 patients, 289 responded to the survey. In the nonoperative group (n = 233), 20% had persistent or new onset of hemangioma-associated symptoms, including potentially life-threatening complications in 2%. In the operative group (n = 56), perioperative complications occurred in 14%, including potentially life-threatening complications in 7%. None of the operative patients had persistent or new onset of hemangioma-associated symptoms after resection of the dominant hemangioma. In group comparison, the rate of adverse events was similar (20% versus 14%; p = 0.45) with an overall low risk for potentially life-threatening complications (2% versus 7%; p = 0.07). Size of hemangiomas was not associated with adverse events in either group. Subjective health status and quality of life at follow-up were similar in both groups (p > 0.54).

Conclusions.—Clinical observation of patients with giant hemangioma of the liver has a similar rate of complications compared with operative management, but might prevent the need for invasive interventions in some patients. Clinical observation is preferred in most patients and operative treatment should be reserved for patients with severe symptoms or disease-associated complications.

▶ Hepatic hemangiomas are the most common type of liver tumor and most often are small and require no treatment or follow-up. On occasion (17% in this study), hemangiomas are greater than 4 cm in largest dimension and are classified as giant. Frequently, the association of the term giant implies the risk of untoward consequences, namely, rupture and life-threatening hemorrhage, and many surgeons contend that prophylactic resection should be undertaken. Schnelldorfer et al challenged this long-held teaching and examined 289 patients (233 in the observation group and 56 in the operative group) who were followed up for a mean of more than 11 years in the observation group. The results clearly show that observation is prudent in the vast majority of the patients, with only 2% of the nonoperative patients developing life-threatening complications, whereas 7% of patients who underwent resection developed life-threatening postoperative complications. The findings in the nonoperative group clearly show that patients rarely develop new onset symptoms, and, in fact, symptoms may resolve spontaneously. In addition, the size of the hemangioma appeared unimportant since even tumors greater than 10 cm in size did not necessarily produce symptoms. Although few patients sustained abdominal trauma, this often-cited risk for rupture was not evident in this study since no patient with a hepatic hemangioma who sustained abdominal trauma experienced hemangioma rupture. Finally, only 14% of the patients had hemangiomas that increased greater than 1 cm in size during follow-up. Thus, these data suggest that only the infrequent patient requires resection, preferably enucleation, for significantly symptomatic hemangiomas. Of note, this study was funded by the National Center for Research Resources, which funds comparative effectiveness studies, and was an outstanding example of investigating straightforward management questions.

K. E. Behrns, MD

Early Cholecystectomy Safely Decreases Hospital Stay in Patients With Mild Gallstone Pancreatitis: A Randomized Prospective Study

Aboulian A, Chan T, Yaghoubian A, et al (Harbor UCLA Med Ctr, Torrance, CA; et al)
Ann Surg 251:615-619, 2010

Objective.—We hypothesized that laparoscopic cholecystectomy performed within 48 hours of admission for mild gallstone pancreatitis, regardless of resolution of abdominal pain or abnormal laboratory values, would result in a shorter hospital stay.

Summary of Background Data.—Although there is consensus among surgeons that patients with gallstone pancreatitis should undergo cholecystectomy to prevent recurrence, the precise timing of laparoscopic cholecystectomy for mild disease remains controversial.

Methods.—Consecutive patients with mild pancreatitis (Ranson score ≤3) were prospectively randomized to either an early laparoscopic cholecystectomy group (within 48 hours of admission) versus a control laparoscopic cholecystectomy group (performed after resolution of abdominal pain and normalizing trend of laboratory enzymes). The primary end point was hospital length of stay. Secondary end point was a composite of rates of conversion to an open procedure, perioperative complications, and need for endoscopic retrograde cholangiography. The study was designed to enroll 100 patients with an interim analysis after 50 patients.

Results.—At interim analysis, 50 patients were enrolled at a single university-affiliated public hospital. Of them, 25 patients were randomized to the early group and 25 patients to the control group. Patient age ranged from 18 to 74 years with a median duration of symptoms of 2 days upon presentation and a median Ranson score of 1. There were no baseline differences between the groups with regards to demographics, clinical presentation, or the presence of comorbidities. The hospital length of stay was shorter for the early cholecystectomy group (mean: 3.5 [95% CI, 2.7−4.3], median: 3 [IQR, 2−4]) compared with the control group (mean: 5.8 [95% CI, 3.8−7.9], median: 4 [IQR, 4−6] [$P = 0.0016$]). Six patients from the early group required endoscopic retrograde cholangiography, compared with 4 in the control group ($P = 0.72$). There was no statistically significant difference in the need for conversion to an open procedure or in perioperative complication rates between the 2 groups.

Conclusion.—In mild gallstone pancreatitis, laparoscopic cholecystectomy performed within 48 hours of admission, regardless of the resolution of abdominal pain or laboratory abnormalities, results in a shorter hospital length of stay with no apparent impact on the technical difficulty of the procedure or perioperative complication rate.

▶ The symptomatic patient with gallstones in the gallbladder or common bile duct requires careful consideration because, as the study by Reinders et al[1] shows, persistent symptoms after treatment of choledocholithiasis are common. In the not-too-distant past, there was significant enthusiasm for eradication of common duct stones followed by a wait-and-see approach. However, this has fallen by the wayside, and treatment by cholecystectomy to relieve persistent biliary symptoms is warranted. Reinders et al further refine this approach by clearly demonstrating that early cholecystectomy (within 72 hours) after endoscopic bile duct clearance is associated with decreased biliary symptoms when compared with cholecystectomy performed at 6 to 8 weeks. How will these findings change the management of patients with choledochocystolithiasis? Likely, most patients can be treated practically by early cholecystectomy. However, in many instances this may not be possible; thus, the patient may develop recurrent symptoms (at least the complication and conversion rate would be unchanged, given the data presented). However, another option is single-setting treatment by laparoscopic cholecystectomy with common bile duct exploration. This is a very reasonable approach that does, however, have a steep learning curve. However, once the technical skills are acquired, this approach can be applied widely with little increase in operative time and a large reduction in patient treatment time when compared with the need for both endoscopic retrograde cholangiopancreatography and laparoscopic cholecystectomy. Surgeons should embrace laparoscopic cholecystectomy combined with common bile exploration and offer single-stage treatment for choledochocystolithiasis.

K. E. Behrns, MD

Reference

1. Reinders JS, Goud A, Timmer R, et al. Early laparoscopic cholecystectomy improves outcomes after endoscopic sphincterotomy for choledochocystolithiasis. *Gastroenterology.* 2010;138:2315-2320.

Radiofrequency Ablation as First-Line Treatment in Patients With Early Colorectal Liver Metastases Amenable to Surgery

Otto G, Düber C, Hoppe-Lotichius M, et al (Johannes Gutenberg Univ of Mainz, Germany)
Ann Surg 251:796-803, 2010

Objective.—Aiming at avoidance of futile surgery, we have tested whether radiofrequency ablation (RFA) may be used as first-line treatment in patients with colorectal metastases (CRLM) occurring within the first year after colorectal surgery.

Summary Background Data.—Surgical resection is the standard treatment in patients with CRLM. Major retrospective analyses have identified the interval between colorectal surgery and the occurrence of CRLM to be of prognostic importance. So far, it is unknown whether survival of the respective patients is hampered if RFA is used as first-line treatment.

Methods.—According to a clinical pathway, we have treated patients with CRLM detected within the first year after colorectal surgery preferentially by RFA (n = 28). Resection (n = 82) was performed in patients who were deemed not amenable to RFA due to number, size, or location of metastatic lesions. The diameter of lesions differed between the groups.

All other characteristics of patients and lesions were comparable. Local recurrence and new hepatic lesions were treated with repeated RFA or surgery whenever possible.

Results.—Local recurrence at the site of ablation or resection occurred in 32% and 4% ($P < 0.001$), new metastases apart from the site of previous treatment in 50% and 34% ($P = 0.179$), and systemic recurrence in 32% and 37% ($P = 0.820$) of the patients after RFA and surgery, respectively. Time to progression was significantly shorter in patients primarily treated with RFA (203 vs. 416 days; $P = 0.017$). After primary treatment, 9 RFA patients and 8 surgery patients were amenable to repeated RFA or repeated surgery resulting in identical rates of disease-free patients and identical 3-year overall survival in both treatment groups: 67% and 60%, respectively; $P = 0.93$.

Conclusions.—Despite striking differences in local tumor recurrence and shorter time to progression, survival in patients with early CRLM does not depend on the mode of primary hepatic treatment (Fig 1).

▶ Patients with colorectal cancer who present with early (1 year or less after primary diagnosis) liver metastases represent a select subgroup of patients who have difficult-to-treat metastatic disease. As dictated by the primary lesion

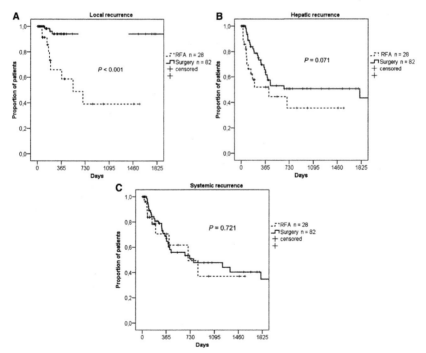

FIGURE 1.—Local (A), hepatic (B), and systemic (C) recurrences in patients treated with RFA versus hepatic resection for early occurring colorectal liver metastases. (Reprinted from Otto G, Düber C, Hoppe-Lotichius M, et al. Radiofrequency ablation as first-line treatment in patients with early colorectal liver metastases amenable to surgery. *Ann Surg.* 2010;251:796-803, with permission from Lippincott Williams & Wilkins.)

with lymph node metastasis, the majority of these patients are also treated with chemotherapy. The treatment of liver metastases in this scenario is traditionally by hepatic resection. In the study by Otto et al, the outcome of patients treated initially by radiofrequency ablation (RFA) was determined. The findings show that survival did not differ compared with patients treated by hepatic resection. As expected, RFA was associated with increased local recurrence, which occurred in a shorter period of time than in patients treated by resection. The authors conclude that a randomized trial of RFA versus surgery is warranted given the potential for nontherapeutic surgery. While this conclusion may be valid, the question is whether any local therapy should be used in patients with a high recurrence rate in the liver and systemically. Clearly, survival is the ultimate goal and, therefore, neither surgery nor RFA is of significant benefit in this high-risk group. Alternative systemic strategies are needed for this group of patients with a high propensity for recurrent disease.

K. E. Behrns, MD

A Multicenter Analysis of Distal Pancreatectomy for Adenocarcinoma: Is Laparoscopic Resection Appropriate?

Kooby DA, Hawkins WG, Schmidt CM, et al (Emory Univ School of Medicine, Atlanta, GA; Washington Univ, St Louis, MO; Indiana Univ, Indianapolis; et al)
J Am Coll Surg 210:779-787, 2010

Background.—As compared with open distal pancreatectomy (ODP), laparoscopic distal pancreatectomy (LDP) affords improved perioperative outcomes. The role of LDP for patients with pancreatic ductal adenocarcinoma (PDAC) is not defined.

Study Design.—Records from patients undergoing distal pancreatectomy (DP) for PDAC from 2000 to 2008 from 9 academic medical centers were reviewed. Short-term (node harvest and margin status) and long-term (survival) cancer outcomes were assessed. A 3:1 matched analysis was performed for ODP and LDP cases using age, American Society of Anesthesiologists (ASA) class, and tumor size.

Results.—There were 212 patients who underwent DP for PDAC; 23 (11%) of these were approached laparoscopically. For all 212 patients, 56 (26%) had positive margins. The mean number of nodes (±SD) examined was 12.6 ± 8.4 and 114 patients (54%) had at least 1 positive node. Median overall survival was 16 months. In the matched analysis there were no significant differences in positive margin rates, number of nodes examined, number of patients with at least 1 positive node, or overall survival. Logistic regression for all 212 patients demonstrated that advanced age, larger tumors, positive margins, and node positive disease were independently associated with worse survival; however, method of resection (ODP vs. LDP) was not. Hospital stay was 2 days shorter in the matched comparison, which approached significance (LDP, 7.4 days vs. ODP, 9.4 days, p = 0.06).

Conclusions.—LDP provides similar short- and long-term oncologic outcomes as compared with OD, with potentially shorter hospital stay.

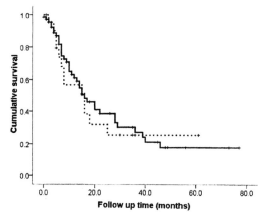

FIGURE 2.—Matched analysis overall survival for patients undergoing open (solid line, n = 70, median survival 16 months) versus laparoscopic (dotted line, n = 23, median survival 16 months) distal pancreatectomy for adenocarcinoma, in the 3:1 matched analysis (p = 0.71, log rank). (Reprinted from Journal of American College of Surgeons, Kooby DA, Hawkins WG, Schmidt CM, et al. A multicenter analysis of distal pancreatectomy for adenocarcinoma: is laparoscopic resection appropriate? *J Am Coll Surg.* 2010;210:779-787. Copyright © 2010, with permission from the American College of Surgeons.)

These results suggest that LDP is an acceptable approach for resection of PDAC of the left pancreas in selected patients (Fig 2).

▶ Kooby et al answer the important question of whether laparoscopic resection is an appropriate approach for surgical resection of the distal pancreas for adenocarcinoma. The answer is a resounding yes! This trial, although small in number, definitively shows that laparoscopic resection is associated with equivalent survival to open distal pancreatectomy for adenocarcinoma (Fig 2). This study shows that in addition to similar long-term survival, laparoscopic distal pancreatectomy results in equivalent lymph node harvest and margin-free resection. However, margin-free resection remains problematic for both open and laparoscopic distal pancreatectomy since multiple studies show that a positive margin adversely affects survival and this study, like others, demonstrates a margin-positive rate of approximately 25%. Clearly, all pancreatic resections should strive for a margin-negative resection since this variable is of prime importance in long-term survival.

K. E. Behrns, MD

Impact of Acute Care Surgery on Biliary Disease
Britt RC, Bouchard C, Weireter LJ, et al (Eastern Virginia Med School, Norfolk)
J Am Coll Surg 210:595-601, 2010

Background.—We introduced an acute care surgery (ACS) service in July 2007 to address all new consults. This study examines the impact on treatment of biliary disease.

Study Design.—A retrospective review was done of a prospective database of all inpatient operative biliary disease treated in a tertiary care hospital 1 year before and 2 years after implementation of an ACS service. Data collected included diagnosis, time from admission to operation, time of operation, length of stay, comorbidities, and complications.

Results.—There were 54 patients in the pre-ACS group and 132 in the post-ACS group, with no difference in percentage of females, comorbidities, and diagnosis. The post-ACS group had a trend toward a shorter time from consult to operating room (59.9 vs 68.7 hours, p = 0.45) and shorter hospital length of stay (5.5 vs 6.7 days, p = 0.27). In the acute cholecystitis post-ACS cohort, there was also a trend toward shorter time to operating room (39.8 vs 45.5 hours, p = 0.55) and shorter length of stay (4.6 vs 5.7 days, p = 0.39). The second year of ACS showed continued improvement in time to operating room (30.9 hours) compared with both pre-ACS and the first year of ACS. There was no significant difference in laparoscopic versus open surgery or complications between the groups.

Conclusions.—There is a trend toward improvement in timeliness of care for complex inpatient biliary disease with implementation of an ACS service, especially as the service matures. There remains wide variability in patient complexity, which affects timeliness of care.

▶ The development of acute care surgery (ACS) services has resulted in improved patient access for surgical treatment for multiple, acute gastrointestinal diseases. Britt et al describe their model of the ACS service and the positive effects noted on the treatment of biliary disease. Indeed, the authors demonstrate that patients in the post-ACS period had a trend to a shorter period of time to operating room treatment. Importantly, the patients in this group also had a shorter length of stay, which was associated with cost savings. There was no difference in the complication rates in the 2 groups. The introduction of ACS services in some institutions has caused consternation about which group of surgeons is best suited to deliver care to patients with acute diseases. This conflict is improperly focused on the surgeon's perspective when we should be focused on patient-centered care. The commitment to our patients is to deliver timely high-quality care as demonstrated in this article. The surgeon-patient relationship should be the same whether the care is delivered by an ACS surgeon, a hepatobiliary-pancreatic surgeon, or a general surgeon. We owe it to our patients to deliver the most timely and expert care! Implicit in this surgeon-patient agreement is that we will recognize our practice domain and engage the assistance of experts as required by the patient's condition. Clearly, the use of endoscopic retrograde cholangiopancreatography in the patients presented in this article represents the engagement of experts to assess complex biliary disease. The introduction of ACS services has permitted timely care for acute gastrointestinal diseases while at the same time allowing surgeons with elective schedules to render timely care to their patients. Undoubtedly, this structure is a benefit to many patients who receive timely care. The surgical community needs to retain and reinforce the commitment to patient-centered care as noted in this article.

K. E. Behrns, MD

Choledochoceles: Are They Choledochal Cysts?
Ziegler KM, Pitt HA, Zyromski NJ, et al (Indiana Univ School of Medicine, Indianapolis)
Ann Surg 252:683-690, 2010

Objective.—The aim of this analysis was to report a multidisciplinary series comparing choledochoceles to Todani Types I, II, IV, and V choledochal cysts.

Summary Background Data.—Choledochoceles have been classified as Todani Type III choledochal cysts. However, most surgical series of choledochal cysts have reported few choledochoceles because they are managed primarily by endoscopists.

Methods.—Surgical, endoscopic, and radiologic records were reviewed at the Riley Children's Hospital and the Indiana University Hospitals to identify patients with choledochal cysts. Patient demographics, presenting symptoms, radiologic studies, associated abnormalities, surgical and endoscopic procedures as well as outcomes were reviewed.

Results.—A total of 146 patients with "choledochal cysts" including 45 children (31%) and 28 with choledochoceles (18%) were identified, which represents the largest Western series. Patients with choledochoceles were older (50.7 vs. 29.0 years, $P < 0.05$) and more likely to be male (43% vs. 19%, $P < 0.05$), to present with pancreatitis (48% vs. 24%, $P < 0.05$) rather than jaundice (11% vs. 30%, $P < 0.05$) or cholangitis (0% vs. 21%, $P < 0.05$), to have pancreas divisum (38% vs. 10%, $P < 0.01$), and to be managed with endoscopic therapy (79% vs. 17%, $P < 0.01$). Two patients with choledochoceles (7%) had pancreatic neoplasms.

Conclusions.—Patients with choledochoceles differ from patients with choledochal cysts with respect to age, gender, presentation, pancreatic ductal anatomy, and their management. The association between choledochoceles and pancreas divisum is a new observation. Therefore, we conclude that classifications of choledochal cysts should not include choledochoceles.

▶ The root of understanding surgical management stems from a complete understanding of anatomy and embryology and the consequent physiology. Thus, as surgical trainees have been told many times, form and function dictate surgical management. This work by Ziegler et al is a superb example of how surgeons should continue to question the form and function of long-held anatomic and physiologic teachings. Clearly, based on the results of this study, choledochoceles are different than choledochal cysts and should not be included in the classification of choledochal cysts. Furthermore, the data here indicate that patients with choledochoceles are at risk for pancreatitis and that the risk of malignancy is low. Furthermore, an association between choledochoceles and pancreas divisum is not infrequent. Obviously, given these associations, the real question is "How many patients with choledochoceles are truly symptomatic, and in what proportion of these patients are symptoms directly attributable to the choledochocele?" This is a difficult question to answer, but this study sheds significant light on the type of symptoms and associated abnormalities and, therefore, management of choledochoceles should be based on data generated in this study. A few years ago, I had the opportunity to serve on a panel of experts discussing complex biliary disease, and a question arose about the treatment of choledochoceles regarding the risk of cancer. I was (and still am) of the opinion that a prophylactic operation (Whipple) was unnecessary in these patients. However, I was astonished that one of the participants on the panel suggested that a pancreatoduodenectomy was appropriate based on the classification scheme (Todani type III) of choledochoceles and the known risk of cholangiocarcinoma. The data in this article add clarification that choledochoceles are likely not a variant of a choledochal cyst and these entities should not be lumped together. Using these data, we should carefully follow patients with choledochoceles and add more information to our database regarding this anatomic variant.

K. E. Behrns, MD

Endoscopic Treatment of Biliary Fistulas After Complex Liver Resection
Farhat S, Bourrier A, Gaudric M, et al (Cochin Hosp, Paris, France)
Ann Surg 253:88-93, 2011

Objective.—The aim of this study was to evaluate the safety and efficacy of endoscopic treatment for biliary fistulas after complex liver resection.

Background.—The role of endoscopy in the treatment of fistulas of the common bile duct is well documented. On the contrary, results of endoscopic procedures for fistulas arising from peripheral bile ducts after liver resections are poorly studied, although more complex hepatectomies are increasingly performed. We analyzed retrospectively the results of these procedures in our experience.

Patients.—Twenty-six patients aged 10 to 74 years were included. Fistulas arose after extended right hepatectomy, n = 14; extended left hepatectomy, n = 2; segmentectomy, n = 7; and split-liver transplantation, n = 3. All patients underwent radiologic or surgical external drainage before endoscopic retrograde cholangiopancreatography (ERCP). Mean bile outflow before endoscopy was 493.1 ± 386.1 mL/24 h (median, 400; range, 100–2000 mL). The mean time from surgery to diagnosis was 29.4 ± 45.5 days.

Results.—The ERCP was performed after a median of 13 days after the diagnosis of biliary fistula. A sphincterotomy was required in 96.1% of patients. A 5F to 10F polyethylene stent bypassing the leaking bile duct was implanted in 21 (80.7%) of 26 patients. Fistulas were dried up completely in 25 (96.1%) of 26 patients. The mean time from initial

TABLE 3.—Time Required to Achieve Success After ERCP (See Methods Section for Definition of Success)

Time to (Days)	Mean ± SD	Median	Range
Clinical success	17.5 ± 12.4	15	2–60
Primary technical success	38 ± 89.4	13	2–428
Final technical success	68.6 ± 52.9	57	6–210

ERCP to running dry of the leaks was 17.5 ± 12.4 days. Procedure-related morbidity was 0%. There was no mortality.

Conclusion.—Biliary fistulas arising from intrahepatic ducts after complex liver resections are more difficult to treat than distal fistulas arising from the common bile duct. However, despite a longer time for cure and the need for repeated ERCP, endoscopic therapy appears efficient and does not induce additional morbidity (Table 3).

▶ Biliary fistula following liver resection is one of the more common and troublesome complications. It is pesky in some patients because despite what appears to be adequate drainage, the leak will not seal. Farhat et al publish their results with the use of endoscopically placed biliary stents with or without endoscopic sphincterotomy in such cases. The results showed that this approach is 95% successful. Furthermore, bile output is decreased markedly in a relatively short period of time (Table 3). These results raise the question, "why not perform endoscopic stenting immediately upon fistula diagnosis?" Personal experience with pancreatic fistulas following distal pancreatectomy suggests that peritoneal drainage along with prompt endoscopic placement of a pancreatic duct stent results in rapid resolution and decreased symptoms in these patients who are often quite uncomfortable with a partially controlled fistula. Although we await data to prove this hypothesis, any measure that provides prompt resolution of symptoms and permit hospital discharge should be used and studied in this difficult-to-treat patient group.

K. E. Behrns, MD

Adverse Outcomes in Patients With Chronic Liver Disease Undergoing Colorectal Surgery

Ghaferi AA, Mathur AK, Sonnenday CJ, et al (Univ of Michigan, Ann Arbor)
Ann Surg 252:345-350, 2010

Objective.—We sought to use a multi-institutional, prospective, clinical database to better understand adverse outcomes in chronic liver disease (CLD) patients undergoing colorectal surgery.

Background.—CLD confers significant perioperative risk. However, there are little population-based data available for prognostication and risk stratification in these patients.

Methods.—We used data from the 2005–2007 American College of Surgeons National Surgical Quality Improvement Project to study 30,927 patients undergoing colorectal resections. We first identified patients with CLD (n = 1565) with any of the following clinical characteristics: ascites, esophageal varices, or total bilirubin greater than 2 mg/dL. Postoperative complications and mortality rates were then compared between CLD and non-CLD patients.

Results.—CLD patients have a nearly 6.5-fold increased risk of mortality following colorectal operations (Relative Risk [RR], 6.53; 3.2% in non-CLD group versus 21.5% in CLD group). Patients with CLD also had significantly higher major complication rates (RR, 2.72; 15.4% vs. 41.9%, respectively). The failure to rescue rate (ie, proportion of deaths following major complications) was also markedly higher in patients with CLD (RR, 2.27; 15.1% vs. 34.2%, respectively). Furthermore, stratification of CLD patients by Model for End-stage Liver Disease (MELD) score demonstrated significantly higher rates of complications (RR, 2.41; 2.31–2.51), failure to rescue (RR, 2.62; 2.35–2.90), and mortality (RR, 8.92; 8.11–9.78) in CLD patients with MELD ≥15 compared with CLD patients with MELD <15.

Conclusions.—Colorectal surgery in CLD patients is associated with significant morbidity and mortality. Furthermore, those who develop major complications have a significantly higher risk of death compared to non-CLD. These very high risks should be discussed at length with patients prior to undertaking major surgical procedures.

▶ Chronic liver disease is a known risk factor for increased mortality and morbidity following abdominal surgery. Quantifying the relative risk of patients with chronic liver disease has been somewhat problematic because of a relatively small number of patients. Ghaferi et al used data from the National Surgical Quality Improvement Program to assess the outcome of patients with chronic liver disease undergoing colorectal surgery. More than 1500 patients with chronic liver disease were included, and liver disease was defined as the presence of ascites, esophageal varices, and a serum bilirubin greater than 2.0 mg/dL. In addition, liver disease was evaluated in the context of the Child-Turcotte-Pugh and Model for End-stage Liver Disease scoring systems. Not surprisingly, patients with liver disease had a 6.5-fold increased risk of death and a 2.7-fold risk of complications. Importantly, the failure to rescue was about 2.3-fold higher in the patients with liver disease. Therefore, colorectal surgery in patients with liver disease has a substantial risk of death, and even if complications are identified the risk of mortality remains high. This study used markers of relatively advanced liver disease—ascites, esophageal varices, and bilirubin greater than 2.0 mg/dL. Mortality is expected in patient populations with these indicators of disease, and perhaps palliative care only should be offered to patients with advanced liver disease. Consideration of palliative care will likely become more important in this era of health care reform. Because surgeons are in the business of saving lives, we too infrequently contemplate palliative care options. Furthermore, we should look for novel biomarkers that will help identify at-risk patients with liver disease who may undergo abdominal surgery. The increasing prevalence of chronic liver injury from hepatitis C infection and nonalcoholic steatohepatitis will increase the likelihood of encountering this difficult clinical situation.

K. E. Behrns, MD

Comparison of outcomes after laparoscopic versus open appendectomy for acute appendicitis at 222 ACS NSQIP hospitals

Ingraham AM, Cohen ME, Bilimoria KY, et al (American College of Surgeons, Chicago, IL; Northwestern Univ Feinberg School of Medicine, Chicago, IL; et al)

Surgery 148:625-637, 2010

Background.—The benefit of laparoscopic (LA) versus open (OA) appendectomy, particularly for complicated appendicitis, remains unclear. Our objectives were to assess 30-day outcomes after LA versus OA for acute appendicitis and complicated appendicitis, determine the incidence of specific outcomes after appendectomy, and examine factors influencing the utilization and duration of the operative approach with multi-institutional clinical data.

Methods.—Using the American College of Surgeons National Surgical Quality Improvement Program (ACS NSQIP) database (2005—2008), patients were identified who underwent emergency appendectomy for acute appendicitis at 222 participating hospitals. Regression models, which included propensity score adjustment to minimize the influence of treatment selection bias, were constructed. Models assessed the association between surgical approach (LA vs OA) and risk-adjusted overall morbidity, surgical site infection (SSI), serious morbidity, and serious morbidity/mortality, as well as individual complications in patients with acute appendicitis and complicated appendicitis. The relationships between operative approach, operative duration, and extended duration of stay with hospital academic affiliation were also examined.

Results.—Of 32,683 patients, 24,969 (76.4%) underwent LA and 7,714 (23.6%) underwent OA. Patients who underwent OA were significantly older with more comorbidities compared with those who underwent LA. Patients treated with LA were less likely to experience an overall morbidity (4.5% vs 8.8%; odds ratio [OR], 0.60; 95% confidence interval [CI], 0.54—0.68) or a SSI (3.3% vs 6.7%; OR, 0.57; 95% CI, 0.50—0.65) but not a serious morbidity (2.6% vs 4.2%; OR, 0.86; 95% CI, 0.74—1.01) or a serious morbidity/mortality (2.6% vs 4.3%; OR, 0.87; 95% CI, 0.74—1.01) compared with those who underwent OA. All patients treated with LA were significantly less likely to develop individual infectious complications except for organ space SSI. Among patients with complicated appendicitis, organ space SSI was significantly more common after laparoscopic appendectomy (6.3% vs 4.8%; OR, 1.35; 95% CI,

1.05–1.73). For all patients with acute appendicitis, those treated at academic-affiliated versus community hospitals were equally likely to undergo LA versus OA (77.0% vs 77.3%; $P = .58$). Operative duration at academic centers was significantly longer for both LA and OA (LA, 47 vs 38 minutes [$P < .0001$]; OA, 49 vs 44 minutes [$P < .0001$]). Median duration of stay after LA was 1 day at both academic-affiliated and community hospitals.

Conclusion.—Within ACS NSQIP hospitals, LA is associated with lower overall morbidity in selected patients. However, patients with complicated appendicitis may have a greater risk of organ space SSI after LA. Academic affiliation does not seem to influence the operative approach. However, LA is associated with similar durations of stay but slightly greater operative times than OA at academic versus community hospitals.

▶ Acute appendicitis remains one of the most common conditions addressed by the general surgeon. The treatment of appendicitis has evolved since the introduction of laparoscopy. Multiple nonrandomized studies have compared outcomes of open versus laparoscopic appendectomy, and most have failed to reveal significant differences. However, the study by Ingraham et al demonstrates that more than 75% of patients are treated by the laparoscopic method. Furthermore, this study is unique in that the data are obtained from more than 200 hospitals that have participated in the National Surgical Quality Improvement Program database. Thus, this study reveals the investigative power of this outcome database. The results demonstrate that older patients with comorbidities and complicated appendicitis have open operations. In those patients who underwent laparoscopic appendectomy, overall morbidity is decreased, as is wound infection. Patients with complicated appendicitis have similar outcomes whether treated by the open or laparoscopic method, especially with regard to deep organ space infection. The results of this study demonstrate the multiple advantages of laparoscopic appendectomy. However, refinements in the laparoscopic approach are necessary because deep organ space infection as a result of complicated appendicitis is more common with this approach. Potential alterations would include more frequent use of postoperative drainage. In addition, intraoperative lavage with aspiration of the lavage fluid may be important technical components of the laparoscopic approach in patients with complicated disease. Additional studies focused on the management of patients with complicated appendicitis should help improve the technique and outcomes with the laparoscopic method.

K. E. Behrns, MD

Influence of Histamine Receptor Antagonists on the Outcome of Perforated Appendicitis: Analysis from a Prospective Trial
St Peter SD, Sharp SW, Ostlie DJ (The Children's Mercy Hosp, Kansas City, MO)
Arch Surg 145:143-146, 2010

Hypothesis.—Diphenhydramine blocks the H_1 receptor to treat pruritus or to induce sleep, while ranitidine blocks the H_2 receptor to suppress gastric acid. They are often given to ill patients, such as those with perforated appendicitis. However, these receptors are integral to the inflammatory response, and to our knowledge, the impact of H_1 or H_2 blockade on outcome in the setting of perforated appendicitis has never been evaluated.

Design.—Prospective randomized trial.

Setting.—Referral center.

Patients.—Children undergoing an operation for perforated appendicitis from April 2005 to November 2006.

Main Outcome Measures.—We conducted multivariate analysis with Pearson correlation on data from a prospective randomized trial comparing antibiotic regimen after appendectomy for perforated appendicitis and outcome. Medications with a significant correlation to abscess development were investigated by comparing those receiving the medication with those who did not using the *t* test for continuous variables and χ^2 test for discrete variables. Significance was defined as $P \le .05$.

Results.—Significant correlations were found between the use of ranitidine $(P = .05)$ or diphenhydramine $(P = .03)$ and the development of an abscess. Direct comparison found no differences in patient or operative variables in those given either medication compared with those receiving no doses. Abscess rate in those receiving neither medication $(n = 41)$ was 10%. Those given only ranitidine $(n = 24)$ or diphenhydramine $(n = 17)$ had doubled abscess rates of 17% and 18%, respectively. Those given both medications $(n = 16)$ had a quadrupled abscess rate of 44% $(P = .03)$.

Conclusions.—Ranitidine or diphenhydramine given to patients with perforated appendicitis may increase the risk of postoperative abscess. Therefore, these medications should not be used empirically in this population.

▶ Postoperative order sets include several medications that are prescribed to deliver maximum comfort to the patient in the postoperative period. Frequently, medications are administered to combat the side effects of other very necessary medications such as narcotics. St Peter et al demonstrate that administration of histamine antagonists is associated with the development of postoperative abscess formation in patients who had surgery for perforated appendicitis. The proposed mechanism of histamine antagonist association with postoperative abscess is immune suppression; yet, no data are provided to support this provocative hypothesis. This study demonstrates the unintended consequences of combating side effects of 1 medication with yet another medication.

Furthermore, it is unique in that it examines the interactions between postoperative medications and how this may have a deleterious effect on patients' outcomes; that is, the medications that are administered to provide comfort are associated with an adverse event. As a surgical community, we need more studies like this in which the research question is not profound, but may have a significant impact on a patient's outcome. This research addresses the comparative effectiveness of postoperative medication strategies to provide excellent patient care. This is an important area of research that requires close observation as a starting point. As noted by the authors, this study was a byproduct of an antibiotic trial in which the investigators observed an association between histamine antagonists and abscess formation. Indeed, close observation of patient outcomes will lead to timely investigations of effectiveness of our therapies.

K. E. Behrns, MD

A meta-analysis comparing conservative treatment versus acute appendectomy for complicated appendicitis (abscess or phlegmon)
Simillis C, Symeonides P, Shorthouse AJ, et al (Imperial College, London; Northern General Hosp, Sheffield, UK)
Surgery 147:818-829, 2010

Background.—No standardized approach is available for the management of complicated appendicitis defined as appendiceal abscess and phlegmon. This study used meta-analytic techniques to compare conservative treatment versus acute appendectomy.

Methods.—Comparative studies were identified by a literature search. The end points evaluated were overall complications, need for reoperation, duration of hospital stay, and duration of intravenous antibiotics. Heterogeneity was assessed and a sensitivity analysis was performed to account for bias in patient selection.

Results.—Seventeen studies (16 nonrandomized retrospective and 1 nonrandomized prospective) reported on 1,572 patients: 847 patients received conservative treatment and 725 had acute appendectomy. Conservative treatment was associated with significantly less overall complications, wound infections, abdominal/pelvic abscesses, ileus/bowel obstructions, and reoperations. No significant difference was found in the duration of first hospitalization, the overall duration of hospital stay, and the duration of intravenous antibiotics. Overall complications remained significantly less in the conservative treatment group during sensitivity analysis of studies including only pediatric patients, high-quality studies, more recent studies, and studies with a larger group of patients.

Conclusion.—The conservative management of complicated appendicitis is associated with a decrease in complication and reoperation rate compared with acute appendectomy, and it has a similar duration of hospital stay. Because of significant heterogeneity between studies, additional studies should be undertaken to confirm these findings.

▶ Simillis et al addressed the important topic of the management of advanced acute appendicitis characterized by abscess development or phlegmon formation. Because of the lack of large randomized studies, the authors used the approach of meta-analyses of 16 retrospective and 1 prospective nonrandomized study to pool patient outcomes to determine the outcomes of conservative treatment versus acute appendectomy. Conservative therapy included antibiotic therapy with or without drainage and with or without interval appendectomy. The results indicate that conservative treatment is associated with a decreased rate of complications and a lower rate of reoperation. The pooled analysis examined the outcomes in over 1500 patients and seemingly delivered a sound outcome. However, the authors correctly present a measured conclusion because of the heterogeneity of the studies analyzed. Although a meta-analysis may address important outcome questions in clinical studies in which too few patients are treated to arrive at a statistically significant outcome compared with control, this should not be the case with complicated appendicitis. This would be an excellent topic to study comparative effectiveness of surgery versus conservative therapy, and given the number of patients affected, a randomized multicenter trial is appropriate. This is important research that would have a large impact on many patients and on the health care system. The obvious issue is the sponsor of such research, but this is exactly the type of clinical research that should be funded by the National Institutes of Health and/or private industry or foundations. Surgeons need to become more involved in comparative effectiveness research and lead investigative teams to address these important questions. Importantly, we need to collectively seek funding for these important research topics.

K. E. Behrns, MD

Balancing the Risk of Postoperative Surgical Infections: A Multivariate Analysis of Factors Associated With Laparoscopic Appendectomy From the NSQIP Database

Fleming FJ, Kim MJ, Messing S, et al (Univ of Rochester Med Ctr, NY)
Ann Surg 252:895-900, 2010

Objective.—To establish the relationship between operative approach (laparoscopic or open) and subsequent surgical infection (both incisional and organ space infection) postappendectomy, independent of potential confounding factors.

Background.—Although laparoscopic appendectomy has been associated with lower rates of incisional infections than an open approach, the relationship between laparoscopy and organ space infection (OSI) is not as clearly established.

Methods.—Cases of appendectomy were retrieved from the American College of Surgeons National Surgical Quality Improvement Program

(NSQIP) database for 2005 to 2008. Patient factors, operative variables, and the primary outcomes of incisional infections and OSIs were recorded. Factors associated with surgical infections were identified using logistic regression models. These models were then used to calculate probabilities of OSI in clinical vignettes demonstrating varying levels of infectious risk.

Results.—A total of 39,950 appendectomy cases were included of which 30,575 (77%) were performed laparoscopically. On multivariate analysis, laparoscopy was associated with a lower risk of incisional infection [odds ratio (OR) 0.37, 95% confidence interval (CI) 0.32−0.43] but with an increased risk of OSI after adjustment for confounding factors (OR 1.44, 95% CI 1.21−1.73). For a low-risk patient, probability of OSI was calculated to be 0.3% and 0.4%, respectively, for open versus laparoscopic appendectomy, whereas for a high-risk patient, probabilities were estimated at 8.9% and 12.3%, respectively.

Conclusion.—Laparoscopy was associated with a decreased risk of incisional infection but with an increased risk of OSI. The degree of this increased risk varies depending on the clinical profile of a surgical patient. Recognition of these differences in risk may aid clinicians in the choice of operative approach for appendectomy.

▶ Fleming et al used the powerful National Surgical Quality Improvement Program (NSQIP) database to address the seemingly straightforward question about the incidence of organ space infections after open or laparoscopic appendectomy. With the NSQIP database, they were able to assess over 30 000-patient records and find that laparoscopic appendectomy was associated with a lower risk of surgical site infection, whereas it was associated with a higher risk of organ space infections. The authors elegantly controlled confounding variables and appropriately assessed the circumstances when a laparoscopic appendectomy was converted to an open case. The benefits are potentially remarkable for those patients with an increased number of risk factors. But is conversion to an open procedure the only alternative? After all, laparoscopy is just an approach to an operation, so are there not other alternatives that may lead to decreased organ space infection after laparoscopic appendectomy? This data set does not provide information on drainage. What would the outcomes be if intraperitoneal drainage was used on high-risk cases? Furthermore, what techniques are used during an open operation for complicated appendicitis that are not used during a laparoscopic approach? Certainly these intraoperative techniques can be adopted. Finally, this study importantly narrows down the group that may benefit from a conversion; therefore, a multicenter randomized trial may be the appropriate approach.

K. E. Behrns, MD

Provocative Mesenteric Angiography for Lower Gastrointestinal Hemorrhage: Results from a Single-institution Study

Kim CY, Suhocki PV, Miller MJ Jr, et al (Duke Univ Med Ctr, Durham, NC)
J Vasc Interv Radiol 21:477-483, 2010

Purpose.—To determine the diagnostic capability, complication rate, and potential predictors of success for provocative mesenteric angiography in patients with obscure and recurrent lower gastrointestinal (GI) hemorrhage.

Materials and Methods.—Thirty-four patients (age, 7—92 years; 22 men) underwent 36 provocative mesenteric angiograms between January 2002 and December 2008. Provocative mesenteric angiography consisted of systemic anticoagulation with heparin followed by selective transcatheter injection of vasodilator and tissue plasminogen activator into the arterial distribution of highest suspicion. Medications were administered incrementally until active extravasation was visualized or until the operator deemed the outcome negative. The pertinent clinical, radiologic, surgical, laboratory, and pathologic notes were retrospectively reviewed.

Results.—Among 36 provocative mesenteric angiograms, 11 resulted in angiographically visible extravasation (31%) and an additional procedure resulted in angiographic visualization of an undiagnosed hypervascular mass, resulting in the identification of a source of a hemorrhage in 33% overall. In 10 of the 11 cases with visualized extravasation, transcatheter embolization successfully controlled recurrent hemorrhage, while the hypervascular mass without extravasation was successfully resected. Therefore, a total of 11 of 36 studies (31%) resulted in successful definitive treatment of recurrent hemorrhage. One embolization-related complication occurred, resulting in surgical resection of perforated ischemic bowel. No hemorrhagic complications were identified. Patients with melena and patients admitted for reasons other than acute lower GI hemorrhage were significantly less likely to benefit from provocative mesenteric angiography.

Conclusions.—In this series, provocative mesenteric angiography was safe and effective for eliciting the source of occult lower GI hemorrhage, leading to definitive therapy in about one third of patients.

▶ Lower gastrointestinal hemorrhage of unknown origin is a bedeviling condition that can challenge even the most experienced gastrointestinal clinician. Frequently, surgeons are asked to see these patients who have had multiple lower gastrointestinal bleeds over prolonged periods of time. Typically, these patients have had multiple endoscopies, tagged red blood cell scans, CT and angiography, yet, the source of the bleed remains mysterious. Kim et al present a series of 36 patients who fit the previously described condition. In these complex patients, they used provocative angiography with instillation of heparin, a vasodilator and tissue plasminogen activator to induce bleeding. They noted active extravasation in 11 patients (31%), and in 10 of these 11 patients embolization of the bleeding vessel resulted in long-lasting cessation of bleeding. Only 1 patient had a complication that required surgical therapy. This work represents a careful study of patients with a difficult clinical problem and offers an alternative to surgical therapy. Importantly, the authors note that they had surgical backup on board prior to any intervention. Thus, 10 of these 36 patients were spared surgical therapy, though we do not know the fate of the remaining 25 patients. However, likely many of these patients continued to bleed and some required subtotal colectomy. Many surgeons have experienced the sinking feeling of a recurrent lower gastrointestinal bleed following a subtotal colectomy, despite their best efforts to remove the area of suspected bleeding. This study suggests that we should ask our interventional radiologist to perform these provocative tests and spare patients surgery that may be associated with a high complication rate or, worse yet, a nontherapeutic operation.

K. E. Behrns, MD

A Fast-Track Recovery Protocol Improves Outcomes in Elective Laparoscopic Colectomy for Diverticulitis

Larson DW, Batdorf NJ, Touzios JG, et al (Mayo Clinic, Rochester, MN)
J Am Coll Surg 211:485-489, 2010

Background.—Fast-track (FT) postoperative protocols have been shown to be highly beneficial in open colectomy. Some have questioned the necessity of an FT protocol in the setting of laparoscopic colectomy because hospital stays are short and morbidity is low compared with open surgery. We set out to determine whether an FT protocol has any utility in the setting of elective laparoscopic colectomy.

Study Design.—A retrospective review was conducted on a cohort of 334 patients who underwent elective laparoscopic sigmoid resection for diverticulitis from 1998 to 2008, at Mayo Clinic, a tertiary care center in Rochester, MN. There were 235 patients who were managed with traditional postoperative care, and 99 who were managed with an FT protocol initiated in 2006. The main outcomes measures were time to soft diet, length of stay, overall morbidity, and readmission rate.

Results.—Times to soft diet (mean 2.3 vs 3.6 days), and first bowel movement (mean 2.6 vs 3.5 days) were shorter in the FT group (p < 0.001). The median lengths of stay were 3 days (interquartile range 3 to 4 days) and 5 days (interquartile range 4 to 6 days) for the FT and non-FT groups, respectively (p < 0.001). Morbidity was significantly lower in the FT group compared with the non-FT group (15.2% vs 25.5%, p < 0.03). The 30-day readmission rate was 2.9% for the FT group and 7.6% for the non-FT group (p = NS). There were no deaths in either group.

Conclusions.—Even in patients undergoing laparoscopic colectomy, FT protocols further improve the speed of gastrointestinal recovery, shorten the length of stay, and decrease morbidity.

▶ Laparoscopic colectomy for diverticulitis has proven benefit as have fast-track recovery approaches in open surgery. However, the combination of laparoscopic colon resection and fast-track recovery has not received consider-able attention. Larson et al demonstrate the feasibility and effectiveness of this approach in patients undergoing laparoscopic surgery for diverticulitis. They found that patients in the fast-track group exhibited faster progression to soft diet ingestion and first bowel movement. Importantly, the fast-track group was discharged from the hospital on postoperative day 3 versus postoperative day 5 for conventional therapy. The morbidity and readmission rates were also lower in the fast-track group. These outcomes highlight the importance of applying fast-track principles to laparoscopic surgery. However, several other larger messages of import are evident in this work. First, application of a standardized approach to perioperative care results in improved outcomes. Standardization reduces the variability of care about the mean and permits a larger percentage of patients to recover more readily. In addition, although not studied in this article, standardization of care most often decreases cost of care. Standardization of care, improved outcomes, and reduced costs are components of a nationwide improvement program. How will this be accom-plished? As demonstrated in this work, teamwork is essential to achieving these results. This will require that surgeons throw away their personal bias about care and examine new methods of pre-, intra-, and postoperative care. Widespread adoption of these principles will allow us to study alternative care pathways that will lead to better outcomes for our patients.

K. E. Behrns, MD

Critical Assessment of Risk Factors for Complications After Cytoreductive Surgery and Perioperative Intraperitoneal Chemotherapy for Pseudo-myxoma Peritonei

Saxena A, Yan TD, Chua TC, et al (Univ of New South Wales, Sydney, Australia)
Ann Surg Oncol 17:1291-1301, 2010

Background.—Cytoreductive surgery (CRS) combined with periopera-tive intraperitoneal chemotherapy (PIC) has demonstrated improved survival in selected patients with pseudomyxoma peritonei (PMP). However, this aggressive treatment modality has been consistently associ-ated with variable rates of perioperative mortality between 0% and 18% and morbidity between 30% and 70%.

This study evaluates the clinical and treatment-related risk factors for perioperative morbidity and mortality in PMP patients who underwent CRS and PIC.

Materials and Methods.—A total of 145 consecutive CRS and PIC procedures for PMP performed between January 1996 and March 2009 were evaluated. The association of 12 clinical and 20 treatment-related risk factors with grades III and IV/V morbidity were assessed by univari-able and multivariable analysis.

Results.—The mortality (grade V) rate was 3%. The morbidity rates of grades III and IV were 23% and 22%, respectively. Eight factors were associated with grade IV/V morbidity on univariable analysis: Peritoneal cancer index ≥21 ($P = .034$), ASA score ≥3 ($P = .003$), operation duration ≥10 h ($P < .001$), left upper quadrant peritonectomy procedure ($P = .037$), colonic resection ($P = .012$), ostomy ($P = .005$), ileostomy ($P = .012$), and transfusion ≥6 units ($p = 0.011$). Multivariable analysis showed 2 significant risk factors for grade IV/V morbidity: ASA ≥ 3 ($P = .006$) and an operation length ≥10 h ($P < .001$).

Conclusions.—CRS and PIC has an acceptable rate of perioperative mortality and morbidity in selected patients with PMP. Patients with bulky disease who undergo a long operation are at a particularly high risk of a severe adverse event.

▶ Saxena et al present confirmatory data that demonstrate large operations can be performed for cytoreductive surgery for pseudomyxoma peritonei and that this treatment can also be accompanied by perioperative intraperitoneal chemotherapy with a relatively low mortality of 3%. As demonstrated by Sugarbaker's group, these operations are also associated with prolonged survival.[1] However, the complication rates associated with these operations are high. The data from this investigation reveal that only 14% of patients did not experience a complication. While many of these adverse events were grade 1 or 2, and the focus of the study was grade 3 or 4 events, the significant number of severe complications is associated with increased length of stay and likely substantial consumption of resources. In the last decade or two, the mortality rates for large operations have declined remarkably, demonstrating that improved surgical approaches combined with fastidious critical care can result in meaningful recovery from extensive operative procedures. In addition, surgeons have also improved complication reporting such that complex operations are known to be associated with morbidity rates of 50% or more. Consequently, we know the data and the new frontier in surgical care should lead to a reduction in the rate of adverse events. This endeavor represents a significant challenge that will require new approaches to surgical care and enhanced teamwork with medical and nursing colleagues. This should be an exciting challenge and a team-building journey.

K. E. Behrns, MD

Reference

1. Yan TD, Black D, Savady R, Sugarbaker PH. A systematic review on the efficacy of cytoreductive surgery and perioperative intraperitoneal chemotherapy for pseudomyxoma peritonei. *Ann Surg Oncol.* 2007;14:484-492.

Oncologic Outcomes of Robotic-Assisted Total Mesorectal Excision for the Treatment of Rectal Cancer

Baek J-H, McKenzie S, Garcia-Aguilar J, et al (Gachon Univ of Medicine and Science, Incheon, Korea; City of Hope Natl Med Ctr, Duarte, CA)
Ann Surg 251:882-886, 2010

Objective.—To evaluate local recurrence and survival after robotic-assisted total mesorectal excision (RTME) for primary rectal cancer.

Summary Background Data.—RTME is a novel approach for the treatment of rectal cancer and has been shown to be safe and effective. However, the oncologic results of this approach have not been reported in terms of local recurrence and survival rate.

Methods.—Sixty-four consecutive rectal cancer patients with stage I–III disease treated between November 2004 and June 2008 were analyzed prospectively.

Results.—All patients underwent RTME: 34 had colorectal anastomosis, 18 underwent coloanal anastomosis, and 12 received abdominoperineal resection. Operative mortality rate was 0%. The median operative time was 270 min and median blood loss was 200 mL. The conversion rate was 9.4%. Anastomotic leakage occurred in 4 of 52 (7.7%) patients with anastomosis. Median number of harvested lymph nodes was 14.5. Median distal margin of tumor was 3.4 cm. The circumferential resection margin was negative in all surgical specimens. No port-site recurrence occurred in any patient. Six patients developed recurrence: 2 combined local and distant, and 4 distal alone (mean follow-up of 20.2 months; range, 1.7–52.5). None of the patients developed isolated local recurrence. The mean time to local recurrence was 23 months. The 3-year overall and disease-free survival rates were 96.2% and 73.7%, respectively.

Conclusions.—RTME can be carried out safely and effectively in terms of recurrence and survival rates. Further prospective randomized trials are necessary to better define the absolute benefits and limitations of robotic rectal surgery.

▶ Adoption of robotic approaches to gastrointestinal surgery has been slow and hampered by the cost of the robot itself, the cost of disposable equipment and necessary training, the purported increase in operative time, and the lack of superior outcomes compared with other approaches. Baek et al share the results of 64 patients who underwent robot-assisted rectal surgery for cancer. Their results nicely show that operative parameters and complication rates are similar to those published for laparoscopic approaches. In addition, the oncologic outcome at 3 years compared favorably with large trials of laparoscopic resection of rectal cancer. Thus, they conclude that the technique is feasible, safe, oncologically appropriate, and worthy of a large, randomized trial. While their conclusions are likely justified, this retrospective study provides data only on the robotic-assisted procedures and does not provide data from a historic control group such as laparoscopic proctectomy. Furthermore, only scant data on costs are included, and they are likely not a reflection of the true cost of the procedure. This study, like many others on robotic surgery, essentially converge on the notion that robotic gastrointestinal surgery offers little data-driven advantage in outcomes, but, once mastered, provides a surgeon-friendly approach to a potentially technically difficult operation. So, what is the ease of an operation worth to the surgeon? Furthermore, does marketing the use of a robotic approach bring more patients in the door? These are difficult questions because we have no metrics to compare this technique with others. However, it is clear that a large volume of robotic surgery must be performed to recoup costs. Thus, it is clear that we need to reduce costs associated with robotic surgery and one place to begin is with training. For example, in an academic department of surgery, up to 10 surgeons (colorectal, pediatric, esophageal, and cardiovascular) may want to obtain training on the robot, and these costs can range from $6000 to $20000 per surgeon. Therefore, it may cost a department up to $200000 to train surgeons to do specific robotic cases. This is a large investment that often cannot provide a return, especially if access to the robot is limited.

K. E. Behrns, MD

Recurrence and Impact of Postoperative Prophylaxis in Laparoscopically Treated Primary Ileocolic Crohn Disease

Malireddy K, Larson DW, Sandborn WJ, et al (Mayo Clinic, Rochester, MN)
Arch Surg 145:42-47, 2010

Objectives.—To define risk factors for recurrence and to determine whether postoperative prophylaxis would influence time to recurrence after primary laparoscopic ileocolectomy for Crohn disease.

Design.—Retrospective record review.

Setting.—Tertiary academic medical center.

Patients.—All patients who underwent primary laparoscopic ileocolectomy for terminal ileal Crohn disease between April 28, 1994, and August 3, 2006, at the Mayo Clinic, Rochester, Minnesota.

Main Outcome Measures.—All patients were reviewed for follow-up, recurrence, risk factors for recurrence, and use of postoperative immuno-suppressive prophylaxis.

Results.—One hundred nine patients were identified, of whom 89 were followed up postoperatively at Mayo Clinic with a median follow-up of 3.5 years (range, 1.8 months to 11.9 years). Recurrence was discovered in 54 patients (61%) at a median of 13.1 months (range, 1.3 months to 8.7 years). Forty-four patients (49%) received postoperative immunosup-pressive prophylaxis (37 [42%] received azathioprine, 8 [9%] received 6-mercaptopurine, and 3 [3%] received infliximab). In a multivariate model of various risk factors for recurrence, presence of granulomas was the only significant predictor of recurrence ($P = .01$). The 2-year cumulative recurrence rates in the prophylaxis and nonprophylaxis groups were 37.5% and 52.6%, respectively (log-rank test, $P = .87$).

Conclusions.—Recurrence occurred in more than half of the patients with Crohn disease after primary laparoscopic ileocolectomy. In this highly selected patient population, use of immunosuppressive prophylaxis was not associated with a delay in recurrence. Presence of granulomas was the only significant predictor of recurrence. These findings should be further explored in larger and less selected patient populations.

▶ Surgical treatment of primary ileocolic Crohn disease is satisfying to the patient and the surgeon in the short term, but as this study, from an experienced surgical group, demonstrates, recurrence of disease is frequent over a relatively short period of time. The recurrence rate in this study was 61% at 13 months. Many studies have examined the factors that are associated with recurrence, and in this retrospective analysis, the presence of granulomas in the specimen was identified more commonly in those patients who developed a recurrence. Over the last 2 decades, several randomized multicenter trials have assessed the benefits of pharmacologic prophylaxis with acetylsalicylic acid-based therapies, purine analogs, antibiotics, or combination therapy. The results of these trials have been mixed, with some investigations demonstrating decreased recurrence with prophylaxis and others failing to confirm these findings. This study too fails to demonstrate a benefit of prophylactic medical therapy. However, close inspection of Fig 2 in the original article does show divergence of the curves (prophylaxis vs no prophylaxis) from years 1 to 3. Does this suggest that there may be some advantage to short-term treatment? Likely little benefit is achieved with prophylaxis, but modulation of the immune system via various mechanisms may alter recurrence and deserves further investigation. Perhaps the presence of granulomas suggests that patients should receive prophylaxis.

K. E. Behrns, MD

Complete Mesocolic Excision With Central Vascular Ligation Produces an Oncologically Superior Specimen Compared With Standard Surgery for Carcinoma of the Colon

West NP, Hohenberger W, Weber K, et al (Univ of Leeds, UK; Leeds General Infirmary, UK; Univ Hosp of Erlangen, Germany)
J Clin Oncol 28:272-278, 2010

Purpose.—The plane of surgery in colonic cancer has been linked to patient outcome although the optimal extent of mesenteric resection is still unclear. Surgeons in Erlangen, Germany, routinely perform complete mesocolic excision (CME) with central vascular ligation (CVL) and report 5-year survivals of higher than 89%. We aimed to further investigate the importance of CME and CVL surgery for colonic cancer by comparison with a series of standard specimens.

Methods.—The fresh photographs of 49 CME and CVL specimens from Erlangen and 40 standard specimens from Leeds, United Kingdom, for primary colonic adenocarcinoma were collected. Precise tissue morphometry and grading of the plane of surgery were performed before comparison to histopathologic variables.

Results.—CME and CVL surgery removed more tissue compared with standard surgery in terms of the distance between the tumor and the high vascular tie (median, 131 *v* 90 mm; $P < .0001$), the length of large bowel (median, 314 *v* 206 mm; $P < .0001$), and ileum removed (median, 83 *v* 63 mm; $P = .003$), and the area of mesentery (19,657 *v* 11,829 mm^2; $P < .0001$). In addition, CME and CVL surgery was associated with more mesocolic plane resections (92% *v* 40%; $P < .0001$) and a greater lymph node yield (median, 30 *v* 18; $P < .0001$).

Conclusion.—Surgeons in Erlangen routinely practicing CME and CVL surgery remove more mesocolon and are more likely to resect in the mesocolic plane when compared with standard excisions. This, along with the associated greater lymph node yield, may partially explain the high 5-year survival rates reported in Erlangen.

▶ West et al present a compelling argument for planar surgery in the resection of colon cancer by demonstrating that the amount of tissue removed by their Erlangen technique is increased and results in a higher lymph node yield. Although not shown directly in this study, they cite additional work that indicates planar resection produces a 15% increase in survival. Planar surgery is an intuitive concept to which most surgeons aspire; however, the execution of pristine planar surgery requires not only meticulous technique but also time. Careful dissection in the operating room should not be rushed and, definitely, must be carefully taught to our next generation of surgeons. Too often, hurried surgical resection results in planar violation, potential contamination of the peritoneal cavity with tumor, and excess blood loss. Furthermore, adequate exposure is a requisite for good mesenteric exposure and appropriate resection. In open surgery, this may require a longer incision. The discussion section of this article also notes that laparoscopic resection may result in the removal of less potential tumor-bearing tissue. Further refinement of laparoscopic techniques may be required to ensure resection of an appropriate volume of mesentery. This article is an important reminder of the necessity for planar surgery and an excellent technique, both of which seemingly have received less attention in recent years given the introduction of minimally invasive surgery. Regardless of the approach to the peritoneal cavity, planar surgery and meticulous technique remain important principles of surgical therapy.

K. E. Behrns, MD

Long-Term Consequences of Not Closing the Mesenteric Defect After Laparoscopic Right Colectomy

Cabot JC, Lee SA, Yoo J, et al (New York Presbyterian Hosp-Columbia Campus; Weill Cornell Dept of Surgery, NY; Univ of California, Los Angeles)
Dis Colon Rectum 53:289-292, 2010

Purpose.—The controversy regarding closing the mesenteric defect after laparoscopic right colectomy remains a subject of debate. This study describes the consequences of not closing the mesenteric defect.

Methods.—A 7-year prospective database revealed 530 consecutive patients who underwent laparoscopic right colectomy for neoplasia. No mesenteric defects were closed. Small bowel obstruction was determined by clinical assessment and diagnostic imaging. Statistical analysis included the Student t test and Mann-Whitney U test.

Results.—On average, the 530 patients (44% male) were 69.6 years old ± 12.5 years with American Society of Anesthesiologists' category 2, body mass index 26.6 ± 5.7, operative time 175 ± 65 minutes, incision length 5.7 ± 3.0 cm. Thirty-six patients (6.8%) were converted. Median length of stay was 5 days (interquartile range 4—7). Median follow-up was 20 months (interquartile range 8—45). Four patients (0.8%) had complications attributed to the mesenteric defect: 2 had small bowel obstruction due to internal herniation and 2 had torsion of the anastomosis through the defect. Twenty-six patients (4.9%) had a small bowel obstruction during the follow-up period. Nonoperative treatment was successful in 12 patients. In the 14 patients who were operated on, small bowel obstruction was due to adhesions (4), incarcerated abdominal wall hernias (4), mesenteric defect (4), and cancer recurrence (2). The small bowel obstruction group (n = 26) had a significantly higher percentage of males than the non-small bowel obstruction group (n = 504; 69% vs 43%; $P = .008$).

Conclusions.—These data do not support routinely closing the mesenteric defect after laparoscopic right colectomy for neoplasia. Additional studies with extended long-term follow-up are needed.

▶ The widespread dissemination of laparoscopic surgery has resulted in significant improvement in postoperative pain, hospital length of stay, and earlier return to normal activities. However, minimally invasive surgery has resulted in a few technical challenges, which generally are overcome by advances in instrumentation or changes in the skill set of operating surgeons. However, Cabot et al studied an important technical component of laparoscopic right colectomy that has not been adequately addressed—closure of the mesenteric defect. They studied 530 patients who underwent laparoscopic right colectomy for neoplasia without closure of the mesenteric defect. During the follow-up period, they identified only 4 patients who developed internal hernias as a result of the open defect. Unfortunately, one of these patients succumbed, the only patient to do so in their large series. Two of the patients with internal hernias had twisted anastomoses, and 3 of the 4 patients presented within small bowel obstruction within 10 days of the laparoscopic procedure. While closure of the mesenteric defect may be technically difficult, these data, though few in number, suggest that performing the mental exercise of replacing the bowel appropriately into the abdominal cavity and critically examining the defect at the conclusion of the operation may have prevented 1 or 2 of these episodes. These data highlight a critical detail that is not yet ingrained in the surgical community—the debriefing at the conclusion of an operation. We are better at performing the time-out and checklist at the beginning of an operation, but infrequently do we pause at the end of the case to mentally review the conduct of the operation. This 30-second exercise should be part of all operations.

K. E. Behrns, MD

Surgical Warranties to Improve Quality and Efficiency in Elective Colon Surgery
Fry DE, Pine M, Jones BL, et al (Michael Pine and Associates, Chicago, IL)
Arch Surg 145:647-652, 2010

Background.—Uncomplicated surgical care has highly variable costs. High costs of complications have led payers to deny additional payments even for predictable complications.

Hypothesis.—A payment warranty indexed to effective and efficient hospitals can promote quality and economic stewardship in surgical care.

Design.—Analysis of hospital costs for elective colon surgery in the Healthcare Cost and Utilization Project's National Inpatient Sample from 2002 through 2005.

Setting.—A 20% sample of acute care hospitals in the United States.

Patients and Methods.—Data for elective colon resections were used to create predictive models for adverse outcomes (AOs) and costs. Total hospital costs were determined using cost-to-charge ratios. Costs of AOs were computed as total costs minus predicted costs of uncomplicated care. Surgical warranties were computed as the probability of AOs times per-case predicted costs of AOs. Final predictive models were calibrated using data only from effective and efficient hospitals.

Results.—We studied 51 602 cases from 632 hospitals. There were 4048 (7.8%) AOs with 505 deaths (1.0%); 19 hospitals had excessive AOs and 95 hospitals had excessive costs. For 518 effective and efficient hospitals, total per-case costs for routine care were $9843 with an average warranty of $1294 and a $276 stop-loss allocation. This cost model would reduce national expenditures for colon surgery by 6%.

Conclusions.—Complications and costs of care can be indexed to quality performing hospitals. Warranties for surgical care can reward effective and efficient care and preclude the need for additional payments for complications.

▶ The need to deliver high-quality, efficient, and effective healthcare has never been greater, and with the upcoming implementation of the Patient Protection and Affordable Care Act, the scrutiny over high-quality care will likely become even more intense. Surgeons will need to focus on appropriate patient selection, decreased complications, and performing operations on reasonable-risk patients so that high quality is maintained. One concept that has gathered attention is that of warranties in surgical care. Fry et al examined this concept with the use of the National Inpatient Sample (NIS), an administrative database that covers approximately 20% of the acute care hospitals nationwide. Using these data and complex statistical analysis, the authors identified effective and efficient hospitals in which the warranty costs for an elective colorectal surgery case was nearly $1300. In ineffective or inefficient hospitals, the warranty costs ranged from $2000 to more than $2300. Thus, the cost of an adverse outcome is quite high. To derive these costs, an adverse outcome rate of 7.8% was determined. This rate of complications in colorectal surgery seems far too low, especially when the rate of wound infection in this cohort of patients approaches 15%. In fact, the NIS is known to have frequent missing data points and likely the low rate of complications is related to administrative abstracting of clinical data. However, the concept of a surgical warranty and shared risk for payment is important and likely will gain traction. Surgeons should become familiar with shared risk models of payment and how complications will impact reimbursement that will likely be bundled with hospital payment.

K. E. Behrns, MD

The Presence of Large Serrated Polyps Increases Risk for Colorectal Cancer
Hiraoka S, Kato J, Fujiki S, et al (Okayama Univ Graduate School of Medicine, Dentistry, and Pharmaceutical Sciences; Tsuyama Central Hosp, Okayama; et al)
Gastroenterology 139:1503-1510, 2010

Background & Aims.—There is evidence that serrated polyps (serrated adenomas and hyperplastic polyps) have different malignant potential than traditional adenomas. We used a colonoscopy database to determine the association between the presence of serrated colorectal polyps and colorectal neoplasia.

Methods.—We performed a multicenter observational study of 10,199 subjects who underwent first-time colonoscopies. Data collected on study subjects included age and sex and the location, size, and histology of polyps or tumors found at colonoscopy. Serrated polyps were defined as those diagnosed by the pathologists in the participating hospitals as a serrated lesion (a lesion given the term of "classical hyperplastic polyp," "traditional serrated adenoma," "sessile serrated adenoma," or "mixed serrated polyp"). Large serrated polyps (LSPs) were defined as those ≥ 10 mm.

Results.—There were 1573 patients (15.4%) with advanced neoplasia, 708 patients (6.9%) with colorectal cancer (CRC), and 140 patients (1.4%) with LSPs in our cohort. Multivariate analysis associated the

TABLE 6.—Characteristics of Large Serrated Polyps and Risk of Colorectal Neoplasia

	Distal Advanced Neoplasia, Adjusted OR (95% CI)[a]	Proximal Advanced Neoplasia, Adjusted OR (95% CI)[a]	Distal Cancer, Adjusted OR (95% CI)[b]	Proximal Cancer, Adjusted OR (95% CI)[b]
Proximal LSP	3.41 (2.04–5.53)[c]	4.25 (2.33–7.31)[d]	2.10 (0.96–4.08)	5.36 (2.40–10.8)[d]
Distal LSP	2.57 (1.45–4.38)[c]	2.93 (1.46–5.45)[c]	2.44 (1.11–4.76)[e]	4.12 (1.55–9.19)[c]
Flat-type LSP	3.97 (2.49–6.21)[d]	2.99 (1.61–5.18)[d]	2.74 (1.42–4.86)[c]	2.66 (1.01–5.86)[e]
Protruded LSP	1.62 (0.76–3.17)	5.24 (2.63–9.82)[d]	1.75 (0.60–4.09)	9.00 (2.75–19.2)[d]
Number of LSP ≥2	3.42 (1.15–9.12)[e]	2.70 (0.60–8.66)	3.15 (0.72–9.89)	4.65 (0.70–18.0)

[a]Relative risk adjusted for age, gender, and number of small adenomas.
[b]Relative risk adjusted for age, gender, number of adenomas, and the presence of adenoma (≥10 mm).
[c]$P < .01$.
[d]$P < .001$.
[e]$P < .05$.

presence of LSPs with advanced neoplasia (odds ratio [OR], 4.01; 95% confidence interval [CI], 2.83–5.69) and CRC (OR, 3.34; 95% CI, 2.16–5.03). The presence of LSPs was the greatest risk factor for CRC, particularly for proximal CRC (OR, 4.79; 95% CI, 2.54–8.42). Proximal and protruded LSPs were the highest risk factors for proximal CRC (OR, 5.36; 95% CI, 2.40–10.8 and OR, 9.00; 95% CI, 2.75–19.2, respectively).

Conclusions.—The presence of LSPs is a risk factor for CRC, particularly CRC of the proximal colon (Table 6).

▶ The adenoma-to-carcinoma morphologic and genetic sequences for the development of colorectal carcinoma have been beautifully revealed over a number of years by a series of elegant translational studies. This paper by Hiraoka et al adds additional morphologic findings related to the examination of serrated polyps. The findings of this work are tremendously important because heretofore we have considered many of these small hyperplastic polyps as insignificant growths. In this data set, large (> 10 mm) serrated adenomas were a risk factor for the development of proximal and distal advanced neoplasia and colorectal cancer. Obviously, large is a relative term, and likely endoscopists worldwide have skipped over many 1-cm hyperplastic polyps. Therefore, identification of these lesions as a marker for colorectal cancer is a significant finding. Furthermore, it appears that these lesions are markers for colorectal cancer throughout the colon; thus, a predilection for a site of cancer development is not a consideration (Table 6). These data will likely shed new light on the genetic alterations that occur in the development of colorectal neoplasia. Furthermore, the concept of surveillance in the presence of serrated adenomas may need to be reexamined. Likely, the current guidelines will remain in place; however, for those patients with serrated adenomas, longitudinal follow-up will be important.

K. E. Behrns, MD

A Characterization of Factors Determining Postoperative Ileus After Laparoscopic Colectomy Enables the Generation of a Novel Predictive Score

Kronberg U, Kiran RP, Soliman MSM, et al (Cleveland Clinic, OH; et al)
Ann Surg 253:78-81, 2011

Background/Objective.—Postoperative ileus (POI) after colorectal surgery is associated with prolonged hospital stay and increased costs. The aim of this study is to investigate pre-, intra-, and postoperative risk factors associated with the development of POI in patients undergoing laparoscopic partial colectomy.

Methods.—Patients operated between 2004 and 2008 were retrospectively identified from a prospectively maintained database, and clinical, metabolic, and pharmacologic data were obtained. *Postoperative ileus* was defined as the absence of bowel function for 5 or more days or the need for reinsertion of a nasogastric tube after starting oral diet in the absence of mechanical obstruction. Associations between likelihood of POI and study variables were assessed univariably by using χ^2 tests, Fisher exact tests, and logistic regression models. A scoring system for prediction of POI was constructed by using a multivariable logistic regression model based on forward stepwise selection of preoperative factors.

Results.—A total of 413 patients (mean age, 58 years; 53.5% women) were included, and 42 (10.2%) of them developed POI. Preoperative albumin, postoperative deep-vein thrombosis, and electrolyte levels were associated with POI. Age, previous abdominal surgery, and chronic preoperative use of narcotics were independently correlated with POI on multivariate analysis, which allowed the creation of a predictive score. Patients with a score of 2 or higher had an 18.3% risk of POI (*P* < 0.001).

Conclusion.—Postoperative ileus after laparoscopic partial colectomy is associated with specific preoperative and postoperative factors. The likelihood of POI can be predicted by using a preoperative scoring system. Addressing the postoperative factors may be expected to reduce the incidence of this common complication in high-risk patients.

▶ Intestinal surgery results in relatively long hospital stays largely because the surgeon and patient are anxiously awaiting return of bowel function. Though some studies have suggested that patients who have had intestinal resection may be dismissed earlier on a clear liquid diet, a subset of patients fail this approach because of the development of postoperative ileus. Numerous studies have attempted a variety of therapeutic interventions to treat ileus, but these have universally failed. One reason for the difficulty in finding a reliable treatment is patient selection. Not all patients with bowel resection will develop an ileus, and thus, treatment is not directed toward high-risk patients only. This is complicated by the fact that little research exists on the amelioration of ileus after laparoscopic surgery. The study by Kronberg et al, however, addresses both issues. They studied a large group of patients who had laparoscopic colectomy and identified 3 variables associated with the onset of ileus.

Age, previous abdominal surgery, and chronic use of preoperative narcotics were all associated with postoperative ileus. The authors developed a predictive scoring system based on these 3 independent variables. Therefore, patients at risk may be identified by this straightforward scoring system. However, some caution should be exercised because this study does not prove that this scoring system is truly predictive. Only a prospective trial examining these variables will confidently address the utility of this scoring system. Nonetheless, the identification of these variables paves the way for this important study. General and gastrointestinal surgeons worldwide are anxious to alleviate postoperative ileus.

K. E. Behrns, MD

Fibrin Glue Is Effective Healing Perianal Fistulas in Patients with Crohn's Disease

Grimaud J-C, the Groupe d'Etude Thérapeutique des Affections Inflammatoires du Tube Digestif (GETAID) (Université Méditerranée, Marseille; et al)
Gastroenterology 138:2275-2281, 2010

Background & Aims.—Fibrin glue is a therapeutic for fistulas that activates thrombin to form a fibrin clot, which mechanically seals the fistula tract. We assessed the efficacy and safety of a heterologous fibrin glue that was injected into the fistula tracts of patients with Crohn's disease (ClinicalTrials.gov No. NCT00723047).

Methods.—This multicenter, open-label, randomized controlled trial included patients with a Crohn's disease activity index ≤250 and fistulas between the anus (or low rectum) and perineum, vulva, or vagina, that drained for more than 2 months. Magnetic resonance imaging or endosonography was performed to assess fistula tracts and the absence of abscesses. Patients were stratified into groups with simple or complex fistulas and randomly assigned to receive fibrin glue injections (n = 36) or only observation (n = 41) after removal of setons. The primary end point was clinical remission at week 8, defined as the absence of draining, perianal pain, or abscesses. At week 8, a fibrin glue injection was offered to patients who were not in remission.

Results.—Clinical remission was observed in 13 of the 34 patients (38%) of the fibrin glue group compared with 6 of the 37 (16%) in the observation group; these findings demonstrate the benefit of fibrin glue (odds ratio, 3.2; 95% confidence interval: 1.1–9.8; $P = .04$). The benefit seemed to be greater in patients with simple fistulas. Four patients in the fibrin glue group and 6 in the observation group had adverse events.

Conclusions.—Fibrin glue injection is a simple, effective, and well-tolerated therapeutic option for patients with Crohn's disease and perianal fistula tracts.

▶ Grimaud et al present breakthrough results of a prospective, multicenter, randomized trial studying the effectiveness of fibrin glue in healing of perianal fistulas in Crohn disease (CD). The results showed that patients with fistulas treated with fibrin glue obtained clinical remission in 38% of cases versus only 16% in the observation group with an odds ratio of 3.2. Toxicity was minimal. At first glance, even though the results of the trial favor the experimental arm, a 38% remission rate is not awe inspiring. However, the study included patients with simple and complex fistula tracks, and, not surprisingly, the complex fistulas appeared to respond less well. Surgical experience tells us that complex fistula tracks often harbor small amounts of purulent material that will continue to drive a relatively indolent inflammatory process and preclude complete healing. Clearly, the authors attempted to select patients in whom the inflammatory process has largely abated, as determined by the low CD activity index and extensive imaging. If the fistulous disease is extensive, did the patients receive a diverting ostomy? Also, has the patient been treated with antitumor necrosis factor (TNF) therapy and, if so, when? So where does this trial lead us? A more comprehensive study of these patients would include treatment with anti-TNF therapy preceding fibrin glue treatment. Perhaps patients with complex fistulas should undergo diversion, followed by anti-TNF therapy and then fibrin glue treatment. Finally, the data are clear that if fibrin glue therapy is unsuccessful, there is no need for a second attempt. This important study will likely serve as a platform for further studies examining the combination of anti-TNF therapy and fibrin glue.

K. E. Behrns, MD

Mucosal Advancement Flap Anoplasty for Chronic Anal Fissure Resistant to Conservative Therapy
Ouaïssi M, Giger U, Sielezneff I, et al (Hôpital Timone, Marseille Cedex, France)
World J Surg 35:900-904, 2011

Background.—Sphincter-sparing procedures are increasingly advocated in the treatment of chronic anal fissures (CAF) resistant to conservative management. Herein, we report about our results with sphincter-sparing transanal mucosal advancement flap anoplasty (MAAP) to treat CAF.

Patients and Methods.—The present study was a retrospective single-center analysis of patients in whom conservative management of CAF failed and who subsequently underwent MAAP between January 2003 and December 2008.

Results.—A total of 26 patients with a median age of 46.5 years (range: 17—79 years) had undergone MAAP after suffering with CAF for a median period of 9 months (range: 4—36 months). Surgery was well tolerated in all patients. One patient developed a perianal abscess at the operative site 3 weeks after MAAP, which required excision. At 2, 12, and 24 months follow-up, all patients were free of pain with no fissure recurrence or any worsening of incontinence.

Conclusions.—Mucosal advancement flap anoplasty might be another sphincter-sparing treatment option in patients suffering from CAF. To draw final conclusions about the value of MAAP in the treatment of CAF, more solid data are required.

▶ Ouaïssi et al have advanced the thought process of surgical management of chronic anal fissure by eliminating sphincteroplasty and covering the fissure with a mucosal advancement flap. This approach deviates markedly from the traditional approach that includes sphincterotomy to release the pressure of an overly active internal sphincter with secondary healing of the fissure. With this approach, the internal sphincter is chemically relaxed with botulinum toxin and the fissure is covered with the advancement flap. Thus, this approach includes not only relaxation of the sphincter but also coverage of the chronic wound and often exposed fissure. As the authors point out, this study sets the stage for a randomized clinical trial. However, what question will be answered in the trial? This study raises several questions that challenge long-held concepts. For example, what is the importance sphincterotomy, be it chemical or physical? Is it important to cover the fissure defect, a principle not thought important for many years? These questions are important to address because the design of the trial depends on the priority of these questions, both of which are important. In fact, it is doubtful that both questions could be addressed simultaneously because the number of patients needed to adequately address these questions would be prohibitive. This article is important because although it is straightforward in terms of results, the questions raised are important and markedly alter how we think about the surgical treatment of chronic anal fissures.

K. E. Behrns, MD

Outcomes After Fistulotomy: Results of a Prospective, Multicenter Regional Study
Hyman N, O'Brien S, Osler T (Univ of Vermont, Burlington)
Dis Colon Rectum 52:2022-2027, 2009

Purpose.—This study aimed to determine the outcome sand healing rate after fistula surgery across a broad spectrum of colorectal practices.

Methods.—A prospective, multicenter outcomes registry was created by the New England Regional Chapter of The American Society of Colon and Rectal Surgeons. All consecutive patients undergoing surgical treatment of an anal fistula by a participating surgeon from October 1, 2007 to September 30, 2008, were entered. Demographics, fistula characteristics including Parks' classification, smoking history, previous vaginal deliveries, diagnosis of Crohn's disease, Fecal Incontinence Severity Index, and operations performed were noted. A follow-up datasheet recorded postoperative complications, healing at one and three months, and postoperative continence scores. Factors associated with healing and treatment success were compared by use of Fisher's exact test.

Results.—Twenty-five surgeons at 13 hospitals entered 245 patients (162 male, 83 female) in the registry. Seventy-five patients had recurrent fistulas, 51 had multiple tracts, 62 were smokers, and 24 had Crohn's disease. The overall healing rate was 19.5% at one month and 63.2% at three months. Female gender ($P = 0.04$) and recurrent fistula ($P = 0.03$) were associated with nonhealing, and 28.4% of patients required additional surgery. The best healing rate was associated with fistulotomy (87%), whereas a plug had the worst healing rate (32%, $P = 0.001$).

Conclusions.—Surgical treatment of an anal fistula is associated with a substantial risk of nonhealing at three months. Fistulotomy had a high success rate, whereas the bioprosthetic plug had the lowest success rate. Multicenter studies comparing treatment options for similar fistulas are needed.

▶ Patients with many anal disorders typically experience significant discomfort that is difficult to remedy without surgery, and, therefore, well-executed anorectal surgery can provide significant relief and healing. Anal fistulas are often considered simple problems that can be easily addressed through fistulotomy or use of an anal plug. However, the data by Hyman et al show that treatment of anal fistulas had a disappointing 3-month healing rate of 63%. Despite enthusiasm for the use of plug repair, the healing rate with this modality was only 32% at 3 months. Thus, continued use of this method of treatment should be in the context of a well-constructed trial to provide clear data on which patients, if any, will benefit from this treatment. This study is a good example of consortium data in which 25 surgeons from 13 hospitals treated 245 patients surgically with anal fistulae for 12 months. Collectively, group participation allowed entry of a significant number of patients in a relatively short period of time. While rapid recruitment of patients is an obvious strength of this group approach, the use of standardized protocol of treatment or randomization of treatment would enhance this registry. Furthermore, perhaps because of inconsistencies in defining results or recording data, a data monitoring group that visits the participating sites on a regular basis and reviews results would ensure appropriate designation of outcomes. Nonetheless, this first step in the development of a regional registry once again demonstrates the use of cooperation in reporting results and accruing a significant number of patients in a short period of time.

K. E. Behrns, MD

Natural Orifice Translumenal Endoscopic Surgery Used for Perforated Viscus Repair Is Feasible Using Lower Peritoneal Pressures than Laparoscopy in a Porcine Model

Moran EA, Gostout CJ, McConico AL, et al (Mayo Clinic, Rochester, MN)
J Am Coll Surg 210:474-479, 2010

Background.—Procedure-related complications contribute to 1-year mortality in patients with perforated ulcers. Natural orifice translumenal endoscopic surgery (NOTES) might offer a new repair approach.

Study Design.—Swine were randomized to laparoscopic or NOTES repair. Laparoscopic gastrotomy creation (1 cm) was followed by 4 hours soilage time. After peritoneal cavity irrigation (per group assignment), repair proceeded with a laparoscopic or NOTES approach. For NOTES repair, omentum was endoscopically grasped, pulled into the gastric lumen, and fixed with metallic clips. Feasibility; time to complete procedures; pneumoperitoneal pressures; and clinical parameters, including necropsy and peritoneal culture at 2 weeks, were recorded.

Results.—NOTES repair failed in 1 animal (technical); repair was completed laparoscopically, and data were analyzed as intention to treat. Specific NOTES repair time (minutes) was comparable with laparoscopy (36 versus 46; p = 0.2). Mean abdominal pressure (mmHg) required to complete NOTES repair was lower than in laparoscopy (4 versus 12; p < 0.001). Nineteen of 23 animals thrived until necropsy at 2 weeks. Three animals succumbed to airway compromise in recovery; 1 NOTES animal failed to thrive on postoperative day 7. No intra-abdominal cause for these deaths was found. At necropsy all repairs were intact, and peritoneal cultures revealed a small and equivalent amount of colony-forming units in each group.

Conclusions.—Endoscopic ulcer repair appears technically feasible with similar clinical and infectious outcomes to laparoscopy. The lower required pneumoperitoneal pressures used in these NOTES techniques are recognizable different outcomes from laparoscopy and can be advantageous in critically ill patients.

▶ Perforated gastroduodenal ulcer disease is increasingly uncommon with the introduction of histamine antagonists, proton pump inhibitors, and *Helicobacter pylori* treatment; however, the surgical treatment remains unchanged in principle. Regardless of the method of peritoneal lavage and closure of the defect, the mortality and morbidity of surgery for perforated ulcer disease remain high. The introduction of laparoscopic techniques, though not widely adopted, has limited wound complications and represents an advance in patient treatment. In this article, Moran et al report on the use of natural orifice translumenal endoscopic surgery (NOTES) in a porcine model of perforation. The results of this study demonstrate that NOTES compares favorably with laparoscopic repair of a gastric perforation, and this technique could potentially provide an alternative method of repair. Interestingly, the intra-abdominal pressure required to repair the ulcer via NOTES was markedly decreased compared with the laparoscopic approach. The decrease in pressure required does not have immediately obvious benefits, but it could impact peritoneal bacterial dissemination. As noted by the authors, even though NOTES may be advantageous in that no abdominal wounds are present, this technique may be difficult in the inflamed peritoneal cavity with a thick omentum that is adhered to peritoneal structures. In addition, the size of the perforation may be a significant limitation in that large perforations may not be closed adequately by an omental pull-through technique. Nonetheless, adoption of NOTES for perforation in select and appropriate cases may allow the development of modified approaches and improved instrumentation. Surgeons would be well advised to develop familiarity and comfort with this approach.

K. E. Behrns, MD

The German Registry for Natural Orifice Translumenal Endoscopic Surgery: Report of the First 551 Patients
Lehmann KS, Ritz JP, Wibmer A, et al (Charité Univ Hosp—Campus Benjamin Franklin, Berlin, Germany; et al)
Ann Surg 252:263-270, 2010

Objective.—To analyze patient outcome in the first 14 months of the German natural orifice translumenal endoscopic surgery (NOTES) registry (GNR).

Summary Background Data.—NOTES is a new surgical concept, which permits scarless intra-abdominal operations through natural orifices, such as the mouth, vagina, rectum, or urethra. The GNR was established as a nationwide outcome database to allow the monitoring and safe introduction of this technique in Germany.

Methods.—The GNR was designed as a voluntary database with online access. All surgeons in Germany who performed NOTES procedures were requested to participate in the registry. The GNR recorded demographical and therapy data as well as data on the postoperative course.

Results.—A total of 572 target organs were operated in 551 patients. Cholecystectomies accounted for 85.3% of all NOTES procedures. All procedures were performed in female patients using transvaginal hybrid technique. Complications occurred in 3.1% of all patients, conversions to laparoscopy or open surgery in 4.9%. In cholecystectomies, institutional case volume, obesity, and age had substantial effect on conversion rate, operation length, and length of hospital stay, but no effect on complications.

Conclusions.—Despite the fact that NOTES has just recently been introduced, the technique has already gained considerable clinical application. Transvaginal hybrid NOTES cholecystectomy is a practicable and safe alternative to laparoscopic resection even in obese or older patients.

▶ Natural orifice translumenal endoscopic surgery (NOTES) has been under development for over 5 years. It is often advertised as scarless surgery and is the new wave of minimally invasive surgery. However, Lehmann et al and the German Society for General and Visceral Surgery are careful not to repeat the mistakes associated with the introduction of laparoscopic surgery. They developed a voluntary database (German NOTES Registry) such that the members of their organization could record NOTES procedures. The data presented were accrued over a 14-month period. Interestingly, 64 institutions signaled intent to enter data, but only 28 entered results during the study period. It is clear that the 28 reporting institutions have made a significant investment in NOTES but will the return on investment be realized? First, the promise of scarless surgery has not been achieved because almost every patient had a hybrid procedure with a transabdominal trocar inserted, and in some procedures, the mean number of trocars was 3. In addition, as the authors highlight, there is likely a reporting bias, but the bias may not be to report all-inclusive results. For example, the database contains some inconsistencies, including the finding that complications occurred only in cholecystectomy procedures, but over 28% of colectomies were associated with conversion to laparoscopic or open surgery. Finally, most notable is the 3-day length of stay for cholecystectomy. In the United States, approximately two-thirds of laparoscopic cholecystectomies are performed on an outpatient basis. Thus, the hospital stay for cholecystectomy by NOTES represents a regression in care. NOTES remains in development, and likely improved instrumentation will result in ease of performance and, hopefully, improved results. However, to date, the data suggest that NOTES procedures do not represent a clear advance in surgical care.

K. E. Behrns, MD

Open intraperitoneal versus retromuscular mesh repair for umbilical hernias less than 3 cm diameter
Berrevoet F, D'Hont F, Rogiers X, et al (Univ Hosp Med School, Ghent, Belgium)
Am J Surg 201:85-90, 2011

Background.—Mesh techniques are the preferable methods for repair of small ventral hernias, as a primary suture repair shows high recurrence rates. The aim of this prospective study was to compare the retromuscular sublay technique with the intraperitoneal underlay technique for primary umbilical hernias.

Methods.—From February 2004 to April 2007, all patients treated for umbilical hernias with maximum diameters of 3 cm were prospectively followed. During the first period of 15 months, all patients were treated with retromuscular repair using a large pore mesh (Vypro). After that period, for all patients, mesh repair using an intraperitoneal Ventralex patch was performed. All patients underwent general anesthesia. This analysis included 116 patients, of whom 56 had retromuscular repair (group I; mean age, 54.8 years; mean body mass index, 28.2 kg/m^2) and 60 had open intraperitoneal repair (group II; mean age, 48.1 years; mean body mass index, 29.4 kg/m^2). Operating time was evaluated as skin-to-skin time, and drain management was noted for both techniques. Follow-up was ≥2 years for all patients, and both early and late complications were registered, including seroma and hematoma formation, wound infection, fistula formation, and recurrence rates. Preoperative and postoperative pain was evaluated using a visual analogue scale (range, 0–10) on the day of the first outpatient visit; on postoperative days 1, 7, and 21; and after 1 year. Quality of life was estimated using the EQ-5D questionnaire 1 year after surgery. All data were analyzed using SPSS version 15 software. Wilcoxon's rank-sum test was used to analyze continuous variables, and repeated-measures analysis of variance was used for visual analogue scale scores. The χ^2 test and Fisher's exact test were used to assess the differences between categorical data. *P* values < .05 were considered statistically significant.

Results.—The mean operative times were 79.9 minutes in group I and 33.9 minutes in group II (*P* < .001). The mean hospital stay was significantly longer in group I (3.8 vs 2.1 days, *P* < .001). Seromas and superficial wound infections in the early postoperative period were not different between both groups, although seromas occurred more frequent in the retromuscular group. Postoperative visual analogue scale scores were significantly lower with the intraperitoneal technique at all time points (*P* < .003, repeated-measures analysis of variance). However, 3 patients with the Ventralex patch had to be readmitted for severe pain. The recurrence rate was higher with the intraperitoneal repair (n = 5 [8.3%] vs n = 2 [3.6%]) than for the retromuscular mesh repair, but not statistically significant. Quality of life was comparable in the two groups after 1 year.

Conclusions.—The open intraperitoneal technique using a Ventralex mesh for umbilical hernias seems a very elegant and quick technique. However, possibly because of the less controllable mesh deployment, recurrence rates seem higher. In case open mesh repair is the preferred treatment, a retromuscular repair should be the first choice.

▶ The debate over the most appropriate technique to repair small umbilical hernia defects has been ongoing for many years. Should the repairs be performed primarily or with mesh? Should an open or laparoscopic approach be used? What type of mesh should be used? Where should the mesh be placed: onlay, sublay, or intraperitoneal? All of these questions, and the factors associated with these questions, are important to achieve the ultimate goal: a recurrence-free repair. Berrevoet et al seek to provide some incremental information in terms of the type of mesh used and the location of the mesh placement. They examined equally balanced groups of patients with less than 3 cm umbilical hernias and placed mesh in the retromuscular position versus the intraperitoneal position. Unfortunately, they used different mesh materials in each location; thus, complicating the analysis by adding another variable (mesh type) rather than assessing mesh location alone. They found that the intraperitoneal approach was quicker, easier, and better tolerated initially by the patients. However, the recurrence for the intraperitoneal approach was more than twice as high as the retromuscular approach. As the authors correctly note, the recurrence rate is the most important outcome variable. Although this trial is underpowered, it demonstrates the high recurrence rate for the intraperitoneal repair, which is advertised as a quick easy-to-place material and, therefore, appealing to the surgeon. However, ease of placement and surgeon convenience are not primary outcomes; hernia repair that is free of recurrence and excellent patient outcomes are the goals. When analyzing new surgical techniques and materials, we should keep in mind that if the technique seems too easy and too good to be true, then that indeed may be the case. The results of this trial suggest that intraperitoneal mesh placement is little better than primary repair of umbilical hernias. Finally, minimally secured intraperitoneal mesh has a tendency to migrate and result in a failed repair.

K. E. Behrns, MD

A novel approach for the simultaneous repair of large midline incisional and parastomal hernias with biological mesh and retrorectus reconstruction

Rosen MJ, Reynolds HL, Champagne B, et al (Univ Hosps of Cleveland, OH)
Am J Surg 199:416-421, 2010

Introduction.—Patients with concomitant large midline incisional and parastomal hernias present many unique challenges to the reconstructive surgeon.

Methods.—We describe a novel approach of simultaneously repairing the midline incisional and parastomal defect, while prophylactically reinforcing the relocated stoma site with a retrorectus biological graft.

Results.—During the study period, 9 men and 3 women with a mean age of 65 years, body mass index (BMI) 34 kg/m^2, and American Society of Anesthesiologists score (ASA) 3.1 underwent repair. Hernia defects averaged 338 cm^2. Seven patients had a myofascial advancement flap. Mean operative time was 277 minutes. Postoperative complications occurred in 4 patients (33%) and included superficial surgical site infection, transient renal failure, and deep venous thrombosis; in addition, 1 patient died suddenly on postoperative day 3. After a mean follow-up of 14 months, 2 patients have asymptomatic hernia recurrence.

Conclusions.—The use of various advanced abdominal wall reconstructive techniques may offer an acceptable approach to repairing these challenging defects.

▶ Rosen et al present a challenging group of patients who present with concomitant ventral incisional hernias and parastomal fascial defects. This combination of hernias is difficult to address, and the options are often limited by the size of the defect and the need to relocate the stoma, which introduces the possibility of a mesh infection. In addition, many of these patients have significant comorbidities, and this series is especially notable in that the patients were elderly and obese and a quarter had an active infection. The procedure is relatively high risk because 1 patient died. The follow-up in this series was short at 14 months, and 2 patients had asymptomatic hernia recurrences. Nonetheless, the technique described by the authors is intriguing because it uses a retrorectus mesh placement, which is thought to be more physiologic. Furthermore, the use of the component separation provides maximal release of the abdominal wall creating less tension. Complete coverage of the biologic with native tissue is advantageous because a wound infection with exposed biologic can be difficult to address. Despite several advances in the surgical care and availability of techniques, the recurrence rates remain high and suggest that we need to develop additional techniques, adjuvants or improve patient selection.

Certainly, limiting hernia repair to symptomatic patients who are nonobese, nondiabetic, and do not have an active infection may improve results. Moreover, the time to investigate fibrosis-inducing agents or matrix metalloproteinase-inhibiting drugs in the repair of these complex hernias has arrived.

K. E. Behrns, MD

Chronic pain 5 years after randomized comparison of laparoscopic and Lichtenstein inguinal hernia repair
Eklund A, for the Swedish Multicentre Trial of Inguinal Hernia Repair by Laparoscopy (SMIL) study group (Central Hosp, Västerås, Sweden; et al)
Br J Surg 97:600-608, 2010

Background.—Chronic postoperative pain is a major drawback of inguinal hernia repair. This study compared the frequency of chronic pain after laparoscopic (totally extraperitoneal patch, TEP) and open (Lichtenstein) repairs.

Methods.—A randomized multicentre study with 5 years' follow-up was conducted on men with a primary inguinal hernia. Chronic pain was categorized as mild, moderate or severe by blinded observers. A subgroup analysis was performed on 121 patients who experienced moderate or severe pain at any time during follow-up.

Results.—Overall, 1370 of 1512 randomized patients underwent surgery, 665 in the TEP and 705 in the Lichtenstein group. The total incidence of chronic pain was $11 \cdot 0$ *versus* $21 \cdot 7$ per cent at 1 year, $11 \cdot 0$ *versus* $24 \cdot 8$ per cent at 2 years, $9 \cdot 9$ *versus* $20 \cdot 2$ per cent at 3 years and $9 \cdot 4$ *versus* $18 \cdot 8$ per cent at 5 years in the TEP and Lichtenstein groups respectively ($P < 0 \cdot 001$). After 5 years, $1 \cdot 9$ per cent of patients in the TEP and $3 \cdot 5$ per cent in the Lichtenstein group reported moderate or severe pain ($P = 0 \cdot 092$). Of the 121 patients, 72 ($59 \cdot 5$ per cent) no longer reported pain a median of $9 \cdot 4$ (range $6 \cdot 7 - 10 \cdot 8$) years after operation.

Conclusion.—Five years after surgery only a small proportion of patients still report moderate to severe chronic pain. Laparoscopic inguinal hernia repair leads to less chronic pain than open repair. Registration number: NCT00568269 (http://www.clinicaltrials.gov).

▶ Advances in inguinal hernia repair have resulted in less focus on the declining recurrence rates and more concentration on functional outcomes. Chronic inguinal pain has become the focal point of functional outcomes because of the relative frequency of this sometimes bothersome and sometimes disabling outcome after inguinal hernia repair. Eklund et al use the results from a large randomized trial of open Lichtenstein repair versus laparoscopic repair by totally extraperitoneal patch (TEP) to compare the incidence of chronic inguinal pain. The recurrence rate of TEP was higher (yet only 3.5%), but the rate of chronic inguinal pain was markedly lower in TEP compared with Lichtenstein repair at 1, 2, 3, and 5 years. Thus, the functional outcome appears to be improved in the laparoscopic group. However, it should be noted that by 5 years of follow-up, the rate of chronic inguinal pain was low in both groups. This is an important finding that suggests that surgeons should be slow to reintervene in patients with chronic inguinal pain because the rate of spontaneous resolution is high. The experimental design of this study is limited a bit because this study, as part of a larger study, was not powered to study the rate of chronic inguinal pain but the recurrence rate. Therefore, the number of patients available for follow-up at 5 years is low. Nonetheless, this study addresses the important question of chronic inguinal pain, which obviously should be treated by nonoperative means because resolution over time is the norm.

K. E. Behrns, MD

Working With a Fixed Operating Room Team on Consecutive Similar Cases and the Effect on Case Duration and Turnover Time
Stepaniak PS, Vrijland WW, de Quelerij M, et al (Erasmus Univ Rotterdam, the Netherlands; St Franciscus Hosp, Rotterdam, the Netherlands)
Arch Surg 145:1165-1170, 2010

Hypothesis.—If variation in procedure times could be controlled or better predicted, the cost of surgeries could be reduced through improved scheduling of surgical resources. This study on the impact of similar consecutive cases on the turnover, surgical, and procedure times tests the perception that repeating the same manual tasks reduces the duration of these tasks. We hypothesize that when a fixed team works on similar consecutive cases the result will be shorter turnover and procedure duration as well as less variation as compared with the situation without a fixed team.

Design.—Case-control study.

Setting.—St Franciscus Hospital, a large general teaching hospital in Rotterdam, the Netherlands.

Patients.—Two procedures, inguinal hernia repair and laparoscopic cholecystectomy, were selected and divided across a control group and a study group. Patients were randomly assigned to the study or control group.

Main Outcome Measures.—Preparation time, surgical time, procedure time, and turnover time.

Results.—For inguinal hernia repair, we found a significantly lower preparation time and 10 minutes less procedure time in the study group, as compared with the control group. Variation in the study group was lower, as compared with the control group. For laparoscopic cholecystectomy, preparation time was significantly lower in the study group, as compared with the control group. For both procedures, there was a significant decrease in turnover time.

Conclusions.—Scheduling similar consecutive cases and performing with a fixed team results in lower turnover times and preparation times. The procedure time of the inguinal hernia repair decreased significantly

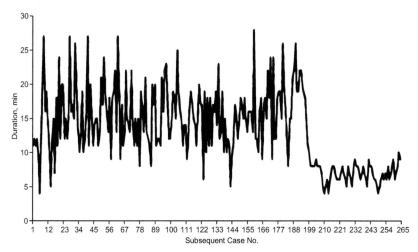

FIGURE.—Preparation time of 200 inguinal hernia repairs prior to starting the study and 68 during the study. (Reprinted from Stepaniak PS, Vrijland WW, de Quelerij M, et al. Working with a fixed operating room team on consecutive similar cases and the effect on case duration and turnover time. *Arch Surg.* 2010;145:1165-1170, with permission from American Medical Association.)

and has practical scheduling implications. For more complex surgery, like laparoscopic cholecystectomy, there is no effect on procedure time (Fig).

▶ As the health care dollars come under tighter control, all practices are examining methods to better use resources. These changes in operational management are most evident where the resources are expensive and time must be used efficiently. Not surprisingly, most hospitals have investigated the efficiency of their operating room. In this study, Stepaniak et al assessed the operating room preparation time, surgical time, and turnover time in the presence or absence of a fixed team of nurses, anesthesiologists, and surgeons. They found that the preparation and turnover times were decreased when a fixed team was employed. Also, for less complex operations, such as inguinal hernia repair, the surgical time was decreased. This study emphasizes the need for standardization in the care of our patients. Reducing the variance (Fig), as this study clearly shows, improves our processes and results in enhanced use of expensive resources, such as the operating room. As health care providers, we need to analyze every step in the delivery of care and standardize the process so that we can most effectively care for our patients. Furthermore, studies have definitively demonstrated that this approach results in better outcomes. Finally, because the surgical time for laparoscopic cholecystectomy was not improved with a fixed team, the question arises, were the steps of this operation standardized?

K. E. Behrns, MD

Immunonutrition in gastrointestinal surgery

Cerantola Y, Hübner M, Grass F, et al (Univ Hosp Vaudois (CHUV), Bugnon, Lausanne, Switzerland)
Br J Surg 98:37-48, 2011

Background.—Patients undergoing major gastrointestinal surgery are at increased risk of developing complications. The use of immunonutrition (IN) in such patients is not widespread because the available data are heterogeneous, and some show contradictory results with regard to complications, mortality and length of hospital stay.

Methods.—Randomized controlled trials (RCTs) published between January 1985 and September 2009 that assessed the clinical impact of perioperative enteral IN in major gastrointestinal elective surgery were included in a meta-analysis.

Results.—Twenty-one RCTs enrolling a total of 2730 patients were included in the meta-analysis. Twelve were considered as high-quality studies. The included studies showed significant heterogeneity with respect to patients, control groups, timing and duration of IN, which limited group analysis. IN significantly reduced overall complications when used before surgery (odds ratio (OR) $0 \cdot 48$, 95 per cent confidence interval (c.i.) $0 \cdot 34$ to $0 \cdot 69$), both before and after operation (OR $0 \cdot 39$, $0 \cdot 28$ to $0 \cdot 54$) or after surgery (OR $0 \cdot 46$, $0 \cdot 25$ to $0 \cdot 84$). For these three timings of IN administration, ORs of postoperative infection were $0 \cdot 36$ ($0 \cdot 24$ to $0 \cdot 56$), $0 \cdot 41$ ($0 \cdot 28$ to $0 \cdot 58$) and $0 \cdot 53$ ($0 \cdot 40$ to $0 \cdot 71$) respectively. Use of IN led to a shorter hospital stay: mean difference $-2 \cdot 12$ (95 per cent c.i. $-2 \cdot 97$ to $-1 \cdot 26$) days. Beneficial effects of IN were confirmed when low-quality trials were excluded. Perioperative IN had no influence on mortality (OR $0 \cdot 90$, $0 \cdot 46$ to $1 \cdot 76$).

Conclusion.—Perioperative enteral IN decreases morbidity and hospital stay but not mortality after major gastrointestinal surgery; its routine use can be recommended (Table 3).

▶ Cerantola et al performed a meta-analysis that examined the effect of immunonutrition (IN) on outcome following gastrointestinal surgery. Several

TABLE 3.—Pooled Data for High-Quality Studies Only

Outcome Measure	Rate		Odds Ratio
	IN	Control	
Complications[2,7,10,12–19,28]	338 of 956	495 of 957	$0 \cdot 46$ ($0 \cdot 38, 0 \cdot 57$)
Infections[2,7,10,12–19,28]	177 of 956	306 of 957	$0 \cdot 47$ ($0 \cdot 38, 0 \cdot 59$)
Length of hospital stay[2,7,10,12–18,28]	—	—	$-2 \cdot 26$ ($-2 \cdot 65, -1 \cdot 88$)*
(1837 patients)			
Mortality[7,10,12–14,16–18,28]	13 of 797	13 of 803	$1 \cdot 01$ ($0 \cdot 46, 2 \cdot 23$)

Values in parentheses are 95 per cent confidence intervals.
Editor's Note: Please refer to original journal article for full references.
*Mean difference. Only trials with a Jadad score of at least 3 were included. IN, immunonutrition.

randomized trials across the world have studied this question with conflicting answers. This meta-analysis pooled the results of the best studies and found that IN was associated with an overall decrease in morbidity, fewer postoperative infections, and decreased length of stay (Table 3). However, IN did not decrease mortality. The findings in this study are similar to other randomized studies that show a benefit for IN but without altering mortality. Several unresolved questions remain regarding IN. For example, which component (arginine, omega-3 fatty acids, RNA) of IN has the beneficial effect? Would administration of omega-3 fatty acids alone result in similar benefits? What is the effective dose of IN? Of course, these questions are of paramount importance in the context of costs of these relatively expensive formulas. The bang for the buck of IN versus conventional enteral nutrition is not clearly evident, so treatment with IN requires justification. Therefore, all trials and studies with IN should be compared with nutrition with less costly isocaloric, isonitrogenous formulas, and costs should be a primary outcome variable. As health care providers, we must focus on the value (effectiveness/costs) for each treatment, and therefore, all trials must assess not only the biologic value of a treatment but also the economic value. Health care reform will clearly have us focus on the value of all treatments, so the time is now for the surgical community to assess the value of our treatment regimens.

K. E. Behrns, MD

11 Oncology

Breast

Changes in the Use and Costs of Diagnostic Imaging Among Medicare Beneficiaries With Cancer, 1999-2006
Dinan MA, Curtis LH, Hammill BG, et al (Duke Clinical Res Inst, Durham, NC; et al)
JAMA 303:1625-1631, 2010

Context.—Emerging technologies, changing diagnostic and treatment patterns, and changes in Medicare reimbursement are contributing to increasing use of imaging in cancer. Imaging is the fastest growing expense for Medicare but has not been examined among beneficiaries with cancer.

Objective.—To examine changes in the use of imaging and how those changes contribute to the overall cost of cancer care.

Design, Setting, and Patients.—Analysis of a nationally representative 5% sample of claims from the US Centers for Medicare & Medicaid Services from 1999 through 2008. Patients were Medicare beneficiaries with incident breast cancer, colorectal cancer, leukemia, lung cancer, non-Hodgkin lymphoma, or prostate cancer.

Main Outcome Measures.—Use and cost of imaging by modality, year, and cancer type.

Results.—There were 100 954 incident cases of breast cancer, colorectal cancer, leukemia, lung cancer, non-Hodgkin lymphoma, and prostate cancer from 1999 through 2006. Significant mean annual increases in imaging use occurred among all cancer types for positron emission tomography (35.9%-53.6%), bone density studies (6.3%-20.0%), echocardiograms (5.0%-7.8%), magnetic resonance imaging (4.4%-11.5%), and ultrasound (0.7%-7.4%). Conventional radiograph rates decreased or stayed the same. As of 2006, beneficiaries with lung cancer and beneficiaries with lymphoma incurred the largest overall imaging costs, exceeding a mean of $3000 per beneficiary within 2 years of diagnosis. By 2005, one-third of beneficiaries with breast cancer underwent bone scans and half of beneficiaries with lung cancer or lymphoma underwent positron emission tomography scans. Mean 2-year imaging costs per beneficiary increased at a rate greater than the increase in mean total costs per beneficiary for all cancer types.

Conclusion.—Imaging costs among Medicare beneficiaries with cancer increased from 1999 through 2006, outpacing the rate of increase in total costs among Medicare beneficiaries with cancer.

▶ This study from the Center for Clinical and Genetic Economics at Duke Clinical Research Institute is an analysis of claims from the US centers for Medicare and Medicaid services looking at imaging utilization among patients with breast cancer, colorectal cancer, leukemia, lung cancer, non-Hodgkin's lymphoma, or prostate cancer. As seen in Fig in the original article, there have been changes over time with increased use of magnetic imaging and positron emission tomography.

Surgeons who are treating any of these diseases (breast cancer, colorectal cancer, lung cancer, and prostate cancer) are responsible for initial screening and staging the disease to determine whether or not patients are eligible for surgical intervention. Therefore, surgeons will be responsible for the increased cost that was seen in this article.

If, under health care reform, we have globalization of reimbursement imaging costs, which is growing faster than other costs in cancer care, it will impact our ability to adequately care for patients with malignancy in the future. Carefully controlled clinical trials to determine not only the most accurate imaging modality but also the most cost-effective utilization of the modality will be necessary. I, therefore, encourage all readers of the *Year Book* to participate in prospective clinical trials so that we may better care for patients with cancer in the future.

T. J. Eberlein, MD

Association of Risk-Reducing Surgery in *BRCA1* or *BRCA2* Mutation Carriers With Cancer Risk and Mortality

Domchek SM, Friebel TM, Singer CF, et al (Univ of Pennsylvania School of Medicine, Philadelphia; Med Univ of Vienna, Austria; et al)
JAMA 304:967-975, 2010

Context.—Mastectomy and salpingo-oophorectomy are widely used by carriers of *BRCA1* or *BRCA2* mutations to reduce their risks of breast and ovarian cancer.

Objective.—To estimate risk and mortality reduction stratified by mutation and prior cancer status.

Design, Setting, and Participants.—Prospective, multicenter cohort study of 2482 women with *BRCA1* or *BRCA2* mutations ascertained between 1974 and 2008. The study was conducted at 22 clinical and research genetics centers in Europe and North America to assess the relationship of risk-reducing mastectomy or salpingo-oophorectomy with cancer outcomes. The women were followed up until the end of 2009.

Main Outcomes Measures.—Breast and ovarian cancer risk, cancer-specific mortality, and overall mortality.

TABLE 1.—Risk-Reducing Mastectomy and Risk of First Occurrence of Breast Cancer[a]

| | | Prior or Concurrent Risk-Reducing Salpingo-oophorectomy | | | | |
| | | Yes | | | No | |
	Total (n = 959)	BRCA1 (n = 617)	BRCA2 (n = 342)	Total (n = 660)	BRCA1 (n = 415)	BRCA2 (n = 245)
Risk-reducing mastectomy						
Yes	172 (17.9)	116 (18.8)	56 (16.4)	75 (11.4)	43 (10.4)	32 (13.1)
Breast cancer diagnosis	0	0	0	0	0	0
No	787 (82.1)	501 (81.2)	286 (83.6)	585 (88.6)	372 (89.6)	213 (86.9)
Breast cancer diagnosis	64 (8.1)	44 (8.8)	20 (7.0)	34 (5.8)	19 (5.1)	15 (7.0)
Age, mean (range), y						
At time of risk-reducing mastectomy	40.7 (22.4-64.6)	40.1 (24.8-62.5)	42.0 (22.4-64.6)	37.9 (22.4-64.6)	36.7 (24.8-52.1)	39.4 (22.4-64.6)
At start of follow-up for those without mastectomy	40.5 (18.3-87.8)	39.5 (18.3-87.8)	42.2 (18.9-79.7)	37.6 (18.3-87.8)	36.7 (18.3-87.8)	39.1 (18.9-79.7)
Follow-up, mean (range), y						
To breast cancer diagnosis	3.1 (0.5-9.3)	3.3 (0.5-9.3)	2.6 (0.6-6.8)	3.1 (0.6-8.7)	3.6 (0.6-8.7)	2.5 (0.6-6.8)
To censoring	3.5 (0.5-13.0)	3.7 (0.5-13.0)	3.0 (0.5-11.5)	2.7 (0.5-13.0)	2.7 (0.5-13.0)	2.5 (0.5-11.5)
Occult breast cancer diagnosis[b]	4 (<1)	3 (<1)	1 (<1)	3 (<1)	2 (<1)	1 (<1)
Breast cancer after risk-reducing mastectomy, HR (95% CI)[c]	NA	NA	NA	NA	NA	NA

Abbreviations: CI, confidence interval; HR, hazard ratio; NA, data cannot be estimated.

[a] Values are expressed as number (percentage) unless otherwise indicated. There were no cases of breast cancer prior to ascertainment or risk-reducing salpingo-oophorectomy. Participants were censored at occurrence of ovarian cancer, death, or last contact.

[b] Cancer was found incidentally at the time of prophylactic mastectomy and excluded from analysis.

[c] There were no cancer events in those with risk-reducing mastectomy so HRs cannot be estimated.

Results.—No breast cancers were diagnosed in the 247 women with risk-reducing mastectomy compared with 98 women of 1372 diagnosed with breast cancer who did not have risk-reducing mastectomy. Compared with women who did not undergo risk-reducing salpingo-oophorectomy, women who underwent salpingo-oophorectomy had a lower risk of ovarian cancer, including those with prior breast cancer (6% vs 1%, respectively; hazard ratio [HR], 0.14; 95% confidence interval [CI], 0.04-0.59) and those without prior breast cancer (6% vs 2%; HR, 0.28 [95% CI, 0.12-0.69]), and a lower risk of first diagnosis of breast cancer in *BRCA1* mutation carriers (20% vs 14%; HR, 0.63 [95% CI, 0.41-0.96]) and *BRCA2* mutation carriers (23% vs 7%; HR, 0.36 [95% CI, 0.16-0.82]). Compared with women who did not undergo risk-reducing salpingo-oophorectomy, undergoing salpingo-oophorectomy was associated with lower all-cause mortality (10% vs 3%; HR, 0.40 [95% CI, 0.26-0.61]), breast cancer-specific mortality (6% vs 2%; HR, 0.44 [95% CI, 0.26-0.76]), and ovarian cancer-specific mortality (3% vs 0.4%; HR, 0.21 [95% CI, 0.06-0.80]).

Conclusions.—Among a cohort of women with *BRCA1* and *BRCA2* mutations, the use of risk-reducing mastectomy was associated with a lower risk of breast cancer; risk-reducing salpingo-oophorectomy was associated with a lower risk of ovarian cancer, first diagnosis of breast cancer, all-cause mortality, breast cancer-specific mortality, and ovarian cancer-specific mortality (Table 1).

▶ This is a prospective multicenter cohort study of almost 2500 women with *BRCA1* or *BRCA2* mutation. It is conducted at 22 clinical and research genetics centers in Europe and North America. As seen in Table 1, no breast cancer events were seen in women who underwent risk-reducing mastectomy during 3 years of prospective follow-up. In contrast, however, 7% of woman without risk-reducing mastectomy had been diagnosed with breast cancer. Similar findings are identified for risk-reducing salpingo-oophorectomy, ovarian cancer and first diagnosis of breast cancer in breast cancer—specific mortality.

It seems in this study that risk-reducing salpingo-oophorectomy was associated with a lower breast cancer risk in *BRCA2* mutation carriers than in *BRCA1* mutation carriers. This is of interest given the fact that *BRCA2* mutation carriers have a high proportion of estrogen receptor—positive breast tumors.

T. J. Eberlein, MD

Utility of the GeneSearch Breast Lymph Node Assay for the Rapid Evaluation of Sentinel Lymph Nodes in Breast Cancer
Funasako Y, Uenosono Y, Hirata M, et al (Kagoshima Univ, Japan)
Cancer 116:4450-4455, 2010

Background.—The potential for reducing the need for second surgery for axillary lymph node dissection (ALND) has made the intraoperative evaluation of sentinel lymph nodes (SLNs) attractive. The goal of the current study was to evaluate the clinical application of the breast lymph node (BLN) assay, a real-time reverse transcriptase-polymerase chain reaction assay for SLN metastases, by comparing this test with routine pathologic examination.

Methods.—A total of 117 patients with breast cancer underwent breast surgery with SLN biopsy. Each SLN was cut in half along the plane of the longest dimension. Half of each lymph node was examined by the 2 markers of the BLN assay, mammaglobin and cytokeratin 19, and the other half was examined by hematoxylin and eosin staining (H&E) and immunohistochemical staining (IHC) for pancytokeratins.

Results.—A total of 204 SLNs were obtained from 117 patients. H&E staining identified metastases in 31 SLNs (15.2%), and IHC staining detected metastases in 6 SLNs; 40 SLNs from 32 patients were found to be positive for metastasis using the BLN assay. The assay results were correlated with the pathologic diagnoses by H&E and IHC staining (P <.001). The sensitivity of the BLN assay compared with pathologic findings classified according to the TNM classification was 95.7% for macrometastases, 60.0% for micrometastases, and 55.6% for isolated tumor cells.

Conclusions.—The 2-marker BLN assay performs in a manner that is comparable to, and analyzes more tissue than, routine pathologic examination. Therefore, clinical intraoperative use of the BLN assay for SLNs may result in a reduction in the need for second surgery for ALND (Table 4).

▶ Evaluation of sentinel lymph nodes, particularly intraoperatively, remains a difficult task. Accurate intraoperative assessment would eliminate the need for patients with positive sentinel lymph nodes from necessitating a second general anesthesia and operation for a completion axillary lymph node dissection. These authors study an intraoperative evaluation of sentinel lymph nodes. The breast lymph node (BLN) assay detects the expression of 2 genes, mammaglobin and cytokeratin 19. Mammaglobin is a marker expressed at high levels in breast tissue, and cytokeratin 19 is an epithelial marker. Neither of these markers is expressed in normal lymph node tissue. As seen in Table 4, BLN assay detects

TABLE 4.—Correlation Between BLN Assay and Pathological Finding of Lymph Node Metastasis

CK	BLN Assay MG	MA	MI	ITC	Negative
+	+	13	2	1	1
+	−	9	1	1	5
−	+	0	0	3	4
−	−	1	2	4	157
Positive rate of BLN assay		95.7%	60.0%	55.6%	6.0%

BLN indicates breast lymph node; CK, cytokeratin, MG, mammaglobin; MA, macrometastasis; MI, micrometastasis; ITC, isolated tumor cells; +, positive; −, negative.

almost 96% of macrometastases and 60% of micrometastases. BLN assay with the double markers of cytokeratin 19 and mammaglobin can be used intraoperatively to assess sentinel lymph nodes. It is faster than messenger RNA quantification. This assay may help alleviate second operations requiring another anesthesia.

T. J. Eberlein, MD

Menstrual Cycle and Surgical Treatment of Breast Cancer: Findings From the NCCTG N9431 Study

Grant CS, Ingle JN, Suman VJ, et al (Mayo Clinic, Rochester, MN; Reproductive Medicine and Infertility Associates, Woodbury, MN; Allegheny Cancer Ctr, Pittsburgh, PA; et al)
J Clin Oncol 27:3620-3626, 2009

Purpose.—For nearly two decades, multiple retrospective reports, small prospective studies, and meta-analyses have arrived at conflicting results regarding the value of timing surgical intervention for breast cancer on the basis of menstrual cycle phase. We present the results of a multi–cooperative group, prospective, observational trial of menstrual cycle phase and outcome after breast cancer surgery, led by the North Central Cancer Treatment Group (NCCTG) in collaboration with the National Surgical Adjuvant Breast and Bowel Project (NSABP) and the International Breast Cancer Study Group (IBCSG).

Patients and Methods.—Premenopausal women age 18 to 55 years, who were interviewed for menstrual history and who were surgically treated for stages I to II breast cancer, had serum drawn within 1 day of surgery for estradiol, progesterone, and luteinizing hormone levels. Menstrual history and hormone levels were used to determine menstrual phase: luteal, follicular, and other. Disease-free survival (DFS) and overall survival (OS) rates were determined by Kaplan-Meier method and were compared by using the log-rank test and Cox proportional hazard modeling.

Results.—Of 1,118 women initially enrolled, 834 women comprised the study cohort: 230 (28%) in luteal phase; 363 (44%) in follicular phase; and 241 grouped as other. During a median follow-up of 6.6 years, and in analysis that accounted for nodal disease, estrogen receptor status, adjuvant radiation therapy or chemotherapy, neither DFS nor OS differed with respect to menstrual phase. The 5-year DFS rates were 82.7%, 82.1%, and 79.2% for follicular, luteal, or other phases, respectively. Corresponding OS survival rates were 91.9%, 92.2%, and 91.8%, respectively.

Conclusion.—When menstrual cycle phases were strictly defined, neither DFS nor OS differed between women who underwent surgery during the follicular phase versus the luteal phase. Nearly 30% of the patients did not meet criteria for either follicular- or luteal-phase categories.

▶ There have been multiple conflicting results regarding the value of timing of surgical intervention in breast cancer based on the patient's menstrual cycle phase. This is a prospective observational phase III clinical trial, where the patient's menstrual cycle was strictly defined. As seen in Fig 2 in the original article and Fig 3 in the original article, there are no differences in disease-free (Fig 2 in the original article) or overall survival (Fig 3 in the original article) in patients who underwent surgery during the follicular phase or luteal phase of their menstrual cycle. It is interesting to note, however, that nearly 30% of the patients did not meet the strict criteria for definition in either follicular or luteal phase category. However, by using very strict biochemical definition of menstrual cycle phase, there appeared to be no advantage to timing of surgery.

T. J. Eberlein, MD

Racial Disparities in the Use of Radiotherapy After Breast-Conserving Surgery: A National Medicare Study
Smith GL, Shih Y-CT, Xu Y, et al (The Univ of Texas M. D. Anderson Cancer Ctr, Houston)
Cancer 116:734-741, 2010

Background.—In prior studies, the use of standard breast cancer treatments has varied by race, but previous analyses were not nationally representative. Therefore, in a comprehensive, national cohort of Medicare patients, racial disparities in the use of radiotherapy (RT) after breast-conserving surgery (BCS) for invasive breast cancer were quantified.

Methods.—A national Medicare database was used to identify all beneficiaries (age >65 years) treated with BCS for incident invasive breast cancer in 2003. Claims codes identified RT use, and Medicare demographic data indicated race. Logistic regression modeled RT use in white, black, and other-race patients, adjusted for demographic, clinical, and socioeconomic covariates.

Results.—Of 34,080 women, 91% were white, 6% were black, and 3% were another race. The mean age of the patients was 76 ± 7 years. Approximately 74% of whites, 65% of blacks, and 66% of other-race patients received RT ($P < .001$). After covariate adjustment, whites were found to be significantly more likely to receive RT than blacks (odds ratio, 1.48; 95% confidence interval, 1.34-1.63 [$P < .001$]). Disparities between white and black patients varied by geographic region, with blacks in areas of the northeastern and southern United States demonstrating the lowest rates of RT use (57% in these regions). In patients age <70 years, racial disparities persisted. Specifically, 83% of whites, 73% of blacks, and 78% of other races in this younger group received RT ($P < .001$).

Conclusions.—In this comprehensive national sample of older breast cancer patients, substantial racial disparities were identified in RT use after BCS across much of the United States. Efforts to improve breast

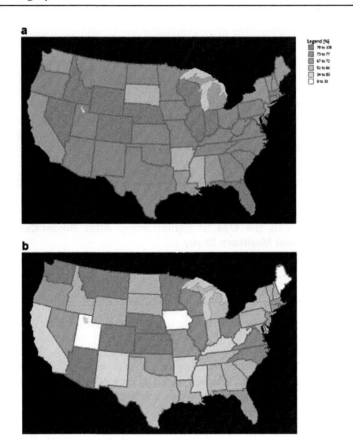

FIGURE 1.—Percentage radiotherapy use in (a) white patients versus (b) black patients is shown. Gray shading indicates that the sample size was too small to provide meaningful data. (Reprinted from Smith GL, Shih Y-CT, Xu Y, et al. Racial disparities in the use of radiotherapy after breast-conserving surgery: a national Medicare study. *Cancer.* 2010;116:734-741. Copyright 2010 American Cancer Society. This material is reproduced with permission of Wiley-Liss, Inc, a subsidiary of John Wiley & Sons, Inc.)

cancer care require overcoming these disparities, which exist on a national scale.

▶ This article is a national Medicare database analysis, which is limited to older patients with breast cancer. As seen in Fig 1, there are substantial racial differences in patients' receipt of radiation therapy. As seen in Fig 1, the percentage of white women that receive radiation therapy is greater than that of black women who receive radiation therapy in many states. Fig 2 shows that this discrepancy is greatest in the South and the Northeast.

Access to care and socioeconomic factors may influence disparities in cancer care. However, the authors made adjustments for physician visits and use of mammography before cancer diagnosis and yet racial disparity persisted.

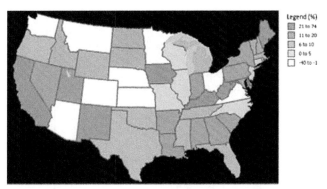

Legend (%)
■ 21 to 74
▨ 11 to 20
▨ 6 to 10
□ 0 to 5
□ -40 to -1

FIGURE 2.—Absolute difference in the rate of radiotherapy (RT) use between white and black patients is shown. An absolute difference <0% indicates that the percentage of black women receiving RT was greater than the percentage of white women. Gray shading indicates that the sample size was too small to provide meaningful data. (Reprinted from Smith GL, Shih Y-CT, Xu Y, et al. Racial disparities in the use of radiotherapy after breast-conserving surgery: a national Medicare study. *Cancer.* 2010;116:734-741. Copyright 2010 American Cancer Society. This material is reproduced with permission of Wiley-Liss, Inc, a subsidiary of John Wiley & Sons, Inc.)

Once again, this study has limitations, but optimizing physician/patient interaction and improving access to high-standard cancer care will help to diminish these racial disparities.

T. J. Eberlein, MD

Colon

Expert Panel Offers Advice to Improve Screening Rates for Colorectal Cancer
Slomski A
JAMA 303:1356-1357, 2010

Physicians who want to use an ESA to treat chemotherapy-related anemia in patients with cancer must register, complete a 15-minute online education course, and document that they have spoken to their patients about the drug and secured the patients' signatures testifying that they were informed of the risks. Physicians who do not register will not be able to prescribe ESAs. The program will be run by Amgen Inc through its APPRISE (Assisting Providers and Center Patients With Risk Information for the Safe Use of ESAs) program.

"This will create new responsibilities for busy health care providers—training, record keeping—however, we are not doing this to make things more difficult for the providers," said Richard Pazdur, MD, director of the FDA's Office of Oncology Drug Products at a February press conference announcing the REMS launch. "We are doing it to make absolutely certain that patients know the risks before they begin their treatment regimens."

TABLE 1.—Colorectal Cancer Screening Recommendations From the United States Preventive Services Task Force (USPSTF) and the American Cancer Society—United States Multisociety Task Force (ACS-USMSTF)

Screening Test	Description	USPSTF	ACS-USMSTF
Fecal occult blood test (FOBT)[a] and fecal immunochemical test (FIT)[a]	Examination of the stool for traces of blood not visible to the naked eye	Recommends highsensitivity FOBT and FIT annually for ages 50-75 y	Age ≥50 y, every year
Sigmoidoscopy[a]	Internal examination of the lower part of the large intestine	Recommends every 5 y with high-sensitivity FOBT annually for ages 50-75 y	Age ≥50 y, every 5 y
Double-contrast barium enema[a]	X-ray examination of the colon	—	Age ≥50 y, every 5 y
Colonoscopy[a]	Internal examination of the entire large intestine	Recommends every 10 y for ages 50-75 y	Age ≥50 y, every 10 y
Computed tomography colonography[a]	Examination of the colon and rectum using pictures obtained using a computed tomography scanner	—	Age ≥50 y, every 5 y
Fecal DNA[a]	Examination of the stool for traces of colorectal cancer DNA	—	Age ≥50 y, interval uncertain

[a]Positive findings require follow-up colonoscopy.

ASCO expressed doubt that this was the best way of handling the safety of ESAs. "Oncologists continually struggle to provide high quality cancer care in the face of dwindling resources and growing administrative burdens. While ASCO supports efforts to raise risk awareness and promote patient safety, we strenuously object to duplicative requirements that further diminish time and resources available for patient care," the professional society wrote in a letter alerting members to the new REMS.

Allen S. Lichter, MD, ASCO's chief executive officer, said he was bothered by the way the FDA developed this REMS. "We were not asked to participate in any way on the design of the program, and we are disappointed in that," Lichter said. "This is in contrast to the FDA's approach for REMS in opioid therapy, where we and the rest of the medical community were given the chance to comment, and we think some of our comments helped improve that program."

In response, the FDA said the opioid REMS was unique in that it involved many different products and manufacturers, while the program for the ESAs involves 2 products and 1 company. The agency went on to say that, in general, REMS are developed through discussions with a drug sponsor and that public meetings or additional input are not customary or required parts of the process.

Lichter is not so sure such exclusion is beneficial, adding that ASCO was preparing a letter to send to the FDA expressing this concern. "Of course we will comply with the REMS, but we hope we can discuss with the FDA and others the value of bringing us into this process to make sure these programs will accomplish what they want them to accomplish without overburdening physicians."

More information on the FDA programs can be found online at http://www.fda.gov/downloads/Drugs/DrugSafety/PostmarketDrugSafety InformationforPatientsandProviders/UCM200104.pdf (for darbepoetin alfa) and http://www.fda.gov/downloads/Drugs/DrugSafety/PostmarketDrug SafetyInformationforPatientsandProviders/UCM200105.pdf (for epoetin alfa) (Table 1).

▶ General surgeons see a preponderance of patients who are at risk for the development of colorectal cancer. Surgeons therefore have an opportunity to influence screening habits of these patients. This article in *JAMA* is a very concise article providing advice, and Table 1 offers concise recommendations that are provided from the US Preventive Services Task Force and the American Cancer Society.

Clearly, balancing cost and effectiveness is key to obtaining best outcomes.

T. J. Eberlein, MD

Rectal

Gene Signature Is Associated with Early Stage Rectal Cancer Recurrence
Kalady MF, Dejulius K, Church JM, et al (Cleveland Clinic, OH)
J Am Coll Surg 211:187-195, 2010

Background.—Despite expected excellent outcomes of surgical resection for early stage rectal cancers, 20% of stage I and II rectal cancers recur. Identifying biologic factors that predict the subset prone to recur could allow more directed therapy. This study identifies a tumor gene expression profile that accurately predicts disease recurrence.

Study Design.—Stage I/II rectal cancer patients treated by surgery alone at a single institution were included and classified as having recurrent or nonrecurrent cancer. Tumor mRNA was isolated from frozen tissue and evaluated for total genome gene expression by microarray analysis. Background-corrected and normalized microarray data were analyzed using BAMarray software. Selected genes were further analyzed using unsupervised clustering and nearest-centroid classification. A balanced K-fold scoring-pair algorithm using 1,000 independent replications was used for gene signature development.

Results.—Sixty-nine patients with disease-free survival and 31 patients with recurrent disease were included at a median follow-up of 105 months (interquartile range 114 months) and 32 months (interquartile range 25 months), respectively. Demographics and tumor characteristics between groups were similar. Fifty-two genes from 43,148 probes were differentially expressed, and a 36-gene signature was found to be statistically associated with recurrence using a scoring-pair algorithm. Accuracy to identify recurrence as measured by area under the receiver operating characteristic curve was 0.803.

Conclusions.—Differential gene expression within rectal cancers is associated with recurrence of early stage disease. A 36-gene signature correlates with an increased risk of more or less aggressive tumor behavior. This information obtainable at biopsy may assist in determining treatment decisions (Fig 4).

▶ This is an article from the Cleveland Clinic that looks at stage I/II rectal cancer patients treated by surgery alone at a single institution. The patients were analyzed for a 36-gene panel as is seen in Fig 4. Increased expression of these 36 genes tended to be associated with recurrence (red bars), whereas underexpression of the same 36 genes tended to be predictive of nonrecurrence (blue bars).

More frequently, we will begin to identify gene signature panels that will correlate with outcome in various carefully defined patient populations. The key, however, is that we carefully define the patient populations and perform the correct statistical methodologies to ensure appropriate interpretation of the data. As in this case, this gene signature panel could help predict disease recurrence for patients who require more aggressive adjuvant therapies instead

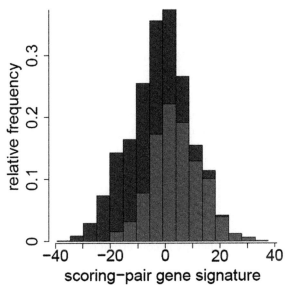

scoring−pair gene signature

FIGURE 4.—Histogram for individual patient score values for the 36-gene signature. Each of the 36 genes in the signature was compared with a control gene and given a score of −1, 0, or +1 depending on decreased, similar, or increased expression, respectively. The 36 values for each patient were summed, allowing a possible range of scores from −36 to +36. Red bars represent patients who developed recurrent disease and blue bars represent patients without recurrent disease. Data are based on test-fold data. Scores on the extremes of this histogram are highly predictive for either recurrence or nonrecurrence. (Reprinted from Journal of American College of Surgeons, Kalady MF, Dejulius K, Church JM, et al. Gene signature is associated with early stage rectal cancer recurrence. *J Am Coll Surg.* 2010;211:187-195. Copyright © 2010, with permission from the American College of Surgeons.)

of just receiving surgery. More importantly, this can be done prospectively in a timely fashion.

T. J. Eberlein, MD

Hepatic Colorectal

Conversion to Resectability Using Hepatic Artery Infusion Plus Systemic Chemotherapy for the Treatment of Unresectable Liver Metastases From Colorectal Carcinoma
Kemeny NE, Huitzil Melendez FD, Capanu M, et al (Memorial Sloan-Kettering Cancer Ctr, NY)
J Clin Oncol 27:3465-3471, 2009

Purpose.—To determine the conversion to resectability in patients with unresectable liver metastases from colorectal cancer treated with hepatic arterial infusion (HAI) plus systemic oxaliplatin and irinotecan (CPT-11).

Patients and Methods.—Forty-nine patients with unresectable liver metastases (53% previously treated with chemotherapy) were enrolled onto a phase I protocol with HAI floxuridine and dexamethasone plus systemic chemotherapy with oxaliplatin and irinotecan.

Results.—Ninety-two percent of the 49 patients had complete (8%) or partial (84%) response, and 23 (47%) of the 49 patients were able to undergo resection in a group of patients with extensive disease (73% with > five liver lesions, 98% with bilobar disease, 86% with ≥ six segments involved). For chemotherapy-naïve and previously treated patients, the median survival from the start of HAI therapy was 50.8 and 35 months, respectively. The only baseline variable significantly associated with a higher resection rate was female sex. Variables reflecting extensive anatomic disease, such as number of lesions or number of vessels involved, were not significantly associated with the probability of resection.

Conclusion.—The combination of regional HAI floxuridine/dexamethasone and systemic oxaliplatin and irinotecan is an effective regimen for the treatment of patients with unresectable liver metastases from colorectal cancer, demonstrating a 47% conversion to resection (57% in chemotherapy-naïve patients). Future randomized trials should compare HAI plus systemic chemotherapy with systemic therapy alone to assess the additional value of HAI therapy in converting patients with hepatic metastases to resectability.

▶ This is a study from Memorial Sloan-Kettering Cancer Center. The institution has used hepatic artery infusion with systemic chemotherapy for the treatment of patients with colorectal cancer. All of these patients had unresectable disease at the outset of their therapy. A number of patients had been treated previously with systemic chemotherapy. Impressively, 47% of the patients were able to undergo resection after response to this combination treatment (resection rate was 57% in chemotherapy-naïve patients). As seen in Fig 3 in the original article, patients who had not received chemotherapy previously tended to have longer median survival.

There are several important points to be emphasized in this trial: First, there was a very detailed description of the initial tumor extent, confirming that patients had truly unresectable disease. Second, the increased response rate may have been due to the selection of agents used in the chemotherapy. Obviously, having technical expertise in managing the hepatic artery catheters and chemotherapy and having cooperation of the medical and surgical oncologists are needed to be able to duplicate these results.

T. J. Eberlein, MD

Improved Survival in Metastatic Colorectal Cancer Is Associated With Adoption of Hepatic Resection and Improved Chemotherapy
Kopetz S, Chang GJ, Overman MJ, et al (The Univ of Texas M. D. Anderson Cancer Ctr, Houston; Mayo Clinic, Rochester, MN)
J Clin Oncol 27:3677-3683, 2009

Purpose.—Fluorouracil/leucovorin as the sole therapy for metastatic colorectal cancer (CRC) provides an overall survival of 8 to 12 months.

With an increase in surgical resections of metastatic disease and development of new chemotherapies, indirect evidence suggests that outcomes for patients are improving in the general population, although the incremental gain has not yet been quantified.

Methods.—We performed a retrospective review of patients newly diagnosed with metastatic CRC treated at two academic centers from 1990 through 2006. Landmark analysis evaluated the association of diagnosis year and liver resection with overall survival. Additional survival analysis of the Surveillance Epidemiology and End Results (SEER) database evaluated a similar population from 1990 through 2005.

Results.—Two thousand four hundred seventy patients with metastatic CRC at diagnosis received their primary treatment at the two institutions during this time period. Median overall survival for those patients diagnosed from 1990 to 1997 was 14.2 months, which increased to 18.0, 18.6, and 29.3 months for patients diagnosed in 1998 to 2000, 2001 to 2003, and 2004 to 2006, respectively. Likewise, 5-year overall survival increased from 9.1% in the earliest time period to 19.2% in 2001 to 2003. Improved outcomes from 1998 to 2004 were a result of an increase in hepatic resection, which was performed in 20% of the patients. Improvements from 2004 to 2006 were temporally associated with increased utilization of new chemotherapeutics. In the SEER registry, overall survival for the 49,459 identified patients also increased in the most recent time period.

Conclusion.—Profound improvements in outcome in metastatic CRC seem to be associated with the sequential increase in the use of hepatic resection in selected patients (1998 to 2006) and advancements in medical therapy (2004 to 2006).

▶ This is a study from M.D. Anderson Cancer Center and the Mayo Clinic. The authors analyze survival in patients with metastatic colorectal cancer. As seen in Fig 1 in the original article, looking at all phase III trials since 1995, there has been a clear improvement in survival. This appears to be likely due to better combination of chemotherapy agents and more aggressive better outcome hepatic resection. As seen in Fig 2 in the original article, there is a clear improvement in overall survival, median overall survival, and 5-year overall survival for these 2 institutions.

More aggressive and better chemotherapy agents will further enhance survival in this patient population. Once again emphasis of a multidisciplinary approach and careful selection of patients is needed to replicate these results. Continued advances in drug development and appropriate use of liver resection will further improve patient survival.

T. J. Eberlein, MD

Long-Term Outcomes After Hepatic Resection for Colorectal Metastases in Young Patients

de Haas RJ, Wicherts DA, Salloum C, et al (AP-HP Hôpital Paul Brousse, Villejuif, France)
Cancer 116:647-658, 2010

Background.—Long-term outcomes after hepatectomy for colorectal liver metastases in relatively young patients are still unknown. The aim of the current study was to evaluate long-term outcomes in patients ≤40 years old, and to compare them with patients >40 years old.

Methods.—All consecutive patients who underwent hepatectomy for colorectal liver metastases at the authors' hospital between 1990 and 2006 were included in the study. Patients ≤40 years old were compared with all other patients treated during the same period. Overall survival (OS), progression-free survival (PFS), and disease-free survival (DFS) rates were determined, and prognostic factors were identified.

Results.—In total, 806 patients underwent hepatectomy for colorectal liver metastases, of whom 56 (7%) were aged ≤40 years. Among the young patients, more colorectal liver metastases were present at diagnosis, and they were more often diagnosed synchronous with the primary tumor. Five-year OS was 33% in young patients, compared with 51% in older patients (*P* = .12). Five-year PFS was 2% in young patients, compared with 16% in older patients (*P* < .001). DFS rates were comparable between the groups (17% vs 23%, *P* = .10). At multivariate analysis, age ≤40 years was identified as an independent predictor of poor PFS.

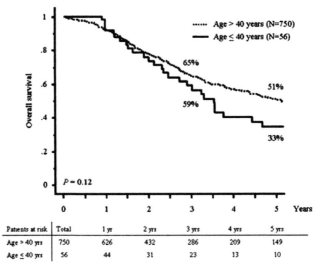

Patients at risk	Total	1 yr	2 yrs	3 yrs	4 yrs	5 yrs
Age > 40 yrs	750	626	432	286	209	149
Age ≤ 40 yrs	56	44	31	23	13	10

FIGURE 1.—Overall survival is shown. (Reprinted from de Haas RJ, Wicherts DA, Salloum C, et al. Long-term outcomes after hepatic resection for colorectal metastases in young patients. *Cancer.* 2010;116:647-658. Copyright 2010 American Cancer Society. This material is reproduced with permission of Wiley-Liss, Inc, a subsidiary of John Wiley & Sons, Inc.)

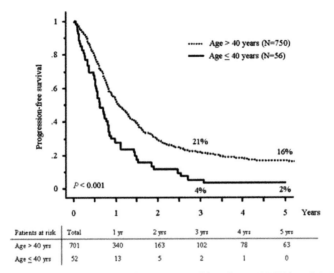

FIGURE 2.—Progression-free survival is shown. (Reprinted from de Haas RJ, Wicherts DA, Salloum C, et al. Long-term outcomes after hepatic resection for colorectal metastases in young patients. *Cancer.* 2010;116:647-658. Copyright 2010 American Cancer Society. This material is reproduced with permission of Wiley-Liss, Inc, a subsidiary of John Wiley & Sons, Inc.)

Conclusions.—In young patients, colorectal liver metastases seem to be more aggressive, with a trend toward lower OS, more disease recurrences, and a significantly shorter PFS after hepatectomy. However, DFS rates were comparable between young and older patients, owing to an aggressive multimodality treatment approach, consisting of chemotherapy and repeat surgery. Therefore, physicians should recognize the poor outcome of colorectal liver metastases in young patients and should consider an aggressive approach to diagnosis and early treatment.

▶ This is a single-institution study from France that maintained a prospective consecutive database and carefully analyzed their results. As seen in Fig 1, overall survival was lower for young patients, but this did not reach statistical significance. However, the 3- and 5-year progression-free survival were significantly lower in younger patients (Fig 2).

These results are somewhat surprising because young patients tend to have fewer comorbidities and better performance status. However, this seeming contradiction could be a result of the fact that young patients present with more advanced stage of disease or even a different disease biology. Using a more aggressive approach in these younger patients may make disease-free survival rates comparable with older patients. Once again, better pharmacologic agents in unique combinations will also improve these patients' survival.

T. J. Eberlein, MD

Gallbladder

Cisplatin plus Gemcitabine versus Gemcitabine for Biliary Tract Cancer

Valle J, for the ABC-02 Trial Investigators (Christie Hosp, Manchester, UK; et al)
N Engl J Med 362:1273-1281, 2010

Background.—There is no established standard chemotherapy for patients with locally advanced or metastatic biliary tract cancer. We initially conducted a randomized, phase 2 study involving 86 patients to compare cisplatin plus gemcitabine with gemcitabine alone. After we found an improvement in progression-free survival, the trial was extended to the phase 3 trial reported here.

Methods.—We randomly assigned 410 patients with locally advanced or metastatic cholangiocarcinoma, gallbladder cancer, or ampullary cancer to receive either cisplatin (25 mg per square meter of body-surface area) followed by gemcitabine (1000 mg per square meter on days 1 and 8, every 3 weeks for eight cycles) or gemcitabine alone (1000 mg per square meter on days 1,8, and 15, every 4 weeks for six cycles) for up to 24 weeks. The primary end point was overall survival.

Results.—After a median follow-up of 8.2 months and 327 deaths, the median overall survival was 11.7 months among the 204 patients in the cisplatin–gemcitabine group and 8.1 months among the 206 patients in the gemcitabine group (hazard ratio, 0.64; 95% confidence interval, 0.52 to 0.80; P<0.001). The median progression-free survival was 8.0 months in the cisplatin–gemcitabine group and 5.0 months in the gemcitabine-only group (P<0.001). In addition, the rate of tumor control among patients in the cisplatin–gemcitabine group was significantly increased (81.4% vs. 71.8%, P = 0.049). Adverse events were similar in the two groups, with the exception of more neutropenia in the cisplatin–gemcitabine group; the number of neutropenia-associated infections was similar in the two groups.

Conclusions.—As compared with gemcitabine alone, cisplatin plus gemcitabine was associated with a significant survival advantage without the addition of substantial toxicity. Cisplatin plus gemcitabine is an appropriate option for the treatment of patients with advanced biliary cancer. (ClinicalTrials.gov number, NCT00262769.) (Fig 2).

▶ This is a randomized, prospective, phase 3 trial that builds on a previous phase 2 study from the United Kingdom, looking at patients with locally advanced or metastatic biliary tract cancer, a common finding for surgeons who treat these types of tumors. The groups are very comparable in this randomized control study. Yet as seen in Fig 2, the cisplatin/gemcitabine combination significantly improves overall survival and progression-free survival. If anything, the group that received gemcitabine alone seemed to have more unexpected serious adverse reactions. This group did not identify

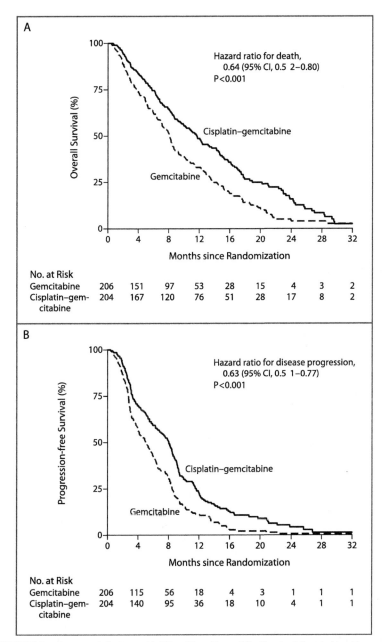

FIGURE 2.—Outcomes in Patients with Biliary Tract Cancer Who Received Gemcitabine Alone versus Cisplatin plus Gemcitabine. Panel A shows Kaplan–Meier estimates of overall survival, and Panel B shows Kaplan–Meier estimates of progression-free survival. CI denotes confidence interval. (Reprinted from Valle J, for the ABC-02 Trial Investigators. Cisplatin plus gemcitabine versus gemcitabine for biliary tract cancer. *N Engl J Med.* 2010;362:1273-1281. Copyright 2010 Massachusetts Medical Society. All rights reserved.)

a correlative predictor of response. Improvement in targeted treatments will be necessary to further impact survival in this disease.

T. J. Eberlein, MD

Pancreatic

A Multicenter Analysis of Distal Pancreatectomy for Adenocarcinoma: Is Laparoscopic Resection Appropriate?

Kooby DA, Hawkins WG, Schmidt CM, et al (Emory Univ School of Medicine, Atlanta, GA; Washington Univ, St Louis, MO; Indiana Univ, Indianapolis; et al)
J Am Coll Surg 210:779-787, 2010

Background.—As compared with open distal pancreatectomy (ODP), laparoscopic distal pancreatectomy (LDP) affords improved perioperative outcomes. The role of LDP for patients with pancreatic ductal adenocarcinoma (PDAC) is not defined.

Study Design.—Records from patients undergoing distal pancreatectomy (DP) for PDAC from 2000 to 2008 from 9 academic medical centers were reviewed. Short-term (node harvest and margin status) and long-term (survival) cancer outcomes were assessed. A 3:1 matched analysis was performed for ODP and LDP cases using age, American Society of Anesthesiologists (ASA) class, and tumor size.

Results.—There were 212 patients who underwent DP for PDAC; 23 (11%) of these were approached laparoscopically. For all 212 patients, 56 (26%) had positive margins. The mean number of nodes (± SD) examined was 12.6 ± 8.4 and 114 patients (54%) had at least 1 positive node. Median overall survival was 16 months. In the matched analysis there were no significant differences in positive margin rates, number of nodes examined, number of patients with at least 1 positive node, or overall survival. Logistic regression for all 212 patients demonstrated that advanced age, larger tumors, positive margins, and node positive disease were independently associated with worse survival; however, method of resection (ODP vs. LDP) was not. Hospital stay was 2 days shorter in the matched comparison, which approached significance (LDP, 7.4 days vs. ODP, 9.4 days, p = 0.06).

Conclusions.—LDP provides similar short- and long-term oncologic outcomes as compared with OD, with potentially shorter hospital stay. These results suggest that LDP is an acceptable approach for resection of PDAC of the left pancreas in selected patients (Figs 1 and 2, Table 3).

▶ This is a multi-institutional series from outstanding hepatopancreatic biliary units. The question asked was, "Could laparoscopic distal pancreatectomy be safely used in patients with adenocarcinoma of the distal pancreatic duct?" In looking at the overall cohort of patients, resection margins predicted outcome with negative margins (Fig 1) having significant improvement in survival compared with positive margins. As seen in Table 3, however, the type of operation did not seem to have an impact with respect to margin and, therefore,

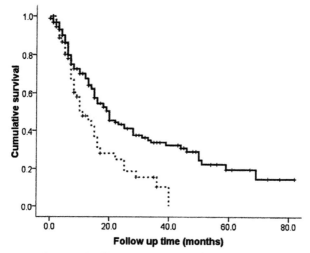

FIGURE 1.—Overall survival for all patients undergoing either margin negative resection (solid line, n = 156, median survival 20 months) or margin positive resection (dotted line, n = 56, median survival 11 months) distal pancreatectomy for adenocarcinoma (p = 0.002, log rank). (Reprinted from Journal of American College of Surgeons, Kooby DA, Hawkins WG, Schmidt CM, et al. A multicenter analysis of distal pancreatectomy for adenocarcinoma: is laparoscopic resection appropriate? *J Am Coll Surg.* 2010;210:779-787. Copyright © 2010, with permission from the American College of Surgeons.)

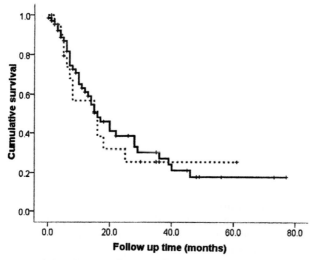

FIGURE 2.—Matched analysis overall survival for patients undergoing open (solid line, n = 70, median survival 16 months) versus laparoscopic (dotted line, n = 23, median survival 16 months) distal pancreatectomy for adenocarcinoma, in the 3:1 matched analysis (p = 0.71, log rank). (Reprinted from Journal of American College of Surgeons, Kooby DA, Hawkins WG, Schmidt CM, et al. A multicenter analysis of distal pancreatectomy for adenocarcinoma: is laparoscopic resection appropriate? *J Am Coll Surg.* 2010;210:779-787. Copyright © 2010, with permission from the American College of Surgeons.)

TABLE 3.—Multivariate Analysis for Factors Contributing to Margin Positive Resection for All 212 Patients Undergoing Distal Pancreatectomy for Pancreatic Ductal Adenocarcinoma

Variable	n	%	Overall Survival p Value	Odds Ratio	95% CI
Age > 65 y	119	56	0.20	1.55	0.79−3.02
Gender (male)	92	43	0.14	1.63	0.86−3.11
ASA > 2	131	62	0.53	1.20	0.63−2.46
BMI > 30 kg/m^2	53	25	0.27	1.25	0.72−3.33
Operation (LDP)	23	11	0.75	1.36	0.46−4.00
Blood loss > 500 mL	126	59	0.01	2.59	1.24−5.43
Tumor size > 4 cm	110	52	0.08	1.82	0.94−3.53
Pancreatic length > 10 cm	101	48	0.60	1.19	0.62−2.27

ASA, American Society of Anesthesiologists classification; BMI, body mass index; LDP, laparoscopic distal pancreatectomy.

overall survival. In fact, this is seen more vividly in Fig 2, which shows no change in the overall survival in patients having open versus laparoscopic distal pancreatectomy.

One of the strengths of this study is its multicenter design. This allows for quite variable experiences in the laparoscopic resection (mimicking what would be done in an individual surgeon's practice). The weakness, however, is its retrospective methodology and lack of surgical and pathologic standardization. Using a prospective randomized trial design, however, would be difficult and, for a single institution, would require an extraordinary length of time.

T. J. Eberlein, MD

Preoperative Biliary Drainage for Cancer of the Head of the Pancreas

van der Gaag NA, Rauws EAJ, van Eijck CHJ, et al (Academic Med Ctr, Amsterdam, the Netherlands; Erasmus Med Ctr, Rotterdam, the Netherlands; et al)
N Engl J Med 362:129-137, 2010

Background.—The benefits of preoperative biliary drainage, which was introduced to improve the postoperative outcome in patients with obstructive jaundice caused by a tumor of the pancreatic head, are unclear.

Methods.—In this multicenter, randomized trial, we compared preoperative biliary drainage with surgery alone for patients with cancer of the pancreatic head. Patients with obstructive jaundice and a bilirubin level of 40 to 250 μmol per liter (2.3 to 14.6 mg per deciliter) were randomly assigned to undergo either preoperative biliary drainage for 4 to 6 weeks, followed by surgery, or surgery alone within 1 week after diagnosis. Preoperative biliary drainage was attempted primarily with the placement of an endoprosthesis by means of endoscopic retrograde cholangiopancreatography. The primary outcome was the rate of serious complications within 120 days after randomization.

Results.—We enrolled 202 patients; 96 were assigned to undergo early surgery and 106 to undergo preoperative biliary drainage; 6 patients were excluded from the analysis. The rates of serious complications were 39% (37 patients) in the early-surgery group and 74% (75 patients) in the biliary-drainage group (relative risk in the early-surgery group, 0.54; 95% confidence interval [CI], 0.41 to 0.71; P < 0.001). Preoperative biliary drainage was successful in 96 patients (94%) after one or more attempts, with complications in 47 patients (46%). Surgery-related complications occurred in 35 patients (37%) in the early-surgery group and in 48 patients (47%) in the biliary-drainage group (relative risk, 0.79; 95% CI, 0.57 to 1.11; P = 0.14). Mortality and the length of hospital stay did not differ significantly between the two groups.

Conclusions.—Routine preoperative biliary drainage in patients undergoing surgery for cancer of the pancreatic head increases the rate of complications. (Current Controlled Trials number, ISRCTN31939699.)

▶ This is a multicenter, randomized, prospective trial. As seen in Fig 2, preoperative biliary drainage (PBD) followed by surgery led to a significant increase in complications. These were frequently related to cholangitis and stent-related issues, such as occlusion or need for exchange. These authors preferred to use

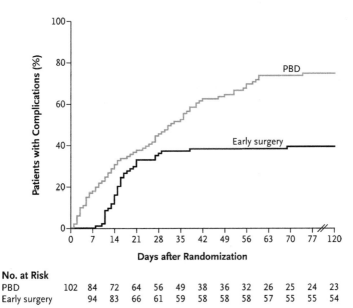

No. at Risk

PBD	102	84	72	64	56	49	38	36	32	26	25	24	23
Early surgery		94	83	66	61	59	58	58	58	57	55	55	54

FIGURE 2.—Proportion of patients with complications. The primary outcome — the rate of serious complications within 120 days after randomization — occurred in 37 patients (39%) who underwent early surgery alone and 75 patients (74%) who underwent preoperative biliary drainage (PBD) followed by surgery (relative risk in the early-surgery group, 0.54; 95% confidence interval [CI], 0.41 to 0.71; P < 0.001). (Reprinted from van der Gaag NA, Rauws EAJ, van Eijck CHJ, et al. Preoperative biliary drainage for cancer of the head of the pancreas. *N Engl J Med*. 2010;362:129-137. Copyright 2010 Massachusetts Medical Society. All rights reserved.)

endoscopic retrograde cholangiopancreatography (ERCP) as a means of drainage when it is needed and only a percutaneous attempt when endoscopy fails.

As neoadjuvant chemotherapies play a larger role in the treatment of patients who present with later stage pancreatic cancer, the authors recommend metal stents instead of plastic stents if PBD is used.

T. J. Eberlein, MD

Gastric

Large-Scale Investigation into Dumping Syndrome after Gastrectomy for Gastric Cancer
Mine S, Sano T, Tsutsumi K, et al (Toranomon Hosp, Tokyo, Japan; Natl Cancer Ctr Hosp, Tokyo, Japan; et al)
J Am Coll Surg 211:628-636, 2010

Background.—The aim of this study was to investigate early and late dumping syndromes in a large number of patients after gastrectomy for gastric cancer.

Study Design.—Responses to questions on a visual analogue scale survey completed by 1,153 gastrectomy patients were analyzed for associations between clinical factors and occurrence of dumping syndrome. Types of gastrectomy included distal gastrectomy with Billroth I or with Roux-Y reconstruction, pylorus preserving gastrectomy, proximal gastrectomy, and total gastrectomy.

Results.—Based on the visual analogue scale rating of symptomatic discomfort, patients were categorized into 1 of 2 groups: symptom-free or symptomatic. Incidences of early or late dumping syndrome in all patients were 67.6% and 38.4%, respectively. Patients in whom early dumping syndrome developed were significantly more likely to experience late dumping syndrome than those in whom it did not develop (p < 0.001). According to multivariate analyses, factors that decreased the risk for developing early dumping syndrome were reduced weight loss (p < 0.01), old age (p < 0.01), pylorus preserving gastrectomy (p < 0.01), distal gastrectomy with Roux-Y reconstruction (p < 0.01), and distal gastrectomy with Billroth I (p = 0.019). In addition, factors that decreased the risk of developing late dumping syndrome were reduced weight loss (p = 0.03), being male (p < 0.01), pylorus preserving gastrectomy (p < 0.01), and distal gastrectomy with Roux-Y reconstruction (p < 0.01). No other clinical factors (lymph node dissection, vagal nerve preservation, and postoperative period) showed a substantial association with the occurrence of dumping syndrome in multivariate analyses.

Conclusions.—Substantially more patients suffered from early dumping syndrome than late dumping syndrome after gastrectomy. Two clinical factors, surgical procedures and amount of body weight loss, associated

TABLE 3.—Associations between Clinical Factors and Early Dumping Syndrome Using Multivariate Analyses

Variables	Adjusted Odds Ratio		P Value	Unadjusted Odds Ratio
Age, 60 y or older	0.471	(0.358−0.619)	<0.0001*	0.56
Surgical procedures				
DGB1	0.58	(0.368−0.913)	0.019*	0.582
DGRY	0.427	(0.288−0.632)	<0.0001*	0.423
PG	0.864	(0.491−1.518)	0.61	0.792
PPG	0.399	(0.254−0.626)	<0.0001*	0.369
Preservation of vagal nerve				
With	0.885	(0.639−1.227)	0.4646	0.682
Postoperative weight loss, %				
<10	0.65	(0.499−0.847)	0.001*	0.631

DGB1, distal gastrectomy with reconstruction in Billroth I; DGRY, distal gastrectomy with reconstruction in Roux-en-Y; PG, proximal gastrectomy; PPG, pylorus preserving gastrectomy.
*p < 0.05.

TABLE 4.—Associations between Clinical Factors and Late Dumping Syndrome Using Multivariate Analyses

Variables	Adjusted Odds Ratio		P Value	Unadjusted Odds Ratio
Male gender	0.651	(0.501−0.846)	0.0013*	0.741
Surgical procedures				
DGB1	0.879	(0.592−1.305)	0.522	0.845
DGRY	0.559	(0.391−0.799)	0.001*	0.588
PG	0.841	(0.52−1.36)	0.48	0.799
PPG	0.438	(0.283−0.677)	<0.0001*	0.386
Extent of LN dissection				
D1	0.792	(0.57−1.101)	0.165	0.637
Preservation of vagal nerve				
With	1.02	(0.726−1.432)	0.9103	0.666
Postoperative weight loss, %				
<10	0.763	(0.594−0.98)	0.0347*	0.696

DGB1, distal gastrectomy with reconstruction in Billroth I; DGRY, distal gastrectomy with reconstruction in Roux-en-Y; LN, lymph node; PG, proximal gastrectomy; PPG, pylorus preserving gastrectomy.
*p < 0.05.

significantly with the occurrence of both early and late dumping syndrome (Tables 3 and 4).

▶ Early and late dumping syndromes are the major causes of morbidity in patients who undergo gastrectomy specifically for gastric cancer. This is a very large study of patients who had undergone different types of gastrectomy with correlation of dumping syndrome and various clinical correlation. As seen in Table 3, patients who underwent pylorus-preserving gastrectomy followed by distal gastrectomy with Roux-en-Y reconstruction had the best results following gastrectomy. Pylorus-preserving gastrectomy had the lowest incidents of late dumping syndrome. Patients who had more than 10% weight loss also had more severe early and late dumping syndromes.

This study is among the first to demonstrate strong correlation between incidents of early and late dumping syndromes. This study showed consistently that pylorus-preserving gastrectomy reduced the incidents of dumping syndrome and bowel reflux. Another important finding in this study was that partial gastrectomy showed nearly the same incidents of early dumping syndrome as other types of gastrectomy. In patients who had distal gastrectomies, Roux-en-Y reconstruction showed lower incidents of dumping syndrome compared with a Billroth I reconstruction.

Considerably more patients suffer from early dumping syndrome than late dumping syndrome. The amount of weight loss and the type of reconstruction can have an influence over these symptoms.

T. J. Eberlein, MD

Role of Imaging in the Preoperative Staging of Small Bowel Neuroendocrine Tumors

Chambers AJ, Pasieka JL, Dixon E, et al (Univ of Calgary and the Tom Baker Cancer Centre, Alberta, Canada)
J Am Coll Surg 211:620-627, 2010

Background.—Imaging studies are important in the preoperative staging of patients with small bowel neuroendocrine tumors (NET) and when selecting patients for cytoreduction procedures for metastatic disease. The purpose of this study was to assess the accuracy of preoperative imaging compared with operative findings in the staging of small bowel NET.

Study Design.—Sixty-four patients with small bowel NET undergoing laparotomy and who had preoperative imaging with combinations of CT, MR, and radionuclide scintigraphy were reviewed. Results of imaging studies were compared with operative findings to assess the ability of these investigations to detect mesenteric, peritoneal, and hepatic metastases.

Results.—Mesenteric nodal metastases were seen on imaging in 47 (73%) patients and were present at laparotomy in 56 (88%) patients. Peritoneal metastases were seen on preoperative imaging in 4 (6%) patients and found at laparotomy in 16 (25%) patients. Hepatic metastases were seen on imaging in 42 patients (66%) and found at laparotomy in 49 (77%). Sensitivity and specificity for detection of hepatic metastases were 77% and 100% for CT, 82% and 100% for MR, 63% and 100% for ^{123}I-meta-iodo-benzylguanadine scintigraphy, and 63% and 100% for ^{111}In-octreotide. Imaging studies failed to detect hepatic metastases in 7 patients and underestimated the extent of hepatic metastatic disease in 17 patients.

Conclusions.—Imaging of small bowel NET, even with combinations of CT, MR, and radionuclide studies, underestimates the extent of peritoneal, mesenteric, and hepatic metastatic disease. Accurate staging of small bowel NET might be best performed at the time of laparotomy (Table 2).

▶ Neuroendocrine tumors (NET) are uncommon malignancies. Surgery plays a primary role in the management of metastatic NET of the small bowel.

TABLE 2.—Performance Characteristics of CT, MR, and Radionuclide Scintigraphy in the Preoperative Detection of Hepatic Metastases Using Operative Findings as the Reference Standard

Imaging Modality	n	Sensitivity, % (95% CI)	Specificity, % (95% CI)	PPV, % (95% CI)	NPV, % (95% CI)	Accuracy, %
CT	61	77 (62−87)	100 (72−100)	100 (88−100)	54 (33−74)	82
MR	27	82 (59−94)	100 (46−100)	100 (78−100)	56 (23−85)	85
^{123}I-mIBG	38	63 (44−78)	100 (52−100)	100 (80−100)	33 (14−59)	68
^{111}In-octreotide	46	63 (45−78)	100 (68−100)	100 (82−100)	46 (26−67)	72

mIBG, meta-iodobenzylguanadine; NPV, negative predictive value; PPV, positive predictive value.

Preoperative imaging of patient with small bowel NET is important to assess resectability. As seen in Table 2, CT, MR, and radionuclide scintigraphy have accuracy ranges from 68% to 85%.

The take-home point of this article is that preoperative radiographic evaluation frequently underestimates the extent of disease. Good surgical judgment is needed, and an aggressive surgical approach can be beneficial to the patient. It appears that intraoperative evaluation and decision making with respect to cytoreduction surgery is best performed intraoperatively.

T. J. Eberlein, MD

Laparoscopic Surgery for Gastric Cancer: A Collective Review with Meta-Analysis of Randomized Trials
Kodera Y, Fujiwara M, Ohashi N, et al (Nagoya Univ Graduate School of Medicine, Aichi; et al)
J Am Coll Surg 211:677-686, 2010

Background.—Laparoscopy has been successfully used to treat cholelithiasis and stage abdominal tumors but is only gradually being introduced to treat gastric cancers. Within the last 10 years laparoscopic resection for colon cancer has produced oncologic outcomes comparable to those with open resection and involve less pain and a shorter hospital stay. However, the laparoscopic approach to gastric cancer surgery is seldom used in Western medicine because resectable disease is rarely encountered. In Eastern countries such as Japan and Korea, early-stage disease is commonly handled surgically, but laparoscopy-assisted gastrectomy is indicated only for stage IA and IB cancers. The current status of laparoscopic surgery for gastric cancer was summarized, noting controversies among Asian surgeons that could alter the standard of care.

Nodal Dissection.—Both the East and West support extended lymph node dissection. D2 dissection that involves en bloc or anatomical dissection of retroperitoneal lymph nodes has been the standard of care in Japan since the 1960s and still achieves superior stage-by-stage survival rates compared to not using D2 dissection. A high proportion of patients who have confirmed retroperitoneal node metastases, which can only be addressed by D2 dissection, are alive 5 years postoperatively. Patients with confirmed N2-stage disease survive only when D2 dissection is performed. D2 lowers the risk for cancer-related death long term. The Japanese Gastric Cancer Guidelines defines D2 as a standard procedure for T2-stage cancer or higher but also permits its use for T1-stage cancer with extensive invasion of the submucosa, when about 20% of patients harbor nodal metastasis. Cancer relapse is rare but possible with suboptimal dissection.

Surgical Training.—In the beginning, laparoscopic surgeons were generally already experts in performing open surgery. They then faced the challenge of using long straight devices with a limited range of motion while dealing with insufficient psychomotor skills and a two-dimensional field of view. Assisted by innovations in surgical instruments such as staplers and vessel sealing systems, the surgeons' determination finally produced surgical quality comparable to that of contemporary open surgery. Lymph node retrieval via laparoscopic approach has consistently equaled that of open surgery. However, the learning curve needed to perform laparoscopic surgery well is considerable.

Outcomes.—Short-term outcomes after laparoscopic gastrectomy demonstrate less blood loss, longer operating time, and no marked increase in morbidity or mortality compared to open surgical outcomes. Fewer surgical complications attend laparoscopic versus open approaches. Looking at long-term data, laparoscopic gastrectomy has achieved excellent results, especially using the modified D2 dissection in patients with mucosal or smaller submucosal cancer. The 5-year disease-free survival rates are 99.8% for stage IA, 98.7% for stage IB, and 85.7% for stage II. These excellent results prompted experienced investigators in Japan and Korea to extend the indications to more advanced cancers. The result was longer operating time, less blood loss, and faster recovery, with lymph node retrieval and short-term survival equal to those with open surgery. Peculiar port-site recurrences have complicated the use of the laparoscopic approach, however.

Controversies.—Port-site recurrence is a troubling complication even though most oncologic outcomes after laparoscopic surgery are comparable to or better than those after open surgery. Patients report less pain, which means better preservation of lung function and physical well-being with the laparoscopic approach. This permits an earlier and/or more intensive use of adjuvant therapies because the patient is stronger.

Research into expanding the indications for laparoscopic gastrectomy is principally conducted in Eastern nations, where earlier-stage cancers are more common. Studies are hampered by comorbidity of patients, lack of experience for the surgeon, small available patient samples, philosophical differences in treatment objectives, and the current wide use of laparoscopy for gastric cancer in Japan that has not waited for evidence-based confirmation. Total gastrectomy is still challenging under laparoscopic guidance with no standardized technique. In Korea gastric cancer surgery

Reference	LADG			ODG			Mean Difference (95% CI)	Mean Difference
	Mean	SD	Total	Mean	SD	Total		
22 Huscher	30	14.9	30	33.4	17.4	29	-3.40 (-11.68~4.88)	
32 Kitano	20.2	3.6	14	24.9	3.5	14	-4.70 (-7.33~-2.07)	
33 Hayashi	28	14	14	27	10	14	1.00 (-8.01~10.01)	
30 Lee	31.8	13.5	24	38.1	15.9	23	-6.30 (-14.75~2.15)	
31 Kim YW	39	11.9	82	45.1	43.8	82	-6.10 (-10.04~-2.16)	
Total			**164**			**162**	**-4.79 (-6.79~-2.79)**	

Heterogeneity: p=0.69, I²=0%

Test for overall effect: z=4.69 (p<0.00001)

-10 -5 0 5 10

Favors ODG   Favors LADG

FIGURE 6.—Forest plot of the weighted mean differences of the number of lymph nodes harvested. The estimates of the weighted mean difference in each trial correspond to the middle of each triangle and horizontal line gives the 95% confidence intervals. The summary mean difference is represented by the middle of the solid diamond. No heterogeneity in data was observed between the groups. The yield was greater for the open distal gastrectomy (ODG) group in 4 of the studies, and the difference was statistically significant in 2, including a study with the largest number of patients enrolled (p = 0.003). Consequently, the difference in lymph node retrieval was significant and in favor of ODG. LADG, laparoscopy-assisted distal gastrectomy; Mean, mean number of lymph nodes retrieved; Total, total number of patients per each treatment group. (Reprinted from Journal of American College of Surgeons, Kodera Y, Fujiwara M, Ohashi N, et al. Laparoscopic surgery for gastric cancer: a collective review with meta-analysis of randomized trials. *J Am Coll Surg.* 2010;211:677-686. Copyright © 2010, with permission from the American College of Surgeons.)

is only available in high-volume hospitals by a few highly trained surgeons. Having evidentiary support for the technique would be readily accepted there.

Conclusions.—Eastern nations are currently at the forefront in investigating the use of the laparoscopic approach to treat early-stage gastric cancer. Because this entity is rarely seen in Western nations, the results may not be widely applicable in Western settings. Support for extending the laparoscopic approach to more advanced cancer does not currently exist but a randomized trial is under way. New techniques are more readily applied when the incidence of gastric cancer is lower and more procedures are done by a few experts located in high-volume hospitals. A program of training is needed to prepare new graduates who have little experience in the open surgical technique (Fig 6).

▶ Minimally invasive surgery is playing an ever greater role in the diagnosis and management of various abdominal malignancies. This is a very nice review in meta-analysis of randomized trials dealing with laparoscopic surgery in gastric cancer. As might be expected, laparoscopic surgery was associated with less blood loss but longer operating time and less morbidity; however, open distal gastrectomies were associated with higher number of lymph nodes harvested (Fig 6).

This article really deals with distal gastrectomy as total gastrectomy remains a challenge using laparoscopic approaches.

Certainly anyone performing many operations for gastric cancer should use this excellent summary analysis.

T. J. Eberlein, MD

Miscellaneous

Hospital Factors and Racial Disparities in Mortality After Surgery for Breast and Colon Cancer

Breslin TM, Morris AM, Gu N, et al (Univ of Michigan, Ann Arbor)
J Clin Oncol 27:3945-3950, 2009

Purpose.—Black patients have worse prognoses than whites with breast or colorectal cancer. Mechanisms underlying such disparities have not been fully explored. We examined the role of hospital factors in racial differences in late mortality after surgery for breast or colon cancer.

Methods.—Patients undergoing surgery after new diagnosis of breast or colon cancer were identified using the Surveillance Epidemiology and End Results—Medicare linked database (1995 to 2005). The main outcome measure was mortality at 5 years. Proportional hazards models were used to assess relationships between race and late mortality, accounting for patient factors, socioeconomic measures, and hospital factors. Fixed and random effects models were used to account for quality differences across hospitals.

Results.—Black patients, compared with white patients, had lower 5-year overall survival rates after surgery for breast (62.1% *v* 70.4%, respectively; *P* < .001) and colon cancer (41.3% *v* 45.4%, respectively; *P* < .001). After controlling for age, comorbidity, and stage, black race remained an independent predictor of mortality for breast (adjusted hazard ratio [HR] = 1.25; 95% CI, 1.16 to 1.34) and colon cancer (adjusted HR = 1.13; 95% CI, 1.07 to 1.19). After risk adjustment, hospital factors explained 36% and 54% of the excess mortality for black patients with breast cancer and colon cancer, respectively. Hospitals with large minority populations had higher late mortality rates independent of race.

Conclusion.—Hospital factors, including quality, are important mediators of the association between race and mortality for breast and colon cancer. Hospital-level quality improvement should be a major component of efforts to reduce disparities in cancer outcomes.

▶ This is an administrative database analysis using the Surveillance Epidemiology and End Results (SEER)—Medicare linked database. The authors looked at mortality. As seen in Fig 1 in the original article, there was significantly reduced survival in black patients for both breast and colon cancer treatment. Black patients tend to present at a younger age, have higher tumor stage, and have lower median household income. With respect to breast cancer, black patients tended to have more comorbidity (Table 1). While there are limitations, for example, this study was limited only to patients older than 65 years (Medicare patients) and there may have been an innate bias because of the utilization of Medicare insurance data in contrast to results that may have been obtained with commercial insurers.

TABLE 1.—Patient and Hospital Characteristics Among Patients Who Underwent Breast and Colon Cancer Procedures

Patient and Hospital Characteristics	Breast Cancer (n = 25,571)			Colon Cancer (n = 22,168)		
	White	Black	P	White	Black	P
Patient population	90.27	9.73		88.24	11.76	
Age, years			.0002			<.0001
65-69	18.74	21.51		12.37	17.65	
70-74	25.57	26.74		20.87	24.14	
75-79	25.11	24.97		24.86	24.64	
80-84	17.9	15.24		21.51	18.15	
85+	12.68	11.54		20.39	15.43	
Sex			NA			.0067
Female				43.78	40.98	
Male				56.22	59.02	
Comorbidity index			< .0001			.09
0	80.57	72.7		66.92	64.77	
1	16.57	22.52		26.99	28.86	
> 2	2.87	4.78		6.1	6.37	
Cancer stage			< .0001			< .0001
I	55.11	41.21		23.47	21.11	
II	36.98	45.03		36.88	34.54	
III	5.63	9.81		27.15	28.2	
IV	2.28	3.94		12.49	16.16	
SES			< .0001			< .0001
$25,000 or less	3.3	26.66		3.89	26.75	
$25,001-$35,000	13.43	31.32		13.54	31.89	
$35,001-$45,000	17.72	21.43		18.12	22.03	
$45,001+	65.55	20.59		64.46	19.34	
Hospital patient volume			< .0001			< .0001
Very low	30.74	30.84		30.97	27.36	
Low	28.5	27.95		31.64	32.92	
Median	19.77	14.52		19.68	14.5	
High	21	26.7		17.71	25.21	
Hospital racial mix			< .0001			< .0001
< 10%	74.78	22.32		74.73	20.76	
10%-19%	15.2	19.02		14.8	17.96	
20%-49%	7.68	24.65		8.73	28.59	
> 50%	2.34	34.02		1.74	32.69	

Abbreviations: NA, not available; SES, socioeconomic status.

This study suggests that where patients obtain treatment after cancer diagnosis is important, and perhaps, directing patients to hospitals and treatment facilities that obtain better results in cancer care may influence public policy and have a potential to reduce racial disparities.

T. J. Eberlein, MD

Adjuvant Therapy With Pegylated Interferon Alfa-2b Versus Observation in Resected Stage III Melanoma: A Phase III Randomized Controlled Trial of Health-Related Quality of Life and Symptoms by the European Organisation for Research and Treatment of Cancer Melanoma Group

Bottomley A, Coens C, Suciu S, et al (European Organisation for Res and Treatment of Cancer Quality of Life Dept and Headquarters, Brussels, Belgium; Institut Jules Bordet, Brussels, Belgium; Istituto Nazionale dei Tumori, Brussels, Belgium; et al)

J Clin Oncol 27:2916-2923, 2009

Purpose.—Interferon (IFN) -based adjuvant therapy in melanoma is associated with significant side effects, which necessitates evaluation of health-related quality of life (HRQOL). Our trial examined the HRQOL effects of adjuvant pegylated IFN-α-2b (PEG-IFN-α-2b) versus observation in patients with stage III melanoma.

Methods.—A total of 1,256 patients with stage III melanoma were randomly assigned after full lymphadenectomy to receive either observation (n = 629) or PEG-IFN-α-2b (n = 627): induction 6 μg/kg/wk for 8 weeks then maintenance 3 μg/kg/wk for an intended total duration of 5 years. The European Organisation for Research and Treatment of Cancer Quality of Life Questionnaire C30 was used to assess HRQOL.

Results.—At 3.8 years of median follow-up, for the primary end point, recurrence-free survival (RFS), risk was reduced by 18% (hazard rate = 0.82; P =.01) in the PEG-IFN-α-2b arm compared with observation. Significant and clinically meaningful differences occurred with the PEG-IFN-α-2b treatment arm compared with the observation group, showing decreased global HRQOL at month 3 (−11.6 points; 99% CI, −8.2 to −15.0) and year 2 (−10.5 points; 99% CI, −6.6 to −14.4). Many of the other scales showed statistically significant differences between scores when comparing the two arms. From a clinical point of view, important differences were found for five scales: two functioning scales (social and role functioning) and three symptom scales (appetite loss, fatigue, and dyspnea), with the PEG-IFN-α-2b arm being most impaired.

Conclusion.—PEG-IFN-α-2b leads to a significant and sustained improvement in RFS. There is an expected negative effect on global HRQOL and selected symptoms when patients undergo PEG-IFN-α-2b treatment.

▶ This is an international multicenter study under the auspices of the European Organisation for Research and Treatment of Cancer. Treating patients with stage III melanoma has remained problematic because of the lack of response to chemotherapy. This study looked at health-related quality of life effects of adjuvant pegylated interferon alpha-2b versus observation in patients with stage III melanoma. While the treatment arm led to improvement in relapse-free survival, there were, clearly, impacts on quality of life in the treatment arm (Fig 4 in the original article). There was decrease in social and role functioning and increase in appetite loss, fatigue, and dyspnea. Social functioning, fatigue, and appetite loss were actually the key factors in this study. Clinicians who treat patients with stage III melanoma should be aware of the impact of interferon treatment, anticipate them, and proactively intervene.

T. J. Eberlein, MD

12 Vascular Surgery

Introduction

Several seminal studies have been published during the past year that have defined the care of vascular surgery patients. Perhaps most notable among these were the ICSS and CREST studies comparing carotid angioplasty and endarterectomy. Similar to EVA-3S and SPACE trials, the early results from the ICSS demonstrated that carotid angioplasty was associated with a higher incidence of adverse events in symptomatic patients. In contrast, CREST reported no difference in the major end points among both symptomatic and asymptomatic patients. The long-term results of the ACST-1 trial comparing immediate carotid endarterectomy to a deferred approach demonstrated that the earlier benefits identified for carotid endarterectomy persisted at 10 years, although the absolute benefit was modest. The long-term results of the DREAM, EVAR-1, and EVAR-2 were also reported and, collectively, were similar to the midterm results. There were no survival advantages for endovascular repair compared with open repair among those patients suitable for either approach, and endovascular repair did not improve survival among the high-risk patients compared with expectant management alone. However, the endovascular approach was consistently associated with increased complications, cost, and need for additional procedures. Lastly, the PIVOTAL trial failed to demonstrate a survival benefit for the endovascular repair of small abdominal aortic aneurysms, although the procedure appeared to be safe. These seminal trials should all be read in their entirety.

Several important papers dealing with aneurysms and acute aortic treatment were included among the selected articles. The Albany Group's approach to the treatment of ruptured abdominal aortic aneurysms using the endovascular approach was detailed and both technical and systems issues identified. An elegant randomized controlled trial demonstrated that closure of the abdominal incision with mesh at the time of abdominal aortic aneurysm repair reduced the incidence of hernias, suggesting that this should be performed routinely. The role of endovascular repair for blunt thoracic aortic injury was examined and, surprisingly, the survival did not appear to be affected by the timing of repair. Lastly, the radiation exposure associated with endovascular aneurysm repair and surveillance was detailed. This collective radiation exposure is significant and should be factored into the treatment and surveillance plan.

One of the "final" papers from the BASIL study comparing bypass and endovascular treatment for patients with infrainguinal occlusive disease and severe limb ischemia was included. The study failed to show a benefit for either treatment in terms of amputation-free survival, but it suggested that patients expected to live longer than 2 years may benefit from bypass. These findings are consistent with the mid-term results of the trial comparing above-knee femoropopliteal bypass with covered stent that failed to demonstrate a difference in patency at 4 years. Two separate studies included among the articles addressed the diameter criteria and harvest technique for the saphenous vein as a conduit for a lower extremity bypass. The early patency rates for saphenous veins 2-3 mm in diameter are comparable to those larger than 3 mm, while the patency rates for endoscopic harvest were inferior to the traditional approach and not associated with a decrease in length of stay or complications. Two systematic reviews examined the role of chemical lysis for acute lower extremity ischemia and thrombosed popliteal artery aneurysms. In the case of acute lower extremity ischemia, it did not appear to provide any benefit over bypass surgery. Lysis did appear to improve bypass graft patency after the treatment of thrombosed popliteal artery aneurysms, but it did not reduce the number of amputations.

Three important articles dealing with hemodialysis access were included in this year's YEAR BOOK selections. A novel technique to salvage massively (4-7 cm) aneurysmal autogenous accesses was described. Although a relatively unusual problem, the success rates were excellent and the procedure reasonable. The largest series of lower extremity prosthetic accesses was reported. Despite the significant infectious complication rates, the patency rates were acceptable and may justify the technique for patients with limited options. Lastly, the outcome of primary balloon angioplasty and balloon-assisted maturation were documented for small veins used to construct autogenous accesses. Despite their diminutive diameter, approximately 85% were ultimately usable for a successful access.

The balance of the articles included in this year's collection address a variety of different topics, helping to define both surgical outcomes and techniques. The incidence of stroke associated with coronary artery bypass was found to be 1.6% among approximately 45,000 patients treated at the Cleveland Clinic. In a separate report from the Vascular Study Group of New England, the use of protamine after carotid endarterectomy was found to reduce the incidence of remedial operation for bleeding, but it did not increase the incidence of ischemic complications. The Johns Hopkins group reported that endovascular treatment may not be necessary before first rib resection for patients with *subacute* and *chronic* axillosubclavian vein thrombosis in contrast to the more traditional approach. A paper describing the technique for anterior spinal exposure for interbody fusion was included and, importantly, the associated complications and predictors of adverse outcome described. Lastly, the management of vascular injuries associated with supracondylar humeral factors was detailed, emphasizing the fact that a "nonpalpable" pulse after reduction of the fracture usually means a vascular injury.

Thomas S. Huber, MD, PhD

Aneurysm

Endovascular versus Open Repair of Abdominal Aortic Aneurysm
The United Kingdom EVAR Trial Investigators (Imperial College, London, UK; et al)
N Engl J Med 362:1863-1871, 2010

Background.—Few data are available on the long-term outcome of endovascular repair of abdominal aortic aneurysm as compared with open repair.

Methods.—From 1999 through 2004 at 37 hospitals in the United Kingdom, we randomly assigned 1252 patients with large abdominal aortic aneurysms (≥5.5 cm in diameter) to undergo either endovascular or open repair; 626 patients were assigned to each group. Patients were followed for rates of death, graft-related complications, re-interventions, and resource use until the end of 2009. Logistic regression and Cox regression were used to compare outcomes in the two groups.

Results.—The 30-day operative mortality was 1.8% in the endovascular-repair group and 4.3% in the open-repair group (adjusted odds ratio for endovascular repair as compared with open repair, 0.39; 95% confidence interval [CI], 0.18 to 0.87; $P = 0.02$). The endovascular-repair group had an early benefit with respect to aneurysm-related mortality, but the benefit was lost by the end of the study, at least partially because of fatal endograft ruptures (adjusted hazard ratio, 0.92; 95% CI, 0.57 to 1.49; $P = 0.73$). By the end of follow-up, there was no significant difference between the two groups in the rate of death from any cause (adjusted hazard ratio, 1.03; 95% CI, 0.86 to 1.23; $P = 0.72$). The rates of graft-related complications and reinterventions were higher with endovascular repair, and new complications occurred up to 8 years after randomization, contributing to higher overall costs.

Conclusions.—In this large, randomized trial, endovascular repair of abdominal aortic aneurysm was associated with a significantly lower operative mortality than open surgical repair. However, no differences were seen in total mortality or aneurysm-related mortality in the long term. Endovascular repair was associated with increased rates of graft-related complications and reinterventions and was more costly. (Current Controlled Trials number, ISRCTN55703451.)

▶ The longer term follow-up (median 6.0 years) of the Endovascular Aneurysm Repair 1 (EVAR 1) trial was reported in the same volume of *The New England Journal of Medicine* as those from the Diabetes REduction Assessment with ramipril and rosiglitazone Medication (DREAM) trial reported above. The results of the EVAR 1 trial also fail to show a difference in long-term mortality between patients undergoing endovascular and open repair among patients suitable for both approaches. These mortality findings are consistent with the midterm results and serve to negate the initial or perioperative mortality benefit demonstrated for the endovascular approach. Unlike the longer term results from the DREAM trial, there were several aneurysm ruptures in the endovascular group that seemed to eliminate the early benefit for aneurysm-related mortality. It is worth emphasizing that the endovascular device technology is a moving target, and it is likely that the newer-generation devices are safer or more secure (and therefore less prone to rupture). Admittedly, this assumption merits further clinical investigation. The increased incidence of graft-related complications and reinterventions in the endovascular group remains a common theme, with the incidence greater by 3- to 4-fold and the annual reintervention rate of approximately 5%. Not surprisingly, the cost associated with the endovascular approach was greater with roughly half of the cost associated with the initial admission and the balance with the subsequent intervention. The authors concede in their discussion that not all of the surveillance and reintervention costs were captured in their analysis and that it is conceivable that the cost differences are even greater. Overall, the longer term results of both the EVAR 1 and DREAM trials demonstrate that the endovascular approach is safe and they will likely be used to further justify the approach. However, the absence of a mortality benefit and the increased cost and reintervention rates could just as easily be used to justify the more traditional open approach depending upon individual bias or available resources.

T. S. Huber, MD, PhD

Long-Term Outcome of Open or Endovascular Repair of Abdominal Aortic Aneurysm

De Bruin JL, for the DREAM Study Group (Vrije Universiteit Med Ctr, Amsterdam, The Netherlands; et al)
N Engl J Med 362:1881-1889, 2010

Background.—For patients with large abdominal aortic aneurysms, randomized trials have shown an initial overall survival benefit for elective endovascular repair over conventional open repair. This survival difference, however, was no longer significant in the second year after the procedure. Information regarding the comparative outcome more than 2 years after surgery is important for clinical decision making.

Methods.—We conducted a long-term, multicenter, randomized, controlled trial comparing open repair with endovascular repair in 351 patients with an abdominal aortic aneurysm of at least 5 cm in diameter who were considered suitable candidates for both techniques. The primary outcomes were rates of death from any cause and reintervention. Survival was calculated with the use of Kaplan—Meier methods on an intention-to-treat basis.

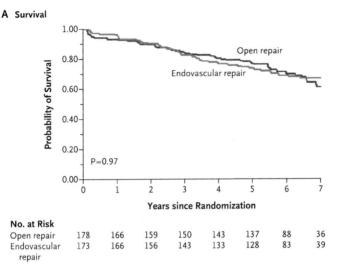

A Survival

B Freedom from Reintervention

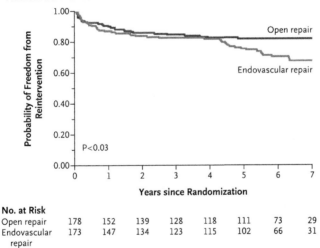

FIGURE 2.—Kaplan—Meier Estimates of Survival (Panel A) and Freedom from Reintervention (Panel B). (Reprinted from De Bruin JL, for the DREAM Study Group. Long-term outcome of open or endovascular repair of abdominal aortic aneurysm. *N Engl J Med.* 2010;362:1881-1889. Copyright © 2010 Massachusetts Medical Society. All rights reserved.)

Results.—We randomly assigned 178 patients to undergo open repair and 173 to undergo endovascular repair. Six years after randomization, the cumulative survival rates were 69.9% for open repair and 68.9% for endovascular repair (difference, 1.0 percentage point; 95% confidence interval [CI], −8.8 to 10.8; P = 0.97). The cumulative rates of freedom from secondary interventions were 81.9% for open repair and 70.4%

for endovascular repair (difference, 11.5 percentage points; 95% CI, 2.0 to 21.0; P = 0.03).

Conclusions.—Six years after randomization, endovascular and open repair of abdominal aortic aneurysm resulted in similar rates of survival. The rate of secondary interventions was significantly higher for endovascular repair. (ClinicalTrials.gov number, NCT00421330 (Fig 2).)

▶ The long-term outcomes of the Dutch Randomized Endovascular Aneurysm Repair (DREAM) trial comparing open with endovascular aneurysm repair (EVAR) are reported. The authors found no difference in survival at 6 years (open, 69.9% vs EVAR, 68.9%), although there was a higher incidence of secondary procedures required in the EVAR group (see Fig 2 A and B). Among the postprocedure deaths, there was only 1 ruptured aneurysm, and this occurred in a patient who had undergone an open repair. Notably, the follow-up rate was almost 100% with a median duration of 6.4 years. These findings from the pivotal DREAM trial suggest that the endovascular approach is as safe as the more traditional open repair, certainly within the midterm time frame. They serve to negate the earlier caveat that the endovascular approach "may not be as durable as open repair." The increased incidence of secondary interventions in the EVAR group is not particularly surprising and serves to underscore the importance of long-term surveillance. Multiple other studies have reported annual remedial intervention rates after EVAR ranging from 5% to 15%. It is worth emphasizing that a significant percentage of patients (18%) required reintervention after open repair with the most frequent procedure being an incisional hernia repair; open repair does not eliminate all aneurysm-related morbidity. Overall, these findings are very reassuring, given the fact that the overwhelming majority of patients opt for EVAR based upon their perception that it is safer and easier.

T. S. Huber, MD, PhD

Endovascular Repair of Aortic Aneurysm in Patients Physically Ineligible for Open Repair

The United Kingdom EVAR Trial Investigators (Imperial College, London, UK; et al)
N Engl J Med 362:1872-1880, 2010

Background.—Endovascular repair of abdominal aortic aneurysm was originally developed for patients who were considered to be physically ineligible for open surgical repair. Data are lacking on the question of whether endovascular repair reduces the rate of death among these patients.

Methods.—From 1999 through 2004 at 33 hospitals in the United Kingdom, we randomly assigned 404 patients with large abdominal aortic aneurysms (≥5.5 cm in diameter) who were considered to be physically ineligible for open repair to undergo either endovascular repair or no repair; 197 patients were assigned to undergo endovascular repair, and 207 were assigned to have no intervention. Patients were followed for rates of death, graft-related complications and reinterventions, and costs until the end of 2009. Cox regression was used to compare outcomes in the two groups.

Results.—The 30-day operative mortality was 7.3% in the endovascular-repair group. The overall rate of aneurysm rupture in the no-intervention group was 12.4 (95% confidence interval [CI], 9.6 to 16.2) per 100 person-years. Aneurysm-related mortality was lower in the endovascular-repair group (adjusted hazard ratio, 0.53; 95% CI, 0.32 to 0.89; $P = 0.02$). This advantage did not result in any benefit in terms of total mortality (adjusted hazard ratio, 0.99; 95% CI, 0.78 to 1.27; $P = 0.97$). A total of 48% of patients who survived endovascular repair had graft-related complications, and 27% required reintervention within the first 6 years. During 8 years of follow-up, endovascular repair was considerably more expensive than no repair (cost difference, £9,826 [U.S. $14,867]; 95% CI, 7,638 to 12,013 [11,556 to 18,176]).

Conclusions.—In this randomized trial involving patients who were physically ineligible for open repair, endovascular repair of abdominal aortic aneurysm was associated with a significantly lower rate of aneurysm-related mortality than no repair. However, endovascular repair was not associated with a reduction in the rate of death from any cause. The rates of graft-related complications and reinterventions were higher with endovascular repair, and it was more costly. (Current Controlled Trials number, ISRCTN55703451.)

▶ The long-term results (median follow-up of 3.1 years until death or study completion) of the Endovascular Aneurysm Repair (EVAR)-2 trial comparing EVAR with expectant management among patients deemed ineligible for open repair are presented. Similar to the earlier EVAR-2 publication, EVAR was not associated with a decrease in all-cause mortality (21.0 vs 22.1 deaths per 100 person-years) but was more costly (difference, US $14 867) and associated with a higher incidence of graft-related complications and interventions. The authors did report a decrease in aneurysm-related mortality in the EVAR group that was not identified during their initial report. Notably, additional patients (N = 66) were randomized after the initial report, and this resulted in a decrease in the overall 30-day operative mortality rate for the EVAR group (9.0% vs 7.3%). Although it appears to support the role of EVAR, aneurysm-related mortality was not the primary end point of the study (end point—all-cause mortality), and I would contend that the cause of death is fairly irrelevant from a patient standpoint and not dying from a ruptured aneurysm is insufficient justification for EVAR in the absence of a survival benefit. Unfortunately, this report suffers from the same criticisms as the initial study in that there was a significant amount of crossover between the study groups. Specifically, 34% (70/207) of the patients in the no-intervention group underwent repair of their aneurysms. The authors did perform a per protocol analysis that showed a trend toward a lower all-cause mortality rate, but the difference did not reach statistical significance ($P = .14$). The report contained several interesting findings that help define the natural history of patients with large aneurysms deemed ineligible for open repair. First, the long-term survival in this group of patients is quite poor (6-year survival: EVAR, 30%; no intervention, 26%), regardless of the type of intervention. Second, the rupture risk of the large aneurysms (baseline diameter 6.7 ± 1.0 cm) in the no-intervention group was 12.4 per 100 person years, although this value must be interpreted with some caution, given the number of crossovers. Third, the risk of graft-related complications and reinterventions was similar between the EVAR-1 and EVAR-2 trials, despite the fact that the patients in EVAR-2 were deemed not to be candidates for EVAR-1 because they couldn't undergo open repair. It is not clear how the results of the study should be used in daily practice. As the authors emphasized in their discussion, the decision to perform EVAR in patients deemed ineligible for open repair is still a balance between the risk of repair and the risk of rupture. EVAR may not improve survival in this group of patients ineligible for open repair, but the determination of ineligibility is somewhat subjective and debatable. The large number of crossovers in the no-intervention group likely reflects the loss of equipoise and the difficulty withholding EVAR.

T. S. Huber, MD, PhD

Endovascular repair compared with surveillance for patients with small abdominal aortic aneurysms

Ouriel K, for the Positive Impact of Endovascular Options for treating Aneurysms Early (PIVOTAL) Investigators (Columbia Univ and NewYork-Presbyterian Hosp; et al)

J Vasc Surg 51:1081-1087, 2010

Background.—Although repair of large abdominal aortic aneurysms (AAAs) is well accepted, randomized clinical trials have failed to demonstrate benefit for early surgical repair of small aneurysms compared with surveillance. Endovascular repair has been shown to be safer than open surgical repair in patients with large aneurysms, prompting a randomized trial of early endovascular repair vs surveillance in patients with small aneurysms.

Methods.—We randomly assigned 728 patients (13.3% women; mean age, 71 ± 8 years) with 4 to 5 cm AAAs to early endovascular repair (366 patients) or ultrasound surveillance (362 patients). Rupture or aneurysm-related death and overall mortality in the two groups were compared during a mean follow-up of 20 ± 12 months.

Results.—Among patients randomized to treatment, 89% underwent aneurysm repair. Among patients randomized to surveillance, 31% underwent aneurysm repair during the course of the study. After a mean follow-up of 20 ± 12 months (range, 0-41 months), 15 deaths had occurred in each group (4.1%). The unadjusted hazard ratio (95% confidence interval) for mortality after early endovascular repair was 1.01 (0.49-2.07, $P = .98$). Aneurysm rupture or aneurysm-related death occurred in two patients in each group (0.6%). The unadjusted hazard ratio was 0.99 (0.14-7.06, $P = .99$) for early endovascular repair.

Conclusions.—Early treatment with endovascular repair and rigorous surveillance with selective aneurysm treatment as indicated both appear to be safe alternatives for patients with small AAAs, protecting the patient from rupture or aneurysm-related death for at least 3 years.

▶ The authors report the results of the randomized controlled Positive Impact of Endovascular Options for Treating Aneurysms Early trial designed to determine whether endovascular aneurysm repair (EVAR) is superior to surveillance for small abdominal aortic aneurysms (4.0-5.0 cm). The study was based upon the premise that the perioperative mortality rate for EVAR is lower than that for open repair and, therefore, early EVAR may be beneficial. It is important to remember that the operative decision making for patients with abdominal aortic aneurysms represents a balance between the operative mortality rate and the risk associated with expectant management (ie, rupture risk and death). The authors reported that EVAR was not associated with a mortality benefit (hazard ratio, 1.01; 95% confidence interval, 0.40-2.07; $P = .98$), although the procedure itself was safe and associated with a mortality rate of <1%. Notably, 31% of the patients randomized to surveillance ultimately underwent aneurysm repair (predominantly EVAR). The perioperative complication rate was 3-fold higher in the EVAR group, although the most common complications were classified as vascular and related to the cannulation site. Based upon these findings, the authors concluded that "early treatment with endovascular repair and rigorous surveillance with selective aneurysm treatment as indicated appear to be safe alternatives..." These conclusions appear to be somewhat biased in favor of EVAR, and I would contend that the most appropriate conclusion might be that EVAR is not indicated for patients with small aneurysms. Despite the elegant study design, the results of the study are not particularly surprising, given the earlier randomized trials that showed no benefit for open repair compared to surveillance for small aneurysms (ie, UK Small Aneurysm trial, Aneurysm Detection and Management) and the comparable survival for open repair and EVAR for larger aneurysms (ie, Dutch Randomized Endovascular Aneurysm Management , EVAR 1, Open Versus Endovascular Repair). The study did underscore 2 important findings from the earlier small aneurysm trials. Specifically, small aneurysms (ie, <5.5 cm) rarely rupture, and most patients with aneurysms in this size range ultimately require repair. Indeed, the important question for patients is not so much if they need to have their aneurysm repaired but rather when. The results of the study have not changed my current clinical practice in terms of the size threshold for intact, asymptomatic abdominal aortic aneurysm repairs (ie, male, 5.5 cm; female, 5.0 cm), but it is reassuring to know that endovascular repair of these smaller aneurysms appears to be safe.

T. S. Huber, MD, PhD

Endovascular aneurysm repair for ruptured abdominal aortic aneurysm: The Albany Vascular Group approach

Mehta M (Albany Med College, NY)

J Vasc Surg 52:1706-1712, 2010

Improvements in endovascular technology and techniques have allowed us to treat patients in ways we never thought possible. Today, endovascular treatment of ruptured abdominal aortic aneurysms is associated with markedly decreased morbidity and mortality compared with the open surgical approach, yet there are several fundamental obstacles in our ability to offer these endovascular techniques to most patients with ruptured aneurysms. This article will focus on the technical aspects of endovascular aneurysm repair for rupture, with particular attention to developing a standardized multidisciplinary approach that will help vascular surgeons deal with not just the technical aspects of these procedures but also address some of the challenges, including the availability of preoperative computed tomography, the choice of anesthesia, the percutaneous vs femoral cutdown approach, use of aortic occlusion balloons, need for bifurcated vs aortouniiliac stent grafts, need for adjunctive procedures, diagnosis and treatment of abdominal compartment syndrome, and conversion to open surgical repair.

▶ Dr Mehta has provided a nice summary of the Albany Vascular Group's approach for ruptured abdominal aortic aneurysm repair using the endovascular aneurysm repair (EVAR) technique, highlighting both system and technical issues. I would strongly encourage everyone performing EVAR for ruptured aneurysms to read the complete article, particularly those contemplating starting a new program. The endovascular approach for ruptured aneurysms represents a significant stride forward in the overall treatment of aneurysmal disease and likely represents the greatest benefit of EVAR in terms of mortality, given the equivocal outcomes in the randomized trials comparing elective open and endovascular repair. Dr Mehta emphasizes several critical system issues required for success, including a multidisciplinary team, a readily available CT scanner, a dedicated hybrid operating room suite suitable for both open and endovascular repairs, sufficient on-the-shelf inventory, and an experienced surgeon. Indeed, the importance of these components must not be underemphasized and provides indirect justification for regionalization of care for ruptured aneurysms and other acute aortic pathologies. The fundamentals of the technique are reviewed in a stepwise fashion with special emphasis on the components critical to the ruptured aneurysm scenario (vs intact). One of the most crucial steps among these is the deployment of an aortic occlusion balloon and the need to place a suitable supporting sheath. Dr Mehta also addresses several more controversial issues surrounding the overall approach to ruptured aneurysms, including the role of preoperative CT scans, choice of anesthesia, access for the endovascular devices, choice of bifurcated or aortouniiliac graft, role of adjunctive procedures, the abdominal compartment syndrome, and conversion to open repair. Based upon the collective experience, it has become clear that most patients are candidates for the endovascular approach and can safely undergo a preoperative planning CT despite the historic surgical dogma that all patients with a ruptured aneurysm need to be taken directly to the operating room. Endovascular repair of ruptured aneurysms may be more complicated than in the elective setting, requiring a low threshold for an aortouniiliac graft and adjunctive techniques to facilitate an adequate proximal seal. The abdominal compartment syndrome is associated with the use of an aortic occlusion balloon, massive transfusions, and coagulopathy. Laparotomy may be justified at the time of EVAR in the presence of abdominal distension and one of the aforementioned factors regardless of whether the bladder pressure is normal. Despite the evolution of the endovascular approach and its application by nonsurgeons, it is important to underscore the fact that a ruptured aneurysm is a surgical emergency that needs to be addressed in an appropriately equipped operating room by skilled surgeons capable of performing both open and endovascular repair.

T. S. Huber, MD, PhD

Randomized clinical trial of mesh *versus* sutured wound closure after open abdominal aortic aneurysm surgery
Bevis PM, Windhaber RAJ, Lear PA, et al (Cheltenham General Hosp, UK; Univ of Bristol, UK; Southmead Hosp, Bristol, UK; et al)
Br J Surg 97:1497-1502, 2010

Background.—Incisional herniation is a common complication of abdominal aortic aneurysm (AAA) repair. This study investigated whether prophylactic mesh placement could reduce the rate of postoperative incisional hernia after open repair of AAA.

Methods.—This randomized clinical trial was undertaken in three hospitals. Patients undergoing elective open AAA repair were randomized to routine abdominal mass closure after AAA repair or to prophylactic placement of polypropylene mesh in the preperitoneal plane.

Results.—Eighty-five patients with a mean age of 73 (range 59—89) years were recruited, 77 (91 per cent) of whom were men. There were five perioperative deaths (6 per cent), two in the control group and three in the mesh group ($P = 0 \cdot 663$), none related to the mesh. Sixteen patients in the control group and five in the mesh group developed a postoperative incisional hernia (hazard ratio $4 \cdot 10$, 95 per cent confidence interval $1 \cdot 72$ to $9 \cdot 82$; $P = 0 \cdot 002$). Hernias developed between 170 and 585 days after surgery in the control group, and between 336 and 1122 days in the mesh group. Four patients in the control group and one in the mesh group underwent incisional hernia repair ($P = 0 \cdot 375$). No mesh became infected, but one was subsequently removed owing to seroma formation during laparotomy for small bowel obstruction.

Conclusion.—Mesh placement significantly reduced the rate of postoperative incisional hernia after open AAA repair without increasing the rate of complications. Registration number: ISRCTN28485581 (http://www. controlled-trials.com).

▶ The authors have performed a simple yet elegant randomized trial examining whether the prophylactic placement of mesh reduces the incidence of incisional hernias after open abdominal aortic aneurysm repair. It is generally well accepted that patients with abdominal aortic aneurysm are at an increased risk for developing both incisional and inguinal hernias, with the incidence of the former approaching 40%. Indeed, the general surgeons at our institution recently implied that the evolution from open to endovascular aneurysm repair has negatively affected their hernia practice. The responsible mechanisms remain unresolved but have been generically attributed to a connective tissue disorder consistent with those for the underlying aneurysm. In this study, the authors reported that the incidence of incisional hernias was lower in the mesh group (37% vs 14%, $P = .02$), although there was no difference in the incidence of remedial hernia repair between the groups (9% vs 3%, $P = .38$). Despite the impressive incidence of hernias in the control group, it is somewhat sobering to reflect that the true incidence may ultimately be higher, given the relative short-term follow-up in the study (< 3 years) and the primary reliance on physical examination for diagnosis (vs ultrasound). The incidence of complications was not different between the groups, and importantly, the mesh did not become infected in any of the cases, although the total number of patients in the experimental group was small ($N = 37$). A total of 4 patients (2 in each group) required laparotomy for a small bowel obstruction, thereby underscoring the fact that patients frequently require remedial procedures and long-term follow-up after both open and endovascular repair. The results of the study beg the question as to whether prophylactic mesh repair should be performed at the time of all open aneurysm repairs. Despite the small sample size, the data suggest that the procedure is safe and effective and does not appear to add much to the procedure in terms of time or expense. Prophylactic repairs certainly merit consideration, particularly because open repair is currently being reserved for patients nonamenable to endovascular treatment with more complex anatomy, potentially associated with more complicated repairs and an increased incidence of postoperative incisional hernias.

T. S. Huber, MD, PhD

The impact of radiation dose exposure during endovascular aneurysm repair on patient safety
Jones C, Badger SA, Boyd CS, et al (Belfast City Hosp, Ireland)
J Vasc Surg 52:298-302, 2010

Objective.—Endovascular aneurysm repair (EVAR) exposes patients to radiation during the procedure and in subsequent follow-up. The study goal was to calculate the radiation dose in our unit and compare it against other published data and national guidelines.

Methods.—All EVAR procedures were identified from a prospectively maintained database. Radiation dose, screening time, and volume of intravenous contrast during the procedure were reviewed. Radiation exposure from subsequent computed tomography (CT) imaging was included in the overall exposure. Results are expressed as mean ± standard deviation.

Results.—From October 1998 to October 2008, 320 elective patients underwent EVAR. Mean screening time was 29.4 ± 23.3 minutes, and the radiation dose was 11.7 ± 7.1 mSv. The EVAR was an emergency in 64 patients. The mean screening time was 22.9 ± 18.2 minutes, and the radiation dose was 13.4 ± 8.6 mSv. During the first postoperative year, follow-up CT scans exposed the patients to 24.0 mSv, with 8.0 mSv in subsequent years. Abdominal radiographs added an additional 1.8 mSv each year.

Conclusion.—EVAR and the follow-up investigations involve substantial amounts of radiation, with well-recognized carcinogenic risks. Because patient safety is paramount, radiation exposure should be minimized. This may be possible by standardizing radiation exposure throughout the United Kingdom by implementing national guidelines and considering other imaging modalities for follow-up.

▶ The report documents the cumulative radiation associated with endovascular aneurysm repair (EVAR) and highlights an important potential risk to patients. The radiation dose associated with an EVAR, both elective and emergent, was approximately 24 mSv, with the follow-up dose roughly the same during the first year and 8 mSv thereafter. Notably, these values were based upon a follow-up protocol that included 3 CT scans during the first year (1, 3, and 12 months) and annual CT scans thereafter, similar to the EVAR trials. Based upon their protocol, the authors estimated a cumulative total radiation exposure of approximately 85 and 135 mSv at 5 and 10 years, respectively. These cumulative dosages are within the lifetime recommended limit of 400 mSv but do represent a risk to patients in light of the carcinogenic potential. Every effort should be made to reduce the radiation exposure to the patient and associated health care providers (including the vascular surgeons). The obvious potential opportunities include reducing the number of postoperative CT scans and/or using duplex ultrasound as a surveillance tool. In our own practice, we obtain postoperative CT scans at 1 month, 12 months and then yearly or biannually thereafter depending upon the appearance of the aneurysm and device. We have used duplex ultrasound alone for patients with contraindications to intravenous contrast (eg, elevated creatinine, allergy), but multiple reports have documented its effectiveness as a routine surveillance tool. Furthermore, we have adopted a best practice in terms of limiting the radiation exposure in the operating room and endovascular suite.

T. S. Huber, MD, PhD

Carotid

Carotid artery stenting compared with endarterectomy in patients with symptomatic carotid stenosis (International Carotid Stenting Study): an interim analysis of a randomised controlled trial

International Carotid Stenting Study investigators (Univ College London, UK; London School of Hygiene and Tropical Medicine, UK; et al)
Lancet 375:985-997, 2010

Background.—Stents are an alternative treatment to carotid endarterectomy for symptomatic carotid stenosis, but previous trials have not established equivalent safety and efficacy. We compared the safety of carotid artery stenting with that of carotid endarterectomy.

Methods.—The International Carotid Stenting Study (ICSS) is a multicentre, international, randomised controlled trial with blinded adjudication of outcomes. Patients with recently symptomatic carotid artery stenosis were randomly assigned in a 1:1 ratio to receive carotid artery stenting or carotid endarterectomy. Randomisation was by telephone call or fax to a central computerised service and was stratified by centre with minimisation for sex, age, contralateral occlusion, and side of the randomised artery. Patients and investigators were not masked to treatment assignment. Patients were followed up by independent clinicians not directly involved in delivering the randomised treatment. The primary outcome measure of the trial is the 3-year rate of fatal or disabling stroke in any territory, which has not been analysed yet. The main outcome measure for the interim safety analysis was the 120-day rate of stroke, death, or procedural myocardial infarction. Analysis was by intention to treat (ITT). This study is registered, number ISRCTN25337470.

Findings.—The trial enrolled 1713 patients (stenting group, n=855; endarterectomy group, n=858). Two patients in the stenting group and one in the endarterectomy group withdrew immediately after randomisation, and were not included in the ITT analysis. Between randomisation and 120 days, there were 34 (Kaplan-Meier estimate $4 \cdot 0\%$) events of disabling stroke or death in the stenting group compared with 27 ($3 \cdot 2\%$) events in the endarterectomy group (hazard ratio [HR] $1 \cdot 28$, 95% CI $0 \cdot 77-2 \cdot 11$). The incidence of stroke, death, or procedural myocardial infarction was $8 \cdot 5\%$ in the stenting group compared with $5 \cdot 2\%$ in the endarterectomy group (72 *vs* 44 events; HR $1 \cdot 69$, $1 \cdot 16-2 \cdot 45$, p=$0 \cdot 006$). Risks of any stroke (65 *vs* 35 events; HR $1 \cdot 92$, $1 \cdot 27-2 \cdot 89$) and all-cause death (19 *vs* seven events; HR $2 \cdot 76$, $1 \cdot 16-6 \cdot 56$) were higher in the stenting group than in the endarterectomy group. Three procedural myocardial infarctions were recorded in the stenting group, all of which were fatal, compared with four, all non-fatal, in the endarterectomy group. There was one event of cranial nerve palsy in the stenting group compared with 45 in the endarterectomy group. There were also fewer haematomas of any severity in the stenting group than in the endarterectomy group (31 *vs* 50 events; p=$0 \cdot 0197$).

Interpretation.—Completion of long-term follow-up is needed to establish the efficacy of carotid artery stenting compared with endarterectomy. In the meantime, carotid endarterectomy should remain the treatment of choice for patients suitable for surgery.

▶ The International Carotid Stenting Study compared carotid angioplasty and stenting in symptomatic patients with high-grade carotid stenosis. The early results (120 days) reported above demonstrate that the incidence of stroke, death, and myocardial infarction were higher after stenting (carotid artery stenting, 8.5% vs carotid endarterectomy [CEA], 5.2%), with the differences largely due to a higher incidence of nondisabling strokes. These results corroborate those from 2 other similar randomized trials (Endarterectomy Versus Angioplasty in Patients with Symptomatic Severe Carotid Stenosis trial and Stent-Protected Angioplasty versus Carotid Endarterectomy), as illustrated by the meta-analysis included in the discussion. The increased incidence of stroke in the stenting group was likely secondary to the instrumentation and manipulation inherent to the procedure itself and could not be easily attributed to bias or a procedural learning curve. Although the procedure requirements for provider inclusion were fairly modest, the incidence of adverse events reported from the experienced centers was surprisingly higher (vs less experienced centers). The inclusion of perioperative myocardial infarction as an end point for carotid revascularization studies has been somewhat controversial and debatable. However, it is worth noting that they did not appear to be a major factor in this study, with only 3 infarctions (3/828) after stenting and 5 after endarterectomy (5/821). Surprisingly, all 3 of the myocardial infarctions after stenting were fatal. The study reported a higher incidence of complications after CEA in women, a consistent finding that merits consideration. Hopefully, the publication of the primary outcome measure (3-year rate of death or disabling stroke in any territory) will help further clarify the role of the carotid stenting for symptomatic patients and resolve the lingering controversy.

T. S. Huber, MD, PhD

Stenting versus Endarterectomy for Treatment of Carotid-Artery Stenosis
Brott TG, for the CREST Investigators (Mayo Clinic, Jacksonville, FL; et al)
N Engl J Med 363:11-23, 2010

Background.—Carotid-artery stenting and carotid endarterectomy are both options for treating carotid-artery stenosis, an important cause of stroke.

Methods.—We randomly assigned patients with symptomatic or asymptomatic carotid stenosis to undergo carotid-artery stenting or carotid endarterectomy. The primary composite end point was stroke, myocardial infarction, or death from any cause during the periprocedural period or any ipsilateral stroke within 4 years after randomization.

Results.—For 2502 patients over a median follow-up period of 2.5 years, there was no significant difference in the estimated 4-year rates of the primary end point between the stenting group and the endarterectomy group (7.2% and 6.8%, respectively; hazard ratio with stenting, 1.11; 95% confidence interval, 0.81 to 1.51; $P = 0.51$). There was no differential treatment effect with regard to the primary end point according to symptomatic status ($P = 0.84$) or sex ($P = 0.34$). The 4-year rate of stroke or death was 6.4% with stenting and 4.7% with endarterectomy (hazard ratio, 1.50; $P = 0.03$); the rates among symptomatic patients were 8.0% and 6.4% (hazard ratio, 1.37; $P = 0.14$), and the rates among asymptomatic patients were 4.5% and 2.7% (hazard ratio, 1.86; $P = 0.07$), respectively. Periprocedural rates of individual components of the end points differed between the stenting group and the endarterectomy group: for death (0.7% vs. 0.3%, $P = 0.18$), for stroke (4.1% vs. 2.3%, $P = 0.01$), and for myocardial infarction (1.1% vs. 2.3%, $P = 0.03$). After this period, the incidences of ipsilateral stroke with stenting and with endarterectomy were similarly low (2.0% and 2.4%, respectively; $P = 0.85$).

Conclusions.—Among patients with symptomatic or asymptomatic carotid stenosis, the risk of the composite primary outcome of stroke, myocardial infarction, or death did not differ significantly in the group undergoing carotid-artery stenting and the group undergoing carotid endarterectomy. During the periprocedural period, there was a higher risk of stroke with stenting and a higher risk of myocardial infarction with endarterectomy. (ClinicalTrials.gov number, NCT00004732.)

▶ The results of the long-awaited Carotid Revascularization Endarterectomy vs Stenting Trial (CREST) demonstrated no difference (carotid-artery stenting, 7.2% vs carotid endarterectomy, 6.8%) in the primary end point (perioperative cerebrovascular accident [CVA], myocardial infarction [MI], death, and ipsilateral CVA with 4 years) with a median follow-up of 2.5 years (see Fig 2A in the original article). Not surprisingly, the perioperative stroke rates were higher among those patients undergoing stenting, while the MI rates were higher for those undergoing endarterectomy. No differences were demonstrated based upon the patient's symptomatic status, although there was an interaction between age and treatment with a crossover at 70 years of age with younger patients favoring stenting and older ones favoring endarterectomy. These secondary analyses are important because Medicare reimbursement for stenting has been restricted to symptomatic patients, and several other studies, including the lead-in data for CREST, have reported a higher complication rate for stenting in elderly patients. Notably, the study encompassed 2502 patients from 117 centers, and enrollment spanned almost 8 years. During this enrollment period, the use of carotid stenting across the country has proliferated and the technique refined. Despite these changing practice patterns, the same stent system (RX Acculink, Abbott Vascular Solutions) and embolic protection devices (RX Accunet, Abbott Vascular Solutions) were used. The overall treatment results for both stenting and endarterectomy are spectacular and, indeed, represent the best ones reported from any of the randomized carotid stenting trials, paralleling those reported for endarterectomy from the Asymptomatic Carotid

Atherosclerosis Study.[1] These excellent results likely reflect the stringent certi-fication criteria for the centers and providers but raise the question about the widespread application of the study results. The main unanswered question is how the CREST data, and carotid stenting itself, should be applied. Although compelling, the current data contradict 3 other well-performed randomized trials (Endarterectomy versus Angioplasty in Patients with Symptomatic Severe Carotid Stenosis, Stent-Protected Angioplasty versus Carotid Endarterectomy, and International Carotid Stenting Study) that failed to support carotid stent-ing. Furthermore, it's debatable whether a perioperative stroke is really equiva-lent to a perioperative MI. However, they do demonstrate that the results in experienced centers are comparable with endarterectomy for appropriately selected patients and likely justify more widespread use of the technique.

T. S. Huber, MD, PhD

Reference

1. Endarterectomy for asymptomatic carotid artery stenosis. Executive Committee for the Asymptomatic Carotid Atherosclerosis Study. *JAMA*. 1995;273:1421-1428.

10-year stroke prevention after successful carotid endarterectomy for asymptomatic stenosis (ACST-1): a multicentre randomised trial
Halliday A, on behalf of the Asymptomatic Carotid Surgery Trial (ACST) Collaborative Group (John Radcliffe Hosp, Oxford, UK; et al)
Lancet 376:1074-1084, 2010

Background.—If carotid artery narrowing remains asymptomatic (ie, has caused no recent stroke or other neurological symptoms), successful carotid endarterectomy (CEA) reduces stroke incidence for some years. We assessed the long-term effects of successful CEA.

Methods.—Between 1993 and 2003, 3120 asymptomatic patients from 126 centres in 30 countries were allocated equally, by blinded minimised randomisation, to immediate CEA (median delay 1 month, IQR $0\cdot3$–$2\cdot5$) or to indefinite deferral of any carotid procedure, and were followed up until death or for a median among survivors of 9 years (IQR 6—11). The primary outcomes were perioperative mortality and morbidity (death or stroke within 30 days) and non-perioperative stroke. Kaplan-Meier percentages and logrank p values are from intention-to-treat anal-yses. This study is registered, number ISRCTN26156392.

Findings.—1560 patients were allocated immediate CEA versus 1560 allocated deferral of any carotid procedure. The proportions operated on while still asymptomatic were $89\cdot7\%$ versus $4\cdot8\%$ at 1 year (and $92\cdot1\%$ *vs* $16\cdot5\%$ at 5 years). Perioperative risk of stroke or death within 30 days was $3\cdot0\%$ (95% CI $2\cdot4$–$3\cdot9$; 26 non-disabling strokes plus 34 disabling or fatal perioperative events in 1979 CEAs). Excluding perioper-ative events and non-stroke mortality, stroke risks (immediate *vs* deferred CEA) were $4\cdot1\%$ versus $10\cdot0\%$ at 5 years (gain $5\cdot9\%$, 95% CI $4\cdot0$—$7\cdot8$)

and 10·8% versus 16·9% at 10 years (gain 6·1%, 2·7—9·4); ratio of stroke incidence rates 0·54, 95% CI 0·43—0·68, p<0·0001. 62 versus 104 had a disabling or fatal stroke, and 37 versus 84 others had a non-disabling stroke. Combining perioperative events and strokes, net risks were 6·9% versus 10·9% at 5 years (gain 4·1%, 2·0—6·2) and 13·4% versus 17·9% at 10 years (gain 4·6%, 1·2—7·9). Medication was similar in both groups; throughout the study, most were on antithrombotic and antihypertensive therapy. Net benefits were significant both for those on lipid-lowering therapy and for those not, and both for men and for women up to 75 years of age at entry (although not for older patients).

Interpretation.—Successful CEA for asymptomatic patients younger than 75 years of age reduces 10-year stroke risks. Half this reduction is in disabling or fatal strokes. Net benefit in future patients will depend on their risks from unoperated carotid lesions (which will be reduced by medication), on future surgical risks (which might differ from those in trials), and on whether life expectancy exceeds 10 years (Fig 3).

▶ The study reports the long-term (median 9 years) follow-up of the Asymptomatic Carotid Surgery Trial 1 comparing immediate and deferred carotid endarterectomy (CEA) for patients with high-grade carotid stenoses. Similar to the initial study, immediate CEA resulted in a significant reduction in perioperative events and stroke at 10 years (13% vs 18%, Fig 3). Notably, the benefits

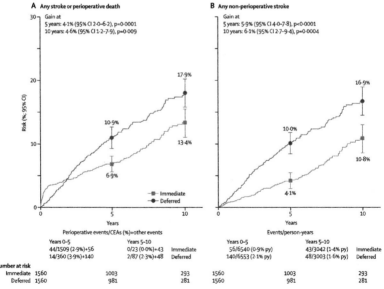

FIGURE 3.—10-year risk of any stroke or perioperative death (A) and any nonperioperative stroke (B) After year 10 there were no perioperative strokes and four immediate versus seven deferred first strokes. CEA=carotid endarterectomy. py=per year. (Reprinted from The Lancet, Halliday A, on behalf of the Asymptomatic Carotid Surgery Trial (ACST) Collaborative Group. 10-year stroke prevention after successful carotid endarterectomy for asymptomatic stenosis (ACST-1): a multicentre randomised trial. *Lancet*. 2010;376:1074-1084. Copyright 2010, with permission from Elsevier.)

identified at 5 years persisted at 10 years. Among the patients randomized to deferred CEA, 34% ultimately underwent the procedure, with approximately one-third of these performed for symptoms. The medical treatment in the 2 groups was essentially the same with most patients on antiplatelets, antihypertensives, and lipid-lowering agents. Notably, the study paralleled the introduction and widespread application of the lipid-lowering agents (ie, statins), with 10% of the patients on these agents at the onset of the study and 80% at completion. Interestingly, the stroke risk was lower in patients with lipid-lower agents in both the immediate and deferred CEA groups, but there was still a benefit for immediate CEA. This is noteworthy since it has been hypothesized to the contrary that the newer lipid-lowering agents may negate the effects of CEA for asymptomatic patients. The results are still somewhat sobering with an absolute stroke reduction of 5% over 10 years and a number needed to treat of approximately 20. Similar to the earlier trials, CEA appears to have benefit for good-risk asymptomatic patients provided that the procedural-associated complication rates are reasonable. It is noteworthy that the perioperative morbidity and mortality rates were approximately 3% and that this rate was not affected for the patients who underwent the deferred CEA. The study does emphasize that the benefit of CEA for asymptomatic lesions is partially dependent on survival and that patients older than 75 years likely derive little benefit.

T. S. Huber, MD, PhD

Temporal Onset, Risk Factors, and Outcomes Associated With Stroke After Coronary Artery Bypass Grafting

Tarakji KG, Sabik JF III, Bhudia SK, et al (Cleveland Clinic, OH)
JAMA 305:381-390, 2011

Context.—Stroke is a devastating and potentially preventable complication of coronary artery bypass graft (CABG) surgery. Better understanding of the timing and risk factors for stroke associated with CABG are needed.

Objectives.—To investigate temporal trends in stroke after CABG and to identify stroke risk factors and association with longitudinal outcomes.

Design, Setting, and Patients.—Prospective study conducted from 1982 through 2009 at a single US academic medical center among 45 432 consecutive patients (mean age, 63 [SD, 10] years) undergoing isolated primary or reoperative CABG surgery. Strokes occurring following CABG were recorded prospectively and classified as having occurred intraoperatively or postoperatively. Complications and survival after stroke were assessed in propensity-matched groups.

Intervention.—CABG performed using 4 different operative strategies (off-pump, on-pump with beating heart, on-pump with arrested heart, on-pump with hypothermic circulatory arrest).

Main Outcome Measures.—Hospital complications; late survival.

Results.—Among 45 432 patients undergoing CABG surgery, 705 (1.6% [95% confidence interval {CI}, 1.4%-1.7%]) experienced a stroke. The prevalence of stroke peaked in 1988 at 2.6% (95% CI, 1.9%-3.4%), then declined at 4.69% (95% CI, 4.68%-4.70%) per year (*P* =.04), despite increasing patient comorbidity. Overall, 279 strokes (40%) occurred intraoperatively and 409 (58%) occurred postoperatively (timing indeterminate in 17 patients). Postoperative stroke peaked at 40 hours, decreasing to 0.055%/d (95% CI, 0.047%-0.065%) by day 6. Risk factors for both intraoperative and postoperative stroke included older age (odds ratio, 8.5 [95% CI, 3.2-22]) and variables representing arteriosclerotic burden. Intraoperative stroke rates were lowest in off-pump CABG (0.14% [95% CI, 0.029%-0.40%]) and on-pump beating-heart CABG (0% [95% CI, 0%-1.6%]), intermediate with on-pump arrested-heart CABG (0.50% [95% CI, 0.41%-0.61%]), and highest with on-pump CABG with hypothermic circulatory arrest (5.3% [95% CI, 2.0%-11%]). Patients with stroke had worse adjusted hospital outcomes, longer intensive care and postoperative stays, and worse downstream survival (mean, 11 [SD, 8.6] years).

Conclusion.—Among patients undergoing CABG surgery at a single center over the past 30 years, the occurrence of stroke declined despite an increasing patient risk profile, and more than half of strokes occurred postoperatively rather than intraoperatively.

▶ The authors have documented the incidence of stroke after coronary artery bypass grafting (CABG) at the Cleveland Clinic in a series spanning almost 3 decades. They reported a stroke risk of 1.6% among over 45 000 patients. They reported that the incidence peaked at 2.6% in 1988 but has gradually decreased since that time despite an increase in the patient risk profile. Somewhat surprisingly, the incidence of postoperative stroke was higher than intraoperative stroke with the peak occurring on the second postoperative day. Several risk factors were identified for both intraoperative and postoperative strokes, including age, presence of peripheral vascular disease, preoperative atrial fibrillation, and the operative technique. New onset postoperative atrial fibrillation did not increase the stroke risk and appeared to be protective. Predictably, stroke was associated with increased perioperative mortality, morbidity, and decreased survival. The findings of the study are particularly noteworthy, given the sheer size of the sample and the duration of the study. Although coronary revascularization is not within the usual purview of most peripheral vascular surgeons, the findings are important given the presence of coronary artery disease among our patients, their frequent need for CABG, and the role that vascular surgeons play in the preoperative and postoperative care of patients undergoing CABG in terms of stroke risk reduction. Unfortunately, this study could not detail whether the strokes were a result of hypoperfusion, thrombosis, or an embolic event, although all were likely contributory. The role of carotid endarterectomy before (or concomitant with) CABG in asymptomatic patients is an ancient unanswered question. It is always disconcerting when a patient with significant known carotid occlusive disease sustains a stroke after CABG, but this is usually related to the burden of atherosclerotic disease in the aortic arch rather than the carotid itself. This concept of atherosclerotic burden is indirectly supported by the stroke risk factors in this study (ie, age, peripheral vascular disease, smoking, diabetes). It is interesting that the stroke risk varied with the operative technique and was greatest for on-pump hypothermic circulatory arrest. These differences justify a patient-specific approach incorporating the identified risk factors.

T. S. Huber, MD, PhD

Protamine reduces bleeding complications associated with carotid endarterectomy without increasing the risk of stroke
Stone DH, for the Vascular Study Group of Northern New England (Dartmouth-Hitchcock Med Ctr, Lebanon, NH; et al)
J Vasc Surg 51:559-564, 2010

Objectives.—Controversy persists regarding the use of protamine during carotid endarterectomy (CEA) based on prior conflicting reports documenting both reduced bleeding as well as increased stroke risk. The purpose of this study was to determine the effect of protamine reversal of heparin anticoagulation on the outcome of CEA in a contemporary multistate registry.

Methods.—We reviewed a prospective regional registry of 4587 CEAs in 4311 patients performed by 66 surgeons from 11 centers in Northern New England from 2003-2008. Protamine use varied by surgeon (38% routine use, 44% rare use, 18% selective use). Endpoints were postoperative bleeding requiring reoperation as well as potential thrombotic complications, including stroke, death, and myocardial infarction (MI). Predictors of endpoints were determined by multivariate logistic regression after associated variables were identified by univariate analysis.

Results.—Of the 4587 CEAs performed, 46% utilized protamine, while 54% did not. Fourteen patients (0.64%) in the protamine-treated group required reoperation for bleeding compared with 42 patients (1.66%) in the untreated cohort (*P* =.001). Protamine use did not affect the rate of MI (1.1% vs 0.91%, *P* =.51), stroke (0.78% vs 1.15%, *P* =.2), or death (0.23% vs 0.32%, *P* =.57) between treated and untreated patients, respectively. By multivariate analysis, protamine (odds ratio [OR] 0.32, 95% confidence interval [CI], 0.17-0.63; *P* =.001) and patch angioplasty (OR 0.46, 95% CI, 0.26-0.81; *P* =.007) were independently associated with diminished reoperation for bleeding. A single center was associated with a significantly higher rate of reoperation for bleeding (OR 6.47, 95% CI, 3.02-13.9; *P* < .001). Independent of protamine use, consequences of reoperation for bleeding were significant, with a four-fold increase in MI, a seven-fold increase in stroke, and a 30-fold increase in death.

Conclusion.—Protamine reduced serious bleeding requiring reoperation during CEA without increasing the risk of MI, stroke, or death, in this large, contemporary registry. In light of significant complications referable to bleeding, liberal use of protamine during CEA appears warranted.

▶ This publication from the Vascular Study Group of New England addresses one of the age-old questions of vascular surgery, specifically whether the use of protamine after carotid endarterectomy (CEA) is beneficial. The proponents of protamine use have pointed to the reduced incidence of bleeding complications, while the opponents have cited the potential increased incidence of thrombotic events. Unfortunately, the available evidence has been limited and somewhat controversial with the single randomized controlled trial (RCT), concluding that protamine was associated with an increased incidence of thrombotic complications.[1] This study, encompassing >4500 CEAs, has demonstrated that the use of protamine was associated with a significantly lower rate of reoperation for bleeding (0.64% vs 1.66%, $P = .001$). Notably, the overall incidence of reoperation for hematoma in both groups was quite small despite the statistical difference. Furthermore, it is worth emphasizing that the adverse bleeding-related end point analyzed was reoperation rather than simply a neck hematoma, although presumably reoperation represents the worse case scenario. Reoperation for hematoma was associated with several adverse events including a higher incidence of myocardial infarction, stroke, and death along with a longer length of stay. However, it is not clear from the data that the reoperation was the cause of these adverse events or a marker for a higher risk patient population. It was interesting to note that the use of a patch closure was also associated with a lower incidence of reoperation. In contrast to its beneficial effects, the use of protamine did not appear to be associated with an increased risk of thrombotic events or complications, although protamine-related events were not specifically recorded among the data. The study has several limitations, as conceded by the authors, including its study design (ie, not an RCT), the lack of a standardized dosing schedule for both heparin and protamine, and the lack of a formal neurologic examination by a neurologist to adjudicate adverse events. However, the data are compelling and support a more liberal use of protamine at the time of CEA.

T. S. Huber, MD, PhD

Reference

1. Fearn SJ, Parry AD, Picton AJ, Mortimer AJ, McCollum CN. Should heparin be reversed after carotid endarterectomy? A randomised prospective trial. *Eur J Vasc Endovasc Surg.* 1997;13:394-397.

Peripheral Arterial Occlusive Disease

Bypass versus Angioplasty in Severe Ischaemia of the Leg (BASIL) trial: An intention-to-treat analysis of amputation-free and overall survival in patients randomized to a bypass surgery-first or a balloon angioplasty-first revascularization strategy
Bradbury AW, on behalf of the BASIL trial Participants (Univ of Birmingham and Vascular and Endovascular Surgery, UK; et al)
J Vasc Surg 51:5S-17S, 2010

Background.—A 2005 interim analysis of the Bypass versus Angioplasty in Severe Ischaemia of the Leg (BASIL) trial showed that in patients with severe lower limb ischemia (SLI; rest pain, ulceration, gangrene) due to infrainguinal disease, bypass surgery (BSX)-first and balloon angioplasty (BAP)-first revascularization strategies led to similar short-term clinical outcomes, although BSX was about one-third more expensive and morbidity was higher. We have monitored patients for a further 2.5 years and now report a final intention-to-treat (ITT) analysis of amputation-free survival (AFS) and overall survival (OS).

Methods.—Of 452 enrolled patients in 27 United Kingdom hospitals, 228 were randomized to a BSX-first and 224 to a BAP-first revascularization strategy. All patients were monitored for 3 years and more than half for >5 years.

Results.—At the end of follow-up, 250 patients were dead (56%), 168 (38%) were alive without amputation, and 30 (7%) were alive with amputation. Four were lost to follow-up. AFS and OS did not differ between randomized treatments during the follow-up. For those patients surviving 2 years from randomization, however, BSX-first revascularization was associated with a reduced hazard ratio (HR) for subsequent AFS of 0.85 (95% confidence interval [CI], 0.5-1.07; $P = .108$) and for subsequent OS of 0.61 (95% CI, 0.50-0.75; $P = .009$) in an adjusted, time-dependent Cox proportional hazards model. For those patients who survived for 2 years after randomization, initial randomization to a BSX-first revascularization strategy was associated with an increase in subsequent restricted mean overall survival of 7.3 months (95% CI, 1.2-13.4 months, $P = .02$) and an increase in restricted mean AFS of 5.9 months (95% CI, 0.2-12.0 months, $P = .06$) during the subsequent mean follow-up of 3.1 years (range, 1-5.7 years).

Conclusions.—Overall, there was no significant difference in AFS or OS between the two strategies. However, for those patients who survived for at least 2 years after randomization, a BSX-first revascularization strategy was associated with a significant increase in subsequent OS and a trend towards improved AFS.

▶ The final results of the Bypass versus Angioplasty in Severe Ischaemia of the Leg (BASIL) trial are presented and represent a follow-up to the 2005 interim analysis. Indeed, the study abstracted above represents one of several final publications from the trial included in a supplement to the *Journal of Vascular Surgery*. In the trial, patients with infrainguinal occlusive disease and severe limb ischemia were randomized to either a bypass surgery (BSX)-first or balloon angioplasty (BAP)-first approach. Severe limb ischemia was defined as ischemic rest pain or tissue loss and differs slightly from the more rigorous definition of chronic limb ischemia that includes a threshold ankle pressure of < 50 mm Hg. Similar to the interim report, there were no differences in the major end points of overall survival and amputation-free survival. These findings support the evolving concept that the outcome in patients with severe limb ischemia is dictated more by the underlying disease process than the choice of treatment. Notably, the Kaplan-Meier estimates for both overall survival (approximately 50%) and amputation-free survival (approximately 40%) at 5 years were quite sobering and reflect the terminal nature of the underlying condition. There was a time-dependent benefit for BSX, and those patients who survived 2 years had an improved overall survival and a trend toward an increased amputation-free survival. The interim results of this seminal trial were criticized on a variety of points (eg, sample size, selection criteria, end points, widespread application, and inclusion of prosthetic grafts), and the authors spent a large part of their discussion addressing these concerns. Despite these potential limitations, the BASIL trial remains the only multicenter randomized trial of its kind, and the data support their recommendations. Specifically, patients expected to survive > 2 years are best treated with BSX using a venous conduit, while those expected to survive < 2 years and those without suitable conduit should undergo BAP. Admittedly, it is not always easy to predict which patients with severe occlusive disease will survive beyond this threshold. A wealth of knowledge is included among the other final reports that comprise the supplement. Among these is an analysis of the trial based upon the actual treatment received (vs intention to treat), demonstrating that BAP is associated with higher failure rate than BSX, most patients undergoing BAP ultimately require BSX, and the outcomes after remedial BSX performed for a failed BAP are worse than those for BSX performed as the initial procedure.[1] However, these latter results must be interpreted with caution because of the inherent selection bias from the fact that the patients did not receive their assigned treatment.

T. S. Huber, MD, PhD

Reference

1. Bradbury AW, Adam DJ, Bell J, et al. Bypass versus Angioplasty in Severe Ischaemia of the Leg (BASIL) trial: analysis of amputation free and overall survival by treatment received. *J Vasc Surg.* 2010;51:18S-31S.

Four-year randomized prospective comparison of percutaneous ePTFE/ nitinol self-expanding stent graft versus prosthetic femoral-popliteal bypass in the treatment of superficial femoral artery occlusive disease
McQuade K, Gable D, Pearl G, et al (Baylor Univ Med Ctr, Dallas, TX; et al)
J Vasc Surg 52:584-591, 2010

Background.—This is a randomized prospective study comparing the treatment of superficial femoral artery occlusive disease percutaneously with an expanded polytetrafluoroethylene (ePTFE)/nitinol self-expanding stent graft (stent graft) versus surgical femoral to above-knee popliteal artery bypass with synthetic graft material.

Methods.—One hundred limbs in 86 patients with superficial femoral artery occlusive disease were evaluated from March 2004 to May 2005. Patient symptoms included both claudication and limb threatening ischemia with or without tissue loss. Trans-Atlantic InterSociety Consensus (TASC II) A (n = 18), B (n = 56), C (n = 11), and D (n = 15) lesions were included. Patients were randomized prospectively into one of two treatment groups; a percutaneous treatment group (group A; n = 50) with angioplasty and placement of one or more stent grafts, or a surgical treatment group (group B; n = 50) with a femoral to above-knee popliteal artery bypass using synthetic conduit (Dacron or ePTFE). Patients were followed for 48 months. Follow-up evaluation included clinical assessment, physical examination, ankle-brachial indices, and color flow duplex sonography at 3, 6, 9, 12, 18, 24, 36, and 48 months.

Results.—Mean total lesion length of the treated arterial segment in the stent graft group was 25.6 cm (SD = 15 cm). The stent graft group demonstrated a primary patency of 72%, 63%, 63%, and 59% with a secondary patency of 83%, 74%, 74%, and 74% at 12, 24, 36, and 48 months, respectively. The surgical femoral-popliteal group demonstrated a primary patency of 76%, 63%, 63%, and 58% with a secondary patency of 86%, 76%, 76%, and 71% at 12, 24, 36, and 48 months, respectively. No statistical difference was found between the two groups with respect to primary ($P = .807$) or secondary ($P = .891$) patency.

Conclusion.—Management of superficial femoral artery occlusive disease with percutaneous stent grafts exhibits similar primary patency at 4-year (48 month) follow up when compared with conventional femoral-popliteal artery bypass grafting with synthetic conduit. This treatment method may offer an alternative to treatment of the superficial femoral artery segment for revascularization when prosthetic bypass is being considered or when autologous conduit is unavailable.

▶ The 4-year results of a single-center randomized trial comparing above-knee femoropopliteal bypass (Dacron or expanded polytetrafluoroethylene [ePTFE]) with an ePTFE-covered nitinol stent graft are presented. Patients with both claudication and limb-threatening ischemia were included in the trial with most patients having Trans-Atlantic InterSociety II A and B lesions (surgery, 66% and stent, 78%). Admittedly, it is unusual that patients with limb-threatening ischemia can be treated with only an above-knee femoropopliteal bypass. There were no differences in the primary (surgery, 58% and stent, 59%) or secondary (surgery, 71% and stent, 74%) patency rates at 4 years, and indeed, these patency rates were quite good overall. A total of 7 patients (surgery, 6 and stent, 1) required amputation, which is disturbing considering the inclusion criteria and the limited bypasses (ie, above the knee). It is important to remember that the goal of treating claudication is to improve lifestyle or walking distances, not to save extremities. The authors addressed the reservation that a failed prosthetic bypass (or covered stent) may lead to a higher grade of ischemia in their discussion and felt that their data did not support this concern. Several recent reports have documented the use of covered stents in a variety of vascular beds, and they appear to represent one of the next magic bullets for endovascular therapy. The covered stent design prevents intimal hyperplasia within the fabric itself, although stenoses (either de novo or recurrent) can develop at the ends of the stent as seen in this study. It is worthwhile to note that the patency rates for the 6 to 7 mm stent grafts appeared to be better than those for the 5 mm grafts, although the trend did not reach statistical significance. These findings are consistent with those reported by Green et al,[1] demonstrating that smaller diameter grafts (< 7 mm) were associated with an increased risk of thrombosis after above-knee femoropopliteal bypass. Overall, these results seem to indicate that covered stents are comparable with above-knee femoropopliteal prosthetic bypasses when both options are feasible. However, these favorable results should be interpreted with some caution, given the small sample size, poor long-term follow-up (loss to follow-up: surgery, 30% and stent, 12%), and industry-funding source. Femoropopliteal bypass with ipsilateral saphenous vein remains the gold standard, albeit a more involved procedure than a percutaneous revascularization.

T. S. Huber, MD, PhD

Reference

1. Green RM, Abbott WM, Matsumoto T, et al. Prosthetic above-knee femoropopliteal bypass grafting: five-year results of a randomized trial. *J Vasc Surg*. 2000;31: 417-425.

Outcome of infra-inguinal bypass grafts using vein conduit with less than 3 millimeters diameter in critical leg ischemia
Slim H, Tiwari A, Ritter JC, et al (King's College Hosp, London, UK)
J Vasc Surg 53:421-425, 2011

Objective.—The purpose of this study was to evaluate the difference in amputation-free survival and patency rates of infra-inguinal bypass grafts in patients with critical leg ischemia (CLI) with vein conduits with an internal diameter <3 mm compared to those with vein conduits with a diameter of ≥3 mm.

Methods.—Retrospective analysis of all consecutive patients with CLI undergoing infra-inguinal bypass. Preoperative duplex scan mapping and measurement of potential vein grafts were performed on all patients. Patients were recruited in a 1-year duplex scan graft surveillance program. Primary end points were amputation-free survival and patency rates at 1 year postoperatively. Kaplan-Meier and χ^2 test were used for statistical analysis.

Results.—Between January 2004 and April 2010, 157 consecutive patients with CLI underwent 171 bypasses using vein conduits (111 men, 46 women; median age, 75 years; range, 45-96 years). Ninety-three bypasses (54.4%) were performed for tissue loss, 44 (25.7%) for gangrene, and for rest pain. Of the 157 patients, 113 (72.0%) had diabetes mellitus, 40 (25.5%) had renal impairment, 131 (83.4%) had hypertension, and 64 (40.8%) had ischemic heart disease. Femoro-popliteal bypass was performed in 38 cases (22.2%), whereas 133 (77.8%) of the bypasses were femoro-distal. Autogenous great saphenous vein (GSV) was used in all cases. All grafts were reversed. The diameter of 31 (18%) vein conduits measured <3 mm (range, 2-2.9 mm) on preoperative duplex scan. One hundred thirty-four grafts had at least 1-year follow-up. The primary, assisted primary, and secondary patency rates at 1 year for vein conduits <3 mm were 51.2%, 82.6%, and 82.6%, respectively, compared to 68.4%, 93.3%, and 95.2%, respectively, in the ≥3 mm group. This was only significant for the secondary patency (*P* =.0392). The amputation-free survival at 48 months was 70.8% for vein conduits <3 mm and 57.3 for vein conduits ≥3 mm.

Conclusion.—This series has shown that primary and assisted primary patency rates in small veins are not significantly different at 1 year but the secondary patency rates are better in the larger veins. Similarly, the amputation-free survival was also comparable. The authors would, therefore, advocate the use of small veins >2 mm in diameter in patients with CLI. Duplex scan surveillance followed by early salvage angioplasty for threatened grafts is needed to achieve good patency rates in both groups.

▶ The authors document their outcome after lower extremity bypass procedures for patients with critical limb ischemia (Rutherford classification 4, 5, or 6) using saphenous vein conduits < 3 mm in diameter. They reported a significant difference in secondary patency (83% for < 3 mm vs 95% for > 3 mm) at 1 year but no differences in the primary (< 3 mm - 51% vs > 3 mm - 68%) or primary-assisted patency (< 3 mm - 83% vs > 3 mm - 93%) rates at the same time point. Furthermore, they failed to demonstrate a difference in amputation-free survival at 4 years (< 3 mm - 71% vs > 3 mm − 57%), the most crucial end point of the study. Based upon these findings, the authors advocated the use of small saphenous veins (> 2 mm) for patients with critical limb ischemia. It is worthwhile to emphasize that there are some inherent inaccuracies in the determination of the vein diameter using duplex ultrasound that may obscure any strict criteria about the suitability of a vein for an arterial conduit. These measurements can vary on a daily basis, likely related to hydration, and it has been my practice to repeat these studies on a separate day if the vein is found to be smaller than the usual threshold diameter. Furthermore, the vein usually dilates over time when used as an arterial conduit as demonstrated in this study. The study helps to answer the critical question about the optimal choice of conduit for infrainguinal bypass in patients in whom adequate saphenous vein (diameter, > 3 mm) is not available. This clinical scenario is quite common and the available alternatives are multiple, including small saphenous vein, arm vein, cryopreserved cadaveric vein, cryopreserved cadaveric artery, a prosthetic graft, and a modified prosthetic graft (eg, anastomotic patch, fistula). It has been my practice to use only autogenous veins > 3 mm, with the choice of procedures being ipsilateral saphenous > contralateral saphenous > arm vein > others. However, this algorithm may merit revision with insertion of smaller diameter saphenous veins, certainly for patients with critical limb ischemia and severe infrainguinal disease. The results of this study must be interpreted with some caution given the relatively small sample size of patients with < 3-mm veins (N = 31), the retrospective study design, and the aggressive strategies to maintain graft patency. These strategies include an intraoperative completion duplex study, anticoagulation in the perioperative period, postoperative antiplatelet agents, postoperative statins, and a graft surveillance protocol (schedule: immediate postoperative and then every 3 months for a year) with relative low thresholds for intervention. Notably, 41% of the patients with small veins required a salvage angioplasty. Indeed, the favorable results may reflect the authors' postoperative management strategies more than the vein diameter threshold.

T. S. Huber, MD, PhD

Thrombolysis for acute arterial occlusion
van den Berg JC (Ospedale Regionale di Lugano, sede Civico, Switzerland)
J Vasc Surg 52:512-515, 2010

Introduction.—Acute leg ischemia is one of the most challenging and dangerous conditions in vascular surgical practice and carries a high risk of amputation and death when left untreated. This article provides an overview of the currently held opinions on the role of catheter-based thrombolytic therapy in patients with acute leg ischemia.

Methods.—A systematic review of literature from 1980 to 2009 was performed. The literature analyzed included randomized trials, large single-center case series, and review articles.

Results.—Three large randomized trials and 14 review articles were identified. Pharmacologic aspects and the results of thrombolytic therapy, as well as indications, contraindications, and complications are described.

Conclusions.—Catheter-directed thrombolysis can be considered a complementary and not a competing technology with surgical or percutaneous revascularization, with an acceptably low complication rate.

▶ The author has performed a systematic review to examine the evidence for catheter-directed thrombolysis in patients with acute lower extremity ischemia. This is a very timely topic in light of the increased emphasis on minimally invasive endovascular therapies that include a variety of pharmacomechanical approaches for both arterial and venous thrombosis. Notably, acute lower extremity ischemia is associated with a significant mortality/morbidity, and these rates have not changed much over the past few decades. In the current review, there did not appear to be a difference in either mortality or amputation rate between surgery or thrombolysis. Not surprisingly, the risk of major hemorrhage (< 5%) was greater in the thrombolysis group with the risk of hemorrhagic stroke being 1% to 2%. The risk of complications associated with thrombolysis, including bleeding, increased fairly dramatically with the duration of therapy and was 8-fold higher after 40 hours relative to 8 hours (4% vs 34%). The overall results of the review should be interpreted with some caution for several reasons. There were only 3 randomized trials in the review and none were published within the current decade. The patients who comprised these trials were fairly heterogeneous in terms of the duration of ischemia and the mechanism (ie, bypass vs native vessel). A Cochrane review on the same topic concluded that the evidence was insufficient to support either surgery or thrombolysis.[1] It is important to emphasize that catheter-directed thrombolysis requires a prolonged period to reverse the ischemia and is not appropriate for patients with type IIb fistulas (threatened-immediate). It has been my impression that thrombolysis is a tool looking for an application and that its role has diminished since the seminal publications highlighted in the review. I would concur with the author that catheter-directed thrombolysis is complementary with surgical and percutaneous revascularization but disagree with his opening statement in the discussion that it can be considered standard of care.

T. S. Huber, MD, PhD

Reference

1. Berridge DC, Kessel D, Robertson I. Surgery versus thrombolysis for initial management of acute limb ischemia. *Cochrane Database Syst Rev.* 2002;(1). CD002784.

Clinical Outcome of Acute Leg Ischaemia Due to Thrombosed Popliteal Artery Aneurysm: Systematic Review of 895 Cases

Kropman RHJ, Schrijver AM, Kelder JC, et al (St Antonius Hosp Nieuwegein, The Netherlands; et al)

Eur J Vasc Endovasc Surg 39:452-457, 2010

Objectives.—A systematic review was performed to summarise outcomes of acute thrombosed popliteal artery aneurysms (PAAs) treated with thrombolysis or thrombectomy followed by bypass.

Methods.—A systematic review was conducted of data on acute thrombosed PAAs dated 1 January 1990 through 30 June 2008 using the Cochrane Library, MEDLINE and EMBASE databases. Primary endpoint was limb salvage; secondary endpoints were mortality and patency of the bypasses.

Results.—Eight prospective studies and 25 retrospective studies with 895 patients presenting with acute ischaemia were included. No randomised trials were included. The mortality rate after surgical repair was 3.2% (95% confidence interval (C.I.) 1.8–4.6). The amputation rate was 14.1% (95% C.I. 11.8–16.4). Thrombolysis before surgery did not result in a significant reduction of the number of amputations, compared with surgery (thrombectomy and bypass) alone. The mean primary patency rates of the bypasses at 1, 3 and 5 years were 79%, 77% and 74%, respectively, in the 'thrombolysis' group and 71% ($P = 0.026$), 54% ($P = 0.164$) and 45% ($P = 0.249$) in the 'thrombectomy' group. No distinction could be made regarding secondary patency and limb-salvage rates between the groups owing to insufficient data.

Conclusions.—Preoperative and intra-operative thrombolyses result in a significant improvement in 1-year primary graft patency rates, but do not result in a significant reduction for amputations compared with surgery alone.

▶ The authors have performed a systematic review to determine the optimal initial treatment (thrombolysis vs open thrombectomy) for patients with acute lower extremity ischemia secondary to thrombosed popliteal artery aneurysms (PAAs). They found that the patency rates were improved with chemical thrombolysis (patency rates at 1, 3, and 5 years are 79% vs 71%, 77% vs 54%, and 74% vs 45%, respectively), but there were no differences in the number of amputations. Patients with acute lower extremity ischemia secondary to thrombosed PAAs are somewhat different from the larger cohort of patients with acute lower extremity ischemia secondary to atherosclerotic occlusive disease. Although atherosclerosis is a systemic process, it is characterized by segmental involvement of the major vessels with intervening normal segments, and it is this segmental distribution that facilitates revascularization or bypass. In contrast, PAAs can act as a source of atheroembolic debris that can lead to the chronic obliteration or pruning off of the tibial vessels and elimination of any suitable bypass targets. Given this potential underlying mechanism, chemical thrombolysis has a tremendous amount of appeal for acute ischemia secondary to thrombosed PAAs because it may dissolve any acute clot and help identify a suitable distal target. One of the inherent limitations of thrombolysis is the obligatory time for the agents to work (ie, lyse the clot) that can range from 6 to 48 hours. Accordingly, thrombolysis is not appropriate for patients with more severe classes of ischemia (ie, Rutherford IIb). The results of this study must be interpreted with some caution, given the inherent selection bias that patients with less severe ischemia (ie, Rutherford IIa) were likely offered initial thrombolysis, while those with more severe ischemia were treated operatively. Indeed, the results of the study may actually reflect the differences in outcome between patients with class IIa and IIb ischemia. I believe that acute lower extremity ischemia secondary to a thrombosed PAA may be one of the more compelling indications for arterial thrombolysis as supported by the authors' data provided that the extremity can tolerate the obligatory delay. Surgical thrombectomy in this setting can be very unsatisfying and ineffective, as reflected by the 14% amputation rate documented in the review.

T. S. Huber, MD, PhD

Long-Term Results of Endoscopic Versus Open Saphenous Vein Harvest for Lower Extremity Bypass

Julliard W, Katzen J, Nabozny M, et al (Univ of Rochester Med Ctr, NY)
Ann Vasc Surg 25:101-107, 2011

Background.—Endoscopic saphenous vein harvest (EVH) has been shown to lower wound infection rates and cost compared with conventional harvest, although long-term patency data are lacking. A small series of studies has recently suggested that patency is inferior to conventionally harvested vein technique, and we thus sought to explore this question by reviewing our cumulative experience with this technique.

Methods.—The short- and long-term outcomes of all lower extremity bypasses (LEBPs) using saphenous vein at one institution over a period of 8.5 years were retrospectively reviewed.

Results.—A total of 363 patients averaging 67 ± 24 to 100 years of age had undergone LEBP and had charts available for review. Of these 363 patients, 170 underwent EVH (90% using a noninsufflation technique) and 193 conventional (by means of continuous or skip incisions); 48% of patients reported tissue loss and no differences in indication for surgery were noted between groups. Mean follow-up was 35.1 (range: <1-105) months. Primary patency rates were worse in the EVH group as compared with conventional at six (63.3% ± 4.0% vs. 77.3% ± 3.3%), 12 (50.4% ± 4.2% vs. 73.7% ± 3.6%), and 36 (42.2% ± 4.5% vs. 59.1% ± 4.9%) months (all $p < 0.001$), although these differences were largely limited to patients with limb-threat and diabetes. However, limb salvage and survival, were identical between groups. Contrary to previous experience, there were no differences in length of stay or wound complication rates.

Conclusions.—The overall results of this study show an inferior long-term patency rate for endoscopically harvested saphenous vein after LEBP in our series as a whole, and do not confirm the short-term benefit previously shown in a selected cohort. These differences were, however, minimal or absent in patients with claudication or absence of diabetes, and EVH may continue to play a role in these cases.

▶ The authors document their experience with endoscopic saphenous vein harvest (EVH) for lower extremity bypass and report that the patency rates were inferior while there were no differences in the perioperative morbidity or length of stay. Notably, these differences in the patency rates were clinically relevant and fairly impressive (ie, 3-year primary patency, 42% vs 59%). However, they were not associated with differences in limb salvage or overall survival and were largely driven by the presence of diabetes and more severe ischemia. These findings are significant, given the earlier results from the same institution touting the advantages of the technique. In the authors' earlier publication, they reported that EVH was cheaper and associated with shorter length of stays and fewer wound complications. The explanation for these apparently contradictory findings is likely multifactorial and includes more liberal application of the technique to patients with advanced ischemia, longer-term follow-up, and improvement in the outcome for patients undergoing open saphenous vein harvest. Furthermore, there was likely a component of publication bias similar to the adoption and dissemination of other technological advances. It is interesting to note that the current findings also support those of Pullat et al[1] and Lopes et al,[2] documenting inferior patency rates after EVH for lower extremity and coronary bypass grafting procedures, respectively. Indeed, Pullat et al[1] compared a single saphenectomy incision with multiple incisions (ie, skip incisions) and EVH, reporting that the patency rates were best in the single incision group. This report begs the question as to the role of EVH for lower extremity bypass. It has been my impression that the technique has not been very widely accepted by vascular surgeons in contrast to cardiac surgeons given the complexity/time-consuming nature of the technique, the need to harvest a long segment of vein, and concerns about longer-term patency. Despite the obvious limitations of a single-center retrospective study, the limited application of the technique among vascular surgeons seems appropriate given the inferior patency rates and absence of a benefit in terms of wound complications. It may have a role for patients without diabetes or with claudication, although the authors' statement that "EVH may not necessarily be worse in non diabetics or patients with claudication" is not a resounding statement of support.

T. S. Huber, MD, PhD

References

1. Pullat R, Brothers TE, Robison JG, Elliot BM. Compromised bypass graft outcomes after minimal-incision vein harvest. *J Vasc Surg.* 2006;44:289-295.
2. Lopes RD, Hafley GE, Allen KB, et al. Endoscopic versus open vein-graft harvesting in coronary-artery bypass surgery. *N Engl J Med.* 2009;361:235-244.

Access

Midterm results of a novel technique to salvage autogenous dialysis access in aneurysmal arteriovenous fistulas

Woo K, Cook PR, Garg J, et al (Scripps Green Hosp, La Jolla, CA; et al)
J Vasc Surg 51:921-925, 2010

Purpose.—Over the last decade, K-DOQI guidelines have increasingly emphasized the importance of autogenous arteriovenous fistulas (AVF) for dialysis access. A complication of AVF is aneurysmal dilatation with a subset developing massive diffuse aneurysm. Treatment of massive aneurysmal AVF generally involves either ligation or resection with use of prosthetic interposition. To maintain an all-autogenous access, we developed a procedure to treat massive aneurysmal AVF in which the luminal diameter is reduced, excess length is resected, and the new reconstructed AVF is re-tunneled for continued use. The purpose of this study is to examine the midterm outcomes of this novel procedure.

Methods.—Over a 4-year period, the reduction/revision procedure was performed on 19 patients with an AVF diameter of 4-7 cm. Indications for operation were thrombosis, skin breakdown, infection, bleeding, and/or poor flow. Revision was performed by resecting redundant length, reducing diameter, and then reconstructing the fistula.

Results.—The median patient age was 47, interquartile range (IQR) 29. There were 13 men and 6 women. The median follow-up was 23 months, IQR 22. The median primary patency was 14 months, IQR 24. The median secondary patency was 16.5 months, IQR 26. Two patients died, one AVF thrombosed, and two were ligated secondary to infection.

Three fistulae developed a stenosis that was treated with percutaneous angioplasty. There are no recurrent aneurysms to date.

Conclusion.—Surgical resection of excess length, reduction of luminal diameter, and reconstruction is a viable option for the treatment of complicated massive diffusely aneurysmal AVF. This technique offers the ability to maintain the benefits of an all autogenous dialysis access while conserving future dialysis sites.

▶ The authors have described a nice technique to salvage aneurysmal autogenous hemodialysis accesses. Notably, these are accesses that are diffusely aneurysmal (diameters, 4-7 cm) with the dilation spanning the whole length of the access, not just a focal segment. Although the series was relatively small (N = 19) and the follow-up short (median, 23 months), the overall success rate in terms of access salvage and midterm patency were noteworthy. Diffuse aneurysmal degeneration of an autogenous access is an uncommon, yet not rare, problem that most access surgeons will encounter over the course of a year. The optimal management of both focal and diffuse aneurysmal degenerations is unclear, and the Kidney Disease Outcomes Quality Initiative guidelines are not all that helpful. The major problem is that the aneurysmal degeneration may lead to erosion of the overlying skin and hemorrhage. Although this can occur, the more common presentation is simply a massively enlarged access with freely mobile uninvolved skin that is not particularly worrisome for rupture. I have taken a similar approach in terms of offering surgical revision in the presence of these massively aneurysmal accesses although I concede that the natural history is poorly defined. The described technique provides an elegant approach to salvage and preserve a functional autogenous access. I have used a similar method but really like the authors' technique of siting the suture line on the lateral aspect of the fistula to avoid having the suture line near the future cannulation sites and rerouting the access through a separate subcutaneous route. In contrast to the authors', my experience with the technique has been somewhat mixed, and the problems that I have encountered were because several of the autogenous accesses were so diffusely degenerated and calcified that it was not possible to simply excise the bad segment and create a new access over a cannula as described. In these instances, I have simply used a large-diameter (ie, 10 mm) expanded polytetrafluoroethylene graft but have been concerned about the potential for wound breakdown and infection. Similar to the authors, I have had a couple of episodes in which the skin broke down over the revised access and bled. This underscores the importance of close conscientious follow-up with further remedial treatment as necessary, including ligation and excision. The underlying mechanism responsible for this diffuse aneurysmal degeneration is unknown. I believe that it is imperative to rule out a venous outflow stenosis as a contributory cause but believe that this abnormal continued dilation may be a patient-specific biologic response.

T. S. Huber, MD, PhD

Prosthetic lower extremity hemodialysis access grafts have satisfactory patency despite a high incidence of infection
Geenen IL, Nyilas L, Stephen MS, et al (Royal Prince Alfred Hosp, Sydney, New South Wales, Australia)
J Vasc Surg 52:1546-1550, 2010

Introduction.—Prosthetic arteriovenous grafts (AVGs) in the lower extremity represent a useful alternative for hemodialysis vascular access when all upper limb access sites have been used or in some patients when freedom of both hands is necessary during dialysis. Reported complications include an increased risk of infection and limb ischemia. This study evaluated our experience with the patency outcomes and complication rates of polytetrafluoroethylene (PTFE) AVGs placed in the thigh.

Methods.—A retrospective outcomes analysis was performed of all femoral AVGs inserted between January 1992 and July 2007. Data were obtained by review of medical records for patient demographics, comorbidities, and AVG-related outcomes. Patency, complication rates, and risk factors for infection were determined.

Results.—A total of 153 prosthetic AVGs were placed in 127 patients (63 men). Mean patient age was 52.7 ± 16.3 years. Median follow-up was 25 months (range, 1-169 months). The most common underlying renal disease was glomerulonephritis in 27 (21%). Hypertension and coronary artery disease were common comorbidities, respectively, in 49 (39%) and 23 patients (18%). The primary and secondary AVG patency rates at 12 months were 53.9% and 75.3%, respectively, and 2- and 5-year patency rates were, respectively, 39.6% and 19.3% (primary) and 63.8% and 50.6% (secondary). The mean AVG survival for all cases was 31.6 months (range, 0-149 months). Surgical thrombectomy was required in 82 (54%), and 22 AVGs (14%) required surgical revision for stenosis. Infection occurred in 41 AVGs (27%), and limb ischemia occurred in 2 (1.3%). Statistical analysis did not reveal a significant risk factor for infection.

Conclusions.—Femoral AVGs are a suitable alternative to upper limb vascular access, with acceptable primary and secondary patency rates. Infection occurred in approximately one-quarter of cases, whereas steal was uncommon.

▶ The authors have documented the largest series of prosthetic hemodialysis accesses in the lower extremity and have reported impressive 1-year primary (54%) and secondary (75%) patency rates, comparable to those reported for prosthetic accesses in the upper extremity. Unfortunately, infectious complications occurred in 27% of the patients and necessitated surgical removal of the entire graft (vs subtotal excision) in most of these cases. The authors concluded that prosthetic lower extremity accesses are suitable alternatives to upper extremity procedures. The sheer size of the sample merits attention although the report is retrospective and spans more than 15 years. It underscores the incidence of infectious complications that represents the major limitation or Achilles heel of this type of access configuration. Indeed, the authors' infectious complications actually seem quite low relative to other published reports and our own institutional experience. Although the authors were able to salvage a significant number of the infected accesses, total excision of an infected lower extremity access is a major undertaking that usually requires repair of the inflow artery (ie, common femoral or superficial femoral) with an autogenous patch. The authors' reported incidence of ischemic complications was actually quite low (< 2%) and likely reflects their patient population and selection process. Despite this low incidence, significant arterial occlusive disease is a relative contraindication to a lower extremity access and should be considered or evaluated during the preoperative process. Unlike the upper extremity, the remedial options for access-associated ischemia in the lower extremity are limited with ligation being the only practical option. The role of lower extremity accesses remains unclear in our own treatment algorithm. We have traditionally exhausted all upper extremity options before considering the lower extremity because of the infectious complications. Furthermore, we have constructed a fair number of autogenous accesses in the lower extremity by transposing the femoral/popliteal vein. It has been our impression that this has reduced the infectious complications, although it is a much larger operative procedure associated with a higher incidence of both ischemic and wound complications. The recent introduction of the HeRO vascular access device (Hemosphere, Eden Prairie, MN) has also impacted our treatment algorithm and approach to lower extremity accesses. This hybrid graft/catheter access device has extended the upper extremity options for patients with severe central venous occlusive disease and may represent a better option than a lower extremity access, although more data in terms of the associated patency rates and infectious risk are necessary.

T. S. Huber, MD, PhD

Primary balloon angioplasty plus balloon angioplasty maturation to upgrade small-caliber veins (<3 mm) for arteriovenous fistulas

De Marco Garcia LP, Davila-Santini LR, Feng Q, et al (North Shore-Long Island Jewish Health System, Manhasset, NY)

J Vasc Surg 52:139-144, 2010

Objective.—Small-diameter veins are often a limiting factor for the successful creation of arteriovenous fistulas (AVFs). This study evaluated the use of intraoperative primary balloon angioplasty (PBA) as a technique to upgrade small-diameter veins during AVF creation. Sequential balloon angioplasty maturation (BAM) was evaluated as a technique to salvage failed fistulas, expedite maturation, and improve the patency of AVFs after PBA.

Methods.—Sixty-two PBAs were performed in 55 patients with an intent-to-treat using an all-autologous policy. PBAs of veins were performed just before AVF creation using 2.5- to 4-mm angioplasty balloons

(1- to 1.5-mm larger than the nominal vein diameter). PBAs were performed through the spatulated end of the vein for a length of up to 8 cm using hydrophilic guidewires and hand inflations without fluoroscopy. BAM was performed in 53 of the 62 PBAs at 2, 4, and 6 weeks after the PBA. Successful outcome was determined as the functional ability to use the fistula for hemodialysis without surgical revision.

Results.—Of the 62 PBAs, 53 (85.4%), comprising 47 of the original AVFs and 6 new site AVFs created at other sites, remained patent and subsequently underwent BAM with a resulting functional AVF. Fifteen of the 47 original AVFs: 14 due to occlusion; one AVF with a steal was ligated. Seven of the 14 fistulas that occluded were salvaged using recanalization techniques during sequential BAMs. Two of the seven fistulas that were not salvaged required AVGs (3%), and five patients underwent redo AVFs using alternative veins. These five cases were also performed using PBAs and BAMs technique. One patient with a functioning fistula underwent intentional ligation for steal syndrome and also underwent an alternative site AVF, PBA, and BAM. At 3 months, 53 AVFs were functional and successfully used for dialysis. Overall, a working AVF was obtained at the initial site in 47 of 55 patients (85.4%), and 53 (96.3%) received working AVFs that were functioning for dialysis access.

Conclusions.—Small or suboptimal veins can undergo PBA and then be matured to create functioning AVFs ≤2 months. Overall, >90% autogenous AVF rates can be achieved using PBA and BAM. BAM can be successfully used to mature AVFs created from small veins and salvage thrombosed AVFs in many cases. The use of these techniques may decrease the number of patients requiring AVGs and indwelling catheters.

▶ The authors describe their use of primary balloon angioplasty (PBA) and balloon angioplasty maturation (BAM) to facilitate maturation of small caliber veins (< 3 mm) for autogenous hemodialysis accesses. Although it was somewhat difficult to follow the authors accounting system, it appears that 85% of the veins were ultimately used for dialysis and that the 12-month secondary patency rates were also approximately 85%. This maturation rate is excellent and exceeds most reports. Indeed, the fistula maturation rate from the National Institutes of Health-funded Dialysis Access Consortium, a randomized trial of clopidogrel to facilitate autogenous access maturation, was less than 40%.[1] The findings are particularly impressive given the small caliber of the veins that was below the normal diameter threshold that most surgeons use and the fact that most of the access configurations were radial artery based. The reported success rate for radial artery based accesses (eg, radiocephalic or Cimino) is actually quite poor, particularly in women, diabetic patients, and the elderly. The specific techniques are nicely described in the article and involve graduated balloon dilation over a wire through the spatulated end of the vein (PBA), the radial artery (BAM), or the proximal aspect of the fistula (BAM). Sequential dilatations were performed as part of the BAM at 2, 4, and 6 weeks postoperatively. The concept of BAM has been previously described, but the current series represents one of the largest, if not the largest, report in the literature. The technique has the potential to increase the incidence and prevalence of autogenous access in keeping with the national initiatives. However, it will be interesting to see if the results can be reproduced at other centers since they seem almost too good to be true.

T. S. Huber, MD, PhD

Reference

1. Dember LM, Beck GJ, Allon M, et al. Effect of clopidogrel on early failure of arteriovenous fistulas for hemodialysis: a randomized controlled trial. *JAMA*. 2008; 299:2164-2171.

Venous

Preoperative thrombolysis and venoplasty affords no benefit in patency following first rib resection and scalenectomy for subacute and chronic subclavian vein thrombosis

Guzzo JL, Chang K, Demos J, et al (The Johns Hopkins Hosp, Baltimore, MD)
J Vasc Surg 52:658-663, 2010

Background.—Axillosubclavian vein thrombosis, also known as Paget-Schroetter syndrome, is a rare presentation of thoracic outlet syndrome (TOS) representing approximately 5% of all cases. Conventional management consists of routine anticoagulation, operative decompression via first rib resection and scalenectomy (FRRS), and, recently, thrombolysis. The purpose of our study was to retrospectively review our experience with this condition and compare the effectiveness of preoperative endovascular intervention with thrombolysis and venoplasty to anticoagulation alone in those undergoing FRRS to preserve subclavian vein patency.

Methods.—A retrospective review was conducted for all venous TOS patients from July 2003 to May 2009 from a prospectively maintained database. Preoperative clinic notes were reviewed to allow stratification into two groups. One group consisted of patients undergoing preoperative endovascular intervention with thrombolysis and venoplasty, while the other group consisted of patients managed medically with anticoagulation alone prior to FRSS. Operative notes, postoperative venograms, and postoperative duplex imaging results were reviewed for presence of recanalization, chronic nonocclusive thrombus, or continued occlusion.

Results.—One hundred three patients had 110 FRRS for subclavian vein thrombosis (53 men, 50 women), seven of which had contralateral FRRS for thrombosis. The cohort averaged 31 years of age (range, 16-54 years) with an overall, mean follow-up time of 16 months (range, 1-52 months). Of the 110 veins evaluated, 45 underwent endovascular intervention (thombolysis, with or without venoplasty) prior to FRRS, and at 1 year, 41 (91%) were patent with improvement of symptoms. In the 65 veins on anticoagulation alone, 59 (91%) ultimately were patent, with symptomatic improvement in all. Overall, 91% (100/110) of subclavian veins were patent in patients completing follow-up, were asymptomatic, and back to their previous active lifestyle.

Conclusions.—Preoperative endovascular intervention offered no benefit over simple anticoagulation prior to FRRS, since the use of thrombolysis prior to FRRS, regardless of need for postoperative venoplasty, had little impact on overall rates of patency. The optimal treatment algorithm may merely be routine anticoagulation for all effort thrombosis patients prior to FRRS followed by venography with venoplasty if needed. The role of thrombolysis for Paget-Schroetter syndrome should be further investigated in randomized trials.

▶ This intriguing report by Freischlag et al questions the role of preoperative endovascular intervention (ie, thrombolysis and venoplasty) for patients with axillosubclavian vein thrombosis secondary to venous thoracic outlet. The authors reviewed their extensive institutional experience for patients presenting with subacute and chronic axillosubclavian vein thrombosis (mean time from symptoms to referral: intervention group, 3.8 months; anticoagulation, 6.3 months) and compared outcomes after first rib resection for those patients treated with some type of endovascular intervention with those that were just anticoagulated. Importantly, neither the endovascular intervention nor anticoagulation was standardized prior to referral, and the outcome or effectiveness of these therapies was poorly documented in the study. The authors reported that 91% of the axillosubclavian veins were patent at 1 year in both groups and that the presenting symptoms were improved after their treatment that included first rib resection, venography with selective intervention at 2 weeks postoperatively, and selective anticoagulation. Notably, almost all of the veins found to be occluded at the time of postoperative venography, as assessed by the inability to pass a wire, were recanalized and were found to be patent on subsequent imaging studies. The results must be interpreted with some caution, given the study limitations that include the retrospective design, patient selection bias, and the poorly controlled treatments prior to referral. However, they do suggest that endovascular intervention before first rib resection may not be necessary. Furthermore, the excellent results suggest that there is no role for additional preoperative endovascular interventions immediately before first rib resection for this subset of patients with subacute or chronic symptoms. Indeed, in our own tertiary practice, we frequently see this subset of patients who were ineffectively treated for some time (ie, weeks to months) prior to referral for definitive treatment. I would wholeheartedly echo the authors' challenge that a randomized trial is necessary to help resolve the optimal treatment options for patients with venous thoracic outlet. There are multiple outstanding fundamental issues as highlighted above.

T. S. Huber, MD, PhD

Miscellaneous

Vascular complications of exposure for anterior lumbar interbody fusion
Garg J, Woo K, Hirsch J, et al (Scripps Green Hosp, La Jolla, CA)
J Vasc Surg 51:946-950, 2010

Objective.—The purpose of this study is to document the incidence of vascular complications during anterior lumbar interbody fusion (ALIF) in 212 consecutive patients treated at the Scripps Clinic and determine what factors adversely affected outcome.

Methods.—We reviewed the prospectively maintained database of all ALIF procedures performed at Scripps Clinic between August 2004 and June 2009. All procedures were performed by a spine surgeon in conjunction with a vascular surgeon who performed the exposure portion of the operation, and protected the vessels from injury during the instrumentation phase of the operation.

Results.—Two hundred twelve ALIF operations were identified. The mean age of the patients was 53.8 years, and 120 (56.6%) were female. The mean body mass index (BMI) was 29.6 (range, 18.1 to 47.8). Twenty-two (10.4%) operations were performed at the L4-5 disc space, 149 (70.3%) at L5-S1, and 41 (19.3%) involved L4-L5 with L5-S1. The mean estimated blood loss (EBL) was 143 milliliters. There was a significant direct correlation between increasing BMI and EBL ($P = .018$). Thirteen (6.1%) vascular injuries occurred of which five were major (38.5%). One major arterial injury (0.5%) occurred and required arterial thrombectomy and stent placement. Four of the major vascular injuries were venous in nature and required a multi-suture repair. The remaining eight injuries (61.5%) were venous, the majority of which required a suture repair. There were no mortalities. There was an increase risk of vascular injury when both L4-L5 and L5-S1 were exposed ($P = .003$) and with the male gender ($P = .013$). Calcification of the aorto-iliac system did not exert an effect on EBL or vascular injury. In four cases, the surgeon was unable to expose the appropriate disc levels.

Conclusions.—Anterior exposure of the spine for ALIF can be performed safely with a team approach that includes a vascular surgeon. Preoperative evaluation by a vascular surgeon is advisable. Patients with increased BMI and bi-level exposures should be approached with caution.

▶ The authors have reported their experience with anterior lumbar exposure for interbody fusion and have documented the complication rates along with providing a nice description of their technique. This is a welcome contribution to the literature given the evolution of clinical practice and the emergence of this approach or procedure as a significant component of most vascular surgeons' practices. The authors reported no perioperative deaths but an overall complication of 11% that included 5 (2%) major vascular injuries. Indeed, it is these major vascular injuries (or more importantly the potential for major vascular injuries) that justify the team approach with the vascular and spine surgeons. Most of the major vascular injuries were venous in nature, although this is not surprising given the anatomic relationship between the confluence of the common iliac veins and the L4–L5 and L5–S1 disc spaces. The authors documented a 4% incidence of retrograde ejaculation among their complications. This is also predictable given the extent of the operative dissection and should be discussed during the preoperative evaluation among the other potential complications. The authors identified male gender, body mass index, and bilevel exposure as predictors of adverse outcome. These preoperative predictors are helpful and potentially allow the surgeon to modify his/her technique in terms of approach or length of incision. My approach is similar to that outlined by the authors, although I must confess that my incision is usually longer than 5 to 6 cm detailed by the authors, particularly in larger patients. Similar to my approach for iliac conduits for endovascular aneurysm repair, I use a curvilinear incision through the anterior rectus fascia and enter the retroperitoneal space caudal to the umbilicus by retracting the rectus muscle medially. I find the Bookwalter retractor invaluable, although I admit that I need to reposition the retractor blades (oriented at 3-, 7-, and 9-o'clock positions with the head being at the 12-o'clock position) several times, serially releasing the tension on the 3-o'clock retractor while increasing the tension on the other 2. Adequate safe exposure of the disc space(s) necessitates mobilizing the common iliac arteries and veins sufficiently so that they can be retracted using pins. This usually requires ligating the medial and lateral sacral veins.

T. S. Huber, MD, PhD

Perfused, Pulseless, and Puzzling: A Systematic Review of Vascular Injuries in Pediatric Supracondylar Humerus Fractures and Results of a POSNA Questionnaire
White L, Mehlman CT, Crawford AH (Univ of Cincinnati College of Medicine, OH)
J Pediatr Orthop 30:328-335, 2010

Background.—Supracondylar humerus fractures that present with a perfused, viable hand yet no pulse continue to be a source of controversy. The purpose of this study was to conduct a systematic review of the literature and perform a Pediatric Orthopaedic Society of North America (POSNA) opinion poll regarding management of pulseless supracondylar humeral fractures in children.

Methods.—A systematic review of the literature was conducted for relevant observational studies concerning neurovascular injuries in supracondylar humerus fractures. Single case reports and non-English language studies were excluded. Data were pooled for defined subgroups and 95% confidence intervals were reported. The results from the literature were then compared to popular opinion via a POSNA-approved survey concerning management of pulseless supracondylar humerus fractures.

Results.—A total of 331 cases of pulseless supracondylar fractures were identified from the literature, irrespective of perfusion status. In all, 157 fractures remained pulseless after closed reduction and stabilization. Of the fractures that continued to be pulseless despite adequate reduction, 82% [95% confidence interval (CI) = 0.82 (0.76-0.88)] were found to have a documented brachial artery injury. POSNA members presumed this number would be 28% [95% CI = 0.28 (0.22-0.34)]. A total of 98 perfused (aka pink) supracondylar fractures were identified. Of these pulseless, perfused fractures, 70% [95% CI = 0.70 (0.58-0.82)] had a documented brachial artery injury. POSNA members speculated that this number would be 17% [95% CI = 0.17 (0.12-0.22). A total of 54 patients had minimum 1 year follow-up data after vascular revascularization, and 91% [95% CI = 0.91 (0.83-0.99)] of these patients had a patent artery based on vascular studies. POSNA members believed this number would be 55% [95% CI = 0.55 (0.48-0.62)].

Conclusions.—Our study revealed that common dogma regarding watchful waiting of pulseless and perfused supracondylar fractures needs to be questioned. In the vast majority of published cases, an absence of pulse is an indicator of arterial injury, even if the hand appears pink and warm, suggesting the need for more aggressive vascular evalvation and vascular exploration and repair in selected cases. Moreover, patency rates for revascularization procedures appear sufficiently high, making this intervention worthwhile.

▶ The management of pediatric vascular injuries is challenging and can be very anxiety provoking for most vascular surgeons considering the diminutive size of the vessels (both arteries and conduit), the potential long-term disability and the apprehension of the parents. The current systematic review and survey addresses treatment of children with supracondylar humerus fractures and a pulseless extremity. Notably, these fractures are the most common ones at the level of the elbow and can be associated with the absence of a pulse in approximately 20% of the cases. The authors found that the pulse returns in about half of the cases after reduction and stabilization of the fracture. However, a frank vascular injury was detected in about 80% of the cases in which the pulse failed to return, regardless of the fact that the hand appeared to be well perfused. Given the high incidence of vascular injury, attributing the pulse deficit to spasm is inappropriate and potentially harmful given the sequelae that include Volkmann ischemic contractures, forearm claudication, cold intolerance, and retarded growth. A definitive diagnosis and aggressive treatment is mandatory. Arterial duplex is the simplest imaging study, given the fact that the test is available in most trauma centers and can be performed portably. There is probably no role for diagnostic catheter-based arteriography, given the diminutive size of the vessels and the obligatory procedure-related delays. Definitive treatment is dictated by the extent of the vascular injury; most focal defects can be repaired with a vein patch while more extensive ones require an interposition graft. Fortunately, these vascular interventions appear to be quite successful as reported from the systematic review with a 90% patency rate at the time of last follow-up visit. The objective results from the systematic review differed significantly from the survey results from the pediatric orthopedic surgeons who grossly underestimated the incidence of vascular injury (28% vs 82%) and the success of revascularization (55% vs 91%). Overall, the results mandate an aggressive treatment for the extremity that remains pulseless after reduction of the supracondylar humerus fracture, presuming the orthopedic surgeons recognize the gravity of the clinical findings and consult a vascular surgeon.

T. S. Huber, MD, PhD

The limitations of thoracic endovascular aortic repair in altering the natural history of blunt aortic injury

Lang JL, Minei JP, Modrall JG, et al (Univ of Texas Southwestern Med Ctr, Dallas)
J Vasc Surg 52:290-297, 2010

Background.—Thoracic endovascular aortic repair (TEVAR) is accepted treatment for blunt aortic injury (BAI). We hypothesized that immediate TEVAR would reduce deaths from aortic rupture in patients with BAI.

Methods.—Review of 81 patients with BAI who arrived alive at a level I trauma center over a 10-year period.

Results.—Twenty-three patients (28%) died within 4 hours of admission, including 12 who died of aortic rupture. Fifty-eight patients (72%) survived beyond 4 hours, and 8 (14%) ultimately died of associated injuries. Forty patients (69%) underwent aortic repair (30 open repair, 10 TEVAR), and 2 died of multisystem organ failure (MSOF). Comparing open repair to TEVAR, there were no differences in the length of hospital stay (33 ± 27 vs 33 ± 31 days), operative complications (77% vs 70%), or mortality (7% vs 0). Ten patients (17%) with minimal BAI were treated with beta blockade and observation; 4 have not healed their aortic injuries and 6 have been lost to follow-up. Thirty-three of the original 81 study patients (41%) ultimately died. Compared with the patients who died, the survivors were younger (37 vs 48 years; $P = .01$) and less likely to develop aortic rupture (0 vs 12; $P < .001$), require intubation in the field (27% vs 49%; $P < .05$), require cardiopulmonary resuscitation (CPR; 2% vs 30%; $P < .001$), or arrive hypotensive (17% vs 67%; $P < .001$). Survivors also had a lower mean injury severity score (34 ± 12 vs 44 ± 12; $P < .001$), fewer associated injuries (3 ± 1 vs 4 ± 3; $P = .02$), and a higher prevalence of aortic repair (79% vs 6%; $P < .001$). Multivariate analysis selected no attempt at aortic repair (odds ratio [OR], 90.9; 95% confidence interval [CI], 10.6-1000) and hypotension on arrival (OR, 6.1; 95% CI, 1.4-27) as the only independent variables associated with death.

Conclusion.—Mortality remains high for patients with BAI, but most patients who arrive alive at the hospital do not experience aortic rupture. Rupture occurs within the first 4 hours of admission, often before the injury is recognized in time for salvage with immediate TEVAR. The decision to repair BAI was based on the extent of associated injuries and on the individual surgeon's judgment. Survival was not influenced by the timing of repair, but further studies are needed to compare the outcome of open repair vs TEVAR in patients who survive beyond 4 hours.

▶ The authors have helped define the natural history of blunt aortic injury (BAI) as framed within the context of thoracic endovascular aortic repair (TEVAR). They hypothesized that immediate TEVAR could reduce deaths from rupture in patients with BAI. In their retrospective single, institutional study, the authors reported that the overall mortality rate for patients with BAI was 41% (33/81). Twenty-eight percent of the patients died within 4 hours of presentation and among this subset, there were 12 deaths from aortic rupture. Although the treatment of the BAI for patients surviving beyond 4 hours was not standardized (open repair vs TEVAR vs expectant management), there were no additional deaths from aortic rupture with the deaths resulting from associated injuries and/or multiple organ dysfunction. Somewhat surprisingly, multivariate analysis demonstrated that no attempt at aortic repair was associated with increased mortality. Based upon their findings, the authors concluded that survival after BAI is not influenced by the timing of repair. Although the study has several limitations (ie, retrospective design, selection bias, small sample size, and inadequate follow-up), it does contribute to our understanding of BAI. It demonstrates that the fatal traumatic aortic ruptures occur shortly after presentation to the emergency room, and the authors estimate that these occurred within 6 hours of the injury itself. Preventing these traumatic ruptures would require immediate diagnosis and definitive treatment. Although this is not outside the realm of possibility, this is likely not feasible given the other associated injuries and the extent of resuscitation required. It is worth emphasizing that the current results were reported from a very sophisticated level 1 trauma center. Among the patients that survive the initial resuscitation, a selective approach to the BAI appears to be safe, although it remains to be determined which injuries merit treatment and which operative approach (ie, open vs TEVAR) is optimal. These are very anxiety-provoking injuries for the surgeon, but the low incidence of rupture beyond the resuscitation phase must be balanced against the early and late complications associated with operative repair. In this study, there were no differences in most of the outcome measures based upon the operative approach, but the number of patients in the TEVAR group was quite small. The trend across the country is clearly to repair these BAIs with TEVAR whenever feasible. However, the TEVAR approach does mandate long-term surveillance, and this is particularly concerning in the trauma population as demonstrated by the fact that 71% of the survivors in this study never returned for any follow-up visit. The results of the multivariate analysis suggesting that mortality was associated with "no attempt at aortic repair" are somewhat misleading because the immediate ruptures were not preventable and no patients surviving the resuscitation phase died from rupture.

T. S. Huber, MD, PhD

13 General Thoracic Surgery

Esophageal Cancer

Novel Treatment for Chylothorax After Esophagectomy With 50% Glucose Pleurodesis

Chen Y, Li C, Xu L, et al (Tian Jin Med Univ, P.R. China; First Hosp of Jilin Univ, Changchun, P.R. China)

Ann Vasc Surg 24:694.e9-694.e13, 2010

Chylothorax is characterized by the presence of chyle in the pleural space and cardiothoracic surgery accounts for nearly half of all the cases. Treatment of chylothorax has traditionally been nonoperative, with alternative medical therapies involving the administration of octreotide or pleurodesis. Pleurodesis with chemical agents has previously been reported, but never with 50% glucose and 0.1% xylocaine. Herein, we report a successful method of intrapleural instillation of 50% glucose and 0.1% xylocaine to treat chylothorax. Five patients treated with this method were all recovered rapidly. This method can generate extensive adherence and prevent the effusion of the chylous fluid with minor side effects.

▶ Chylothorax can be a challenging and frustrating complication of surgery in the thorax. Up to 50% of patients with chylothorax have antecedent surgery as the suspected culprit. Long-term high volume chest tube output from chylothorax leads to a myriad of deleterious consequences, including nutritional, immunologic, and dehydration issues.

Treatment options have focused on ligation of the thoracic duct low in the chest and pleurodesis to remove the potential space for fluid accumulation. The thoracic duct is easily approached via the right hemithorax and is located in the tissue between the aorta, esophagus, and azygous vein at the level of the diaphragm. Often the duct itself cannot be visualized but instead this tissue must be mass ligated in hopes of ligating the thoracic duct. This is particularly unappealing in patients with chylothorax following left thoracotomy, as access to this space from the left chest is challenging.

Surgery is usually considered if the output exceeds 1500 cc/24 hours or the flow persists for 2 weeks. The authors present a novel alternative to be considered prior to surgical intervention. They report their experience with 5 patients with high-volume persistent chylothorax following esophagectomy. All the patients in their series had failed a trial of conservative therapy. They describe their use of a combination of 50% glucose and 0.1% xylocaine as a pleurodesis and potential sclerosis agent. Although they do not quantify the amount of this agent instilled, they do note that it is not diluted in any way. They describe instillation via the chest tube and clamping of the tube for 40 minutes, performed twice per day over 3 days. With this technique, they rapidly achieved success in all 5 of their patients, including 2 who had extremely high-volume outputs prior to the instillation.

Many agents have been reported to successfully achieve chemical pleurodesis. However, each of these agents is also noted to have significant limitations and disadvantages. I believe the novel agent described by the authors may hold promise as an alternative to other means of chemical pleurodesis. However, further study is warranted to better access the reproducibility of the author's results and to better delineate the applicability to other indications for pleurodesis. Additionally, the infectious consequences of instilling high concentrations of glucose into the thorax for other applications requiring pleurodesis require further elucidation.

C. T. Klodell, Jr, MD

Miscellaneous

Nonoperative thoracic duct embolization for traumatic thoracic duct leak: Experience in 109 patients

Itkin M, Kucharczuk JC, Kwak A, et al (Hosp of the Univ of Pennsylvania, Philadelphia; et al)
J Thorac Cardiovasc Surg 139:584-590, 2010

Objective.—To demonstrate the efficacy of a minimally invasive, nonoperative, catheter-based approach to the treatment of traumatic chyle leak.

Methods.—A retrospective review of 109 patients was conducted to assess the efficacy of thoracic duct embolization or interruption for the treatment of high-output chyle leak caused by injury to the thoracic duct.

Results.—A total of 106 patients presented with chylothorax, 1 patient presented with chylopericardium, and 2 patients presented with cervical lymphocele. Twenty patients (18%) had previous failed thoracic duct ligation. In 108 of 109 patients, a lymphangiogram was successful. Catheterization of the thoracic duct was achieved in 73 patients (67%). In 71 of these 73 patients, embolization of the thoracic duct was performed. Endovascular coils or liquid embolic agent was used to occlude the thoracic duct. In 18 of 33 cases of unsuccessful catheterization, thoracic duct needle interruption was attempted below the diaphragm. Resolution of the chyle leak was observed in 64 of 71 patients (90%) post-embolization. Needle interruption of the thoracic duct was successful in 13 of 18 patients (72%). In 17 of the 20 patients who had previous attempts at thoracic duct ligation, embolization or interruption was attempted and successful in 15 (88%). The overall success rate for the entire series was 71% (77/109). There were 3 (3%) minor complications.

Conclusion.—Catheter embolization or needle interruption of the thoracic duct is safe, feasible, and successful in eliminating a high-output chyle leak in the majority (71%) of patients. This minimally invasive, although technically challenging, procedure should be the initial approach for the treatment of a traumatic chylothorax.

▶ Chylothorax remains a challenging and often persistent problem and is often iatrogenic after thoracic surgery, especially esophagectomy. The authors review their experience with relatively uncommon techniques for resolving chylothorax either noninvasively or minimally invasively.

Many still favor an initial conservative approach to chylothorax, with either total parenteral nutrition or medium-chain triglyceride diet. Patients who fail this approach often require surgical ligation of the thoracic duct via either open or thoracoscopic technique. The authors describe a technique of diagnostic pedal lymphangiography followed by transabdominal catheterization of the thoracic duct and embolization. Although several patients required multiple procedures, the ultimate nonoperative success rate was very high. However, the technique they describe is seldomly performed in interventional radiology departments today. Their technique involves a classic pedal lymphangiogram to guide wire access and catheterization of the lymphatic channels. Once the area of the leak is identified by lymphangiography, it is occluded below by a combination of glue and coil embolization. In cases where the thoracic duct could not be cannulated, they next attempted a needle interruption of the thoracic duct below the diaphragm. The combination of these techniques allowed a high success rate in immediately resolving the chylothorax.

Currently, the main limitation to wide adoption of this approach may be the lack of availability of the lymphangiogram. There are both physician and equipment limitations. The older physicians in interventional radiology may have significant experience with this technique, while those contemporarily trained have little to no experience with lymphangiography. Furthermore, many radiology departments no longer have functioning lymphangiogram pumps and equipment to perform this procedure.

Perhaps this report will serve as a nidus to reinvigorate our interventional radiology colleagues to embrace this technique and reconsider it as a viable therapeutic option for chylothorax. Alternatively, given the ongoing blurring of the lines of separation between the different specialties, it may be possible to persuade our vascular and endovascular colleagues to add this procedure to their ever-expanding armamentarium. Given the tremendous success reported by the authors, this technique warrants careful consideration as a noninvasive, or minimally invasive, mechanism to resolve chylothorax.

C. T. Klodell, Jr, MD

Aortic dilatation after endovascular repair of blunt traumatic thoracic aortic injuries

Forbes TL, Harris JR, Lawlor DK, et al (The Univ of Western Ontario, Canada)
J Vasc Surg 52:45-48, 2010

Objective.—Endovascular repair of blunt traumatic thoracic aortic injuries (BTAI) has become routine at many trauma centers despite concerns regarding durability and aortic dilatation in these predominantly young patients. These concerns prompted this examination of thoracic aortic expansion after endovascular repair of a BTAI.

Methods.—The immediate postoperative and most recent computed tomography (CT) scans of patients who had undergone urgent endovascular repair of a BTAI and had at least 1 year of follow-up were reviewed. Diameter measurements were made at four predetermined sites: immediately proximal to the left subclavian artery (D1), immediately distal to the left subclavian artery (D2), distal extent of the endograft (D3), and 15 mm beyond the distal end of the endograft (D4). Split screens permitted direct comparison of measurements between CTs at the corresponding levels.

Results.—During a 6-year period (2001-2007), 21 patients (mean age, 42.9 years; range, 19-81 years) underwent endovascular repair of a BTAI, 17 with at least 1 year of follow-up (mean, 2.6 years; range, 1-5.5 years). No patients required reintervention during this period. The mean rate of dilatation for each level of the thoracic aorta in mm/year was: D1, 0.74 (95% confidence interval [CI], 0.42-1.06); D2, 0.83 (95% CI, 0.55-1.11); D3, 0.63 (95% CI, 0.37-0.89); D4, 0.47 (95% CI, 0.27-0.67). The rate of expansion of D2 differed significantly vs D4 ($P = .025$).

Conclusions.—During the first several years of follow-up, the proximal thoracic aorta dilates minimally after endovascular repair of BTAIs, with the segment just distal to the left subclavian artery expanding at a slightly greater rate. Longer-term follow-up is necessary to determine whether this expansion continues and becomes clinically significant.

▶ The use of modern stent grafts for thoracic endovascular aortic repair (TEVAR) has become widespread for much aortic pathology. As the authors correctly point out, TEVAR for blunt traumatic aortic injuries (BTAIs) has also become commonplace. Several studies have clearly documented the acute advantages of TEVAR over open repair of BTAI. These advantages include lower mortality and stroke rates, as well as dramatically reduced risk of paraplegia. Several questions remain to be answered, including the long-term outcome of the locally injured aorta. The healing of the BTAI once the stent graft has been placed has not yet been fully elucidated. Similarly, the long-term effects of the radial force on the aorta following TEVAR remain unclear.

The authors report close follow-up of 21 patients who underwent TEVAR for BTAI at their institution over a 6-year period, with the intent of better elucidating the potential dilatation of the aorta at the site of repair. All injuries were successfully repaired with TEVAR. In their series, 57% of patients required coverage of the left subclavian artery to have appropriate proximal landing zone during TEVAR. Only 1 patient received concurrent carotid-subclavian bypass. They used a 10% oversize of the graft relative to the aortic size as measured by CT scan. They also report the use of adenosine-induced cardiac asystole early in their experience, with pharmacologically induced hypotension during their later experience.

Our experience mirrors the authors fairly closely. We also have achieved 100% technical success rate when using TEVAR to treat BTAI. We have used carotid-subclavian bypass somewhat more frequently than in the authors' series, based on relative size contributions of the vertebral arteries on CT scan. We have not used adenosine but rely on pharmacologic hypotension or right atrial inflow occlusion in refractory situations. We believe that TEVAR should be used to treat BTAI whenever technically feasible.

The authors raise important points about the ability to longitudinally follow the predominantly young and mobile trauma population. The long-term outcome of the site of injury, both for local healing and potential dilatation, needs to be further studied. With longitudinal follow-up, the true rate of reintervention will become better elucidated. However, I believe it is important to consider that even in patients who do ultimately require reintervention, it will be in a controlled and elective situation far more favorable to successful outcome than during their initial traumatic event.

C. T. Klodell, Jr, MD

The advent of thoracic endovascular aortic repair is associated with broadened treatment eligibility and decreased overall mortality in traumatic thoracic aortic injury

Hong MS, Feezor RJ, Lee WA, et al (Univ of Florida College of Medicine, Gainesville)
J Vasc Surg 53:36-43, 2011

Background.—Aortic injury is the second leading cause of death in trauma. Thoracic endovascular aortic repair (TEVAR) has recently been applied to traumatic thoracic aortic injuries (TTAIs) as a minimally invasive alternative to open surgery. We sought to determine the impact of TEVAR on national trends in the management of TTAI.

Methods.—We queried the Nationwide Inpatient Sample from the years 2001 to 2007 to select patients diagnosed with TTAI (International Classification of Disease-9 code 901.0). Patients were evaluated based on open surgical repair, TEVAR, or nonoperative management, before and after widespread adoption of TEVAR (2001-2005 and 2006-2007). Outcomes of interest were inpatient mortality, length of stay (LOS), and major complications.

Results.—An estimated 1180 annual admissions occurred for TTAI in the United States. Comparing the two time periods, there was an increase in TEVAR ($P < .001$) with a simultaneous decrease in open repair ($P < .001$)

in 2006 to 2007. The overall number of interventions also increased ($P < .001$). Overall mortality decreased (25.0% vs 19.0%; $P < .001$), corresponding to improved survival in the nonoperative group (28.0% vs 23.2%; $P < .001$). There was no improvement in open repair mortality rates between the two time periods. Comparing intervention types, the TEVAR group had a higher percentage of patients with brain injury (26.1% vs 20.6%; $P = .008$), lung injury (25.0% vs 17.7%; $P < .001$), and hemothorax (32.5% vs 21.7%; $P < .001$) than the open surgery group. There were no differences in the number of intra-abdominal injuries or major orthopedic fractures. The open surgery group had more respiratory complications (43.9% vs 54.2%; $P < .001$), whereas TEVAR had a higher stroke rate (1.9% vs 0.7%; $P = .021$). There were no differences in paraplegia or renal failure. Overall in-hospital mortality was 23.2% (nonoperative group 26.7%, open repair 12.4%, and TEVAR 10.6%). Mortality between open repair and TEVAR groups were not significantly different. LOS was shorter among the TEVAR group vs open (15.7 vs 22.9 days; $P < .001$).

Conclusion.—TEVAR has replaced open repair as the primary operative treatment for TTAI and has extended operative treatment to those patients not previously considered candidates for repair. Increased utilization of TEVAR is associated with improved overall mortality. There is no difference in mortality between TEVAR and open repair groups in our study, which likely reflects the multisystem nature of injury and greater preoperative risk in the TEVAR group.

▶ The authors reviewed the national inpatient sample to evaluate the impact of thoracic endograft technology on repair of traumatic thoracic aortic injury. They were able to demonstrate some interesting findings, including that brain injury, intra-abdominal injury, and major orthopedic fractures taken in combination occur in 72% of patients with an aortic injury. This high rate of comorbidities may account for why more patients were treated nonoperatively prior to the advent of stent graft technology. When comparing the patients treated in the thoracic endovascular aortic repair era with those treated by open techniques, they assert that there are a greater number of patients being treated in the current era. This implies that some patients now being deemed as appropriate candidates for new graft techniques were in the past treated nonoperatively because of their high-risk status. This is further supported by the note that the patients with endograft were older, had more severe injuries, and had more concomitant injuries when compared with the open group. In particular, the endograft group had more patients with brain injury and lung injury. This is particularly important when considering the need for anticoagulation with open repair using left atrial-femoral bypass. Most centers are using a selective heparin strategy for patients during endograft placement for traumatic aortic injury, but it is certainly feasible in most cases to perform this procedure with no heparin.

I believe that their findings support that endovascular techniques have essentially replaced open repair as the primary treatment choice for blunt traumatic aortic injury and allows us to extend operative treatment to patients not previously considered candidates for repair. As the device technology continues to evolve, these procedures will become more routine at most centers and I believe are already evolving to be the standard of care for blunt aortic injury.

C. T. Klodell, Jr, MD

Hilar Control in Penetrating Chest Trauma: A Simplified Approach to an Underutilized Maneuver
Van Natta TL, Smith BR, Bricker SD, et al (Harbor-UCLA Med Ctr, Torrance; UC Irvine Med Ctr, Long Beach)
J Trauma 66:1564-1569, 2009

Background.—In both urban and military settings, penetrating thoracic injuries remain a significant source of trauma-related mortality, and many patients require resuscitative thoracotomy. Existing literature emphasizes relief of pericardial tamponade and aortic clamp application as the key therapeutic maneuvers. The purpose of this report is to revisit pulmonary hilar clamping and highlight its application for hemorrhage control, air embolism prevention, and other benefits in the setting of massive hemothorax.

Methods.—Records from an urban, American College of Surgeons verified level I trauma center were evaluated over a six-month period. Patients who underwent early pulmonary hilar clamping were identified.

Results.—Twenty-four patients with trauma presented during the study period required thoracotomy. Of these, three (13%) underwent early pulmonary hilar clamping for massive hemothorax. Trauma mechanism was penetrating in each instance. Injuries included pulmonary lobe destruction, subclavian artery disruption, and internal thoracic artery transection. These cases illustrate the utility of early pulmonary hilar clamping for hemorrhage control, prevention of air embolization, and improved exposure.

Conclusion.—To decrease morbidity and mortality at our institution, a method of pulmonary hilar control has evolved using an organized, "hand-over-hand" approach that controls hemorrhage, prevents fatal air embolism, protects against blood spillage into contralateral airways, and facilitates pulmonary surgery. Several features distinguish our approach from those previously reported.

▶ Penetrating chest trauma management is crucial for all surgeons involved in trauma care and may account for a significant number of lives saved by skilled hands. Thoracostomy tube placement in conjunction with resuscitation and stabilization will suffice in approximately 75% of penetrating chest trauma, with the remainder requiring operative intervention.

In managing surgical thoracic trauma, the basic tenet centers on cross-clamping the descending thoracic aorta and opening the pericardium to relieve any tamponade. This should immediately be followed by hemorrhage control and prevention of air embolism. Lung-sparing techniques are then used to facilitate operative control of both bleeding and air leak, while resuscitation progresses.

The authors describe their technique for control of the pulmonary hilum. It is a 2-person technique involving digital compression of the hilum from the superior approach, while the inferior pulmonary ligament is completely mobilized to the level of the inferior pulmonary vein. This then allows for a hand-over-hand exchange, with the primary digital hilar control now from the inferior aspect of the hilum, which subsequently facilitates the placement of an atraumatic vascular clamp from the superior approach across the hilum. Once the hilum is secured, further repairs and control of hemorrhage can proceed in a controlled fashion without fear of exsanguination or air embolus.

As the authors point out, those facile with pulmonary surgery and thoracic anatomy can often apply the hilar clamp prior to mobilization of the inferior pulmonary ligament. However, the authors' technique is safe and reproducible by the surgeon early out of general surgical training as well as the seasoned thoracic or trauma surgeon.

If available at the time, the surgeon may find it of benefit to use a cable-actuated flexible clamp on the pulmonary hilum. Many find these clamps allow the jaws to be positioned on the pulmonary hilum and closed, with the shaft and handles then flexed out of the way to permit unobstructed access to the remainder of the thoracic cavity. Additionally, it is often useful to disconnect the patient from the ventilator for a brief period and allow the lung to recoil and collapse prior to occluding the bronchus with the clamp. This maneuver permits excellent decompression and exposure, often similar to if a double-lumen endotracheal tube had been used.

Finally, a word of caution about single stapler pneumonectomy using a TA-90 stapler. As a last resort, it may be necessary to perform pneumonectomy in this fashion in an expeditious effort to resuscitate an otherwise dying patient. However, when pneumonectomy is performed in this manner, the bronchial stump is often quite long and may pose a significant long-term risk. Once stabilized, consideration should be given to bronchoscopy to evaluate the remaining bronchial anatomy. In some cases, it may be appropriate to return the patient to the operating room during the same admission when their condition allows for a revision of the mass ligated hilum and appropriate shortening of the bronchial stump to prevent long-term complications.

C. T. Klodell, Jr, MD

Surveyed Opinion of American Trauma, Orthopedic, and Thoracic Surgeons On Rib and Sternal Fracture Repair
Mayberry JC, Ham LB, Schipper PH, et al (Oregon Health and Science Univ, Portland; et al)
J Trauma 66:875-879, 2009

Introduction.—Rib and sternal fracture repair are controversial. The opinion of surgeons regarding those patients who would benefit from repair is unknown.

Methods.—Members of the Eastern Association for the Surgery of Trauma, the Orthopedic Trauma Association, and thoracic surgeons (THS) affiliated with teaching hospitals in the United States were recruited to complete an electronic survey regarding rib and sternal fracture repair.

Results.—Two hundred thirty-eight trauma surgeons (TRS), 97 orthopedic trauma surgeons (OTS), and 70 THS completed the survey. Eighty-two percent of TRS, 66% of OTS, and 71% of THS thought that rib fracture repair was indicated in selected patients. A greater proportion of surgeons thought that sternal fracture repair was indicated in selected patients (89% of TRS, 85% of OTS, and 95% of THS). Chest wall defect/pulmonary hernia (58%) and sternal fracture nonunion (>6 weeks) (68%) were the only two indications accepted by a majority of respondents. Twenty-six percent of surgeons reported that they had performed or assisted on a chest wall fracture repair, whereas 22% of surgeons were familiar with published randomized trials of the surgical repair of flail chest. Of surgeons who thought rib fracture or sternal fracture repair was rarely, if ever, indicated, 91% and 95%, respectively, specified that a randomized trial confirming efficacy would be necessary to change their negative opinion.

Conclusions.—A majority of surveyed surgeons reported that rib and sternal fracture repair is indicated in selected patients; however, a much smaller proportion indicated that they had performed the procedures. The published literature on surgical repair is sparse and unfamiliar to most surgeons. Barriers to surgical repair of rib and sternal fracture include a lack of expertise among TRS, lack of research of optimal techniques, and a dearth of randomized trials.

▶ Although it is well known that most sternal and rib fractures heal without intervention, this is certainly not universally the case. Many believe that extrapolating from other areas of the body that benefit from open reduction and internal fixation would translate to fractures of the ribs and sternum.

Discussions of rib and sternal fracture repair are often very polarizing topics. The authors sought to better elucidate current opinions by surveying thought leaders in trauma surgery, orthopedics, and thoracic surgery. They created an internet-based survey and obtained email addresses for their targeted audience from their respective societies. Ultimately, they obtained responses from 405 surgeons, with the overwhelming majority being trauma surgeons (238 trauma surgeons, 97 orthopedic surgeons, and 70 thoracic surgeons). A very high percentage of respondents from each surgical group were from level 1 trauma centers as well as academic medical centers. While this represents a sampling of the surgeons, the inequitable distribution of responses may have biased the subsequent findings.

Only 26% of the respondents have participated in a rib fracture repair, with the most common technique being metal plates with bicortical screw fixation. Most respondents (58%) agreed that chest wall defect and lung hernia were appropriate for fixation, although only one-third thought that flail chest was an appropriate indication. As the authors appropriately mention, there are 2 randomized trials that support the use of rib fixation for flail chest.

Sternal fractures were similar in opinion, with most agreeing that nonunion at 6 weeks was an indication for fixation. Almost half of the respondents agreed that acute sternal deformity was an indication for repair. The most common repair methods for sternal fractures included wire fixation and metal plating with bicortical screws.

In both rib and sternal fractures, the differences between specialists' experience were dramatic. In both cases, the thoracic surgeons had far greater experiences than either the trauma or orthopedic surgeons. This difference in experience, coupled with the proportions of surgeons sampled, compounds the selection bias inherent to the survey. However, this does not obviate the lessons to be learned from the responses to the survey. It is clear that there needs to be increased awareness of the techniques, especially for indications supported by randomized trials, such as flail chest. Additionally, these results would suggest an opportunity for increased collaboration and cross-pollination of techniques between surgical superspecialists.

C. T. Klodell, Jr, MD

Diagnosis and Treatment of Deep Pulmonary Laceration With Intrathoracic Hemorrhage From Blunt Trauma
Nishiumi N, Inokuchi S, Oiwa K, et al (Tokai Univ School of Medicine, Isehara, Kanagawa)
Ann Thorac Surg 89:232-239, 2010

Background.—Blunt chest trauma resulting in massive hemothorax requires immediate attention. We investigated the diagnostic and prognostic utility of various clinical factors in patients with deep pulmonary laceration caused by blunt chest trauma with a view toward interventional treatment.

Methods.—We reviewed 42 patients with deep pulmonary laceration resulting from blunt chest trauma who were treated between 1988 and 2008. Various clinical factors were compared between survivors and nonsurvivors.

Results.—Of the 42 patients, 29 (69%) survived. Median (25th, 75th percentile) systolic blood pressure at arrival was 102 (76, 121) mm Hg for survivors and 70 (60, 90) mm Hg for nonsurvivors ($p = 0.015$). The median heart rate at arrival was 107 (98, 120) beats/min for survivors and 130 (120, 140) beats/min for nonsurvivors ($p = 0.014$). Respiratory rate, Glasgow Coma Scale score, and arterial blood gas values did not affect prognosis. Blood loss through the chest tube at insertion was 500 (400, 700) mL for survivors and 700 (500, 1000) mL for nonsurvivors ($p = 0.147$) and within 2 hours of arrival was 850 (590, 1100) mm Hg and 1600 (1400, 2000) mL, respectively ($p < 0.001$). Blood loss during thoracotomy was 1170 (600, 1790) mL and 3500 (2000, 6690), respectively ($p < 0.001$).

Conclusions.—In patients with deep pulmonary laceration, hemorrhagic shock with systolic blood pressure less than 80 mm Hg and heart rate more than 120 beats/min leads to a poor prognosis. Emergency thoracotomy and pulmonary lobectomy should be performed before the intrathoracic hemorrhage reaches 1200 mL.

▶ The authors present a retrospective review of 42 patients with deep pulmonary laceration and intrathoracic hemorrhage resulting from blunt trauma. The authors excluded any patient who required emergency room thoracotomy and those with tracheobronchial or direct vascular injury as a source for hemorrhage. The age range of the studied patients spanned children and adolescents and patients in their seventh decade of life. Although this brings to question whether the absolute numbers they use are as valuable as numbers more accurately indexed to body surface area, they may still serve as a guide and springboard for further thought and investigation.

The results of this study demonstrate that the median systolic blood pressure at arrival was greater in survivors (102 vs 70 mm Hg) and the heart rates lower (107 vs 130 beats per minute). Neither the arterial blood gas values nor the interval between the traumatic event and hospital arrival was statistically significant between survivors and nonsurvivors. Additionally, the time from arrival to thoracotomy was not significantly different between groups.

The median initial blood loss at insertion of the chest tube was lower in survivors (500 vs 700 cc) and the blood loss over the first 2 hours of the chest tube drainage (850 vs 1600 cc). Blood loss during the thoracotomy was also significantly lower for survivors (2250 vs 4000 cc).

Most surgeons rely on the advanced cardiac life support (ACLS) guidelines, which include that patients with traumatic hemorrhagic shock receive a rapid infusion of 2 L Ringer's lactate solution, followed by type O blood when indicated. The authors embrace this strategy but then offer a novel approach thereafter. They do not return the shed blood to the patient from the collection chamber after insertion of the chest tube. If greater than 500 cc of blood is drained with chest tube insertion, the authors favor temporary clamping of the chest tube. A repeat chest X-ray is then used to determine the treatment algorithm. Patients with minimal effusion are unclamped to water seal, while those with persistent effusion are prepared for emergency thoracotomy with the chest tube to remain clamped until that procedure. With the combination of clamping of the chest tube and endobronchial occlusion, the thoracic space tamponades the bleeding while not allowing tension pneumothorax to develop as a consequence of the lung injury.

This differs dramatically from the ACLS guidelines which suggest immediate thoracotomy for 1500 cc of output directly after chest tube insertion, continuing blood loss of 200 cc/hr over 2 to 4 hours, or persistent instability following infusion of blood.

The authors' more aggressive approach, including thoracotomy for patients with early output of 500 cc and persistent effusion or those with 800 cc or more within 2 hours of chest tube insertion, warrants additional thought and consideration. Given the considerations that the amount of blood remaining in the chest is often underestimated on plain chest X-ray as well as the time delay in preparing both the patient and the operating room for thoracotomy, this approach may have significant merit in identifying patients with more severe injuries likely to benefit from earlier intervention. Upon entry into the patient's chest, the hilum of the lung should be controlled either with manual compression or with a large clamp. Small lacerations can be closed directly, while larger lacerations often have enough damage to the underlying lung to necessitate lobectomy.

While the authors' approach is significantly more aggressive than the current ACLS guidelines, I believe it has merit in identifying those patients most likely to benefit from early intervention and as such warrants consideration for incorporation into the practice of all surgeons caring for blunt thoracic injuries.

C. T. Klodell, Jr, MD

Laparoscopic diaphragmatic plication for diaphragmatic paralysis and eventration: An objective evaluation of short-term and midterm results
Groth SS, Rueth NM, Kast T, et al (Univ of Minnesota, Minneapolis; et al)
J Thorac Cardiovasc Surg 139:1452-1456, 2010

Objectives.—We sought to objectively assess our outcomes after laparoscopic diaphragmatic plication for symptomatic hemidiaphragmatic paralysis or eventration using a respiratory quality-of-life questionnaire and pulmonary function tests.

Methods.—We performed a retrospective review of all symptomatic patients with hemidiaphragmatic paralysis or eventration who underwent laparoscopic diaphragmatic plication from March 1, 2005, through August 31, 2008. Patients with primary neuromuscular disorders were excluded from our analysis. We collected St George's Respiratory Questionnaire scores (a respiratory quality-of-life questionnaire) and pulmonary function test results preoperatively and at 1 month and 1 year postoperatively. A 2-sided significance level of .05 was used for all statistical testing.

Results.—During the study period, 25 patients underwent laparoscopic diaphragmatic plication (9 right-sided and 16 left-sided plications); 1 patient required conversion to a thoracotomy. St George's Respiratory Questionnaire total scores (59.3 ± 26.8) improved by more than 20 points on average (a reduction of ≥4 points after an intervention is considered a clinically significant improvement). This improvement was statistically significant at 1 month (36.6 ± 15.9, $P = .001$) and maintained significance at 1 year (30.8 ± 18.8, $P = .009$). Similarly, percent predicted maximum forced inspiratory flow (93.2% ± 34.1%) was significantly improved 1 month after plication (113.9% ± 31.8%, $P = .01$) and maintained significance at 1 year (111.5% ± 30.9%, $P = .02$).

Conclusions.—Our objective evaluation of laparoscopic diaphragmatic plication for hemidiaphragmatic paralysis or eventration demonstrated significant short-term and midterm improvements in respiratory quality of life and pulmonary function test results. This approach represents a potential paradigm shift in the surgical management of hemidiaphragmatic paralysis or eventration.

▶ Diaphragmatic paralysis is commonly seen following spinal cord injuries or phrenic nerve injury. It can also commonly be seen from phrenic nerve injuries following cardiac surgery or thymectomy. In contrast, diaphragmatic eventration is a rare congenital defect in the structure of the muscular portion of the diaphragm.

The traditional approach to these conditions has been plication, either with open thoracotomy or minimally invasive thoracoscopic approach. The authors describe a laparoscopic approach to unilateral diaphragmatic plication used in 25 patients and present their results. There was a single conversion to thoracotomy in 1 patient secondary to dense adhesions. They evaluated the patients with a quality-of-life survey and pulmonary function testing.

The authors used a 4-port laparoscopic technique and a very similar surgical approach to both hemidiaphragms, with the exception of mobilization of the falciform ligament when approaching the right diaphragm.

One of the novel aspects of their approach is the creation of a small hole in the diaphragm to allow some of the CO_2 to pass into the thoracic cavity. They report that this maneuver causes the diaphragm to drop down and facilitate the plication. In cases where either hemodynamic or respiratory compromise was encountered, a small chest tube was placed, which they report did not inhibit their exposure or downward displacement of the diaphragm. The authors further highlight that in some cases they made a 5- to 6-cm incision in the diaphragm to release intrathoracic adhesions and allow for safe plication. They used a freehand sewing technique with large pledgeted sutures.

The results of this series seem to compare well with other series using either thoracotomy or thoracoscopic approaches for plication. The patients in this series demonstrated dramatic improvement in the quality-of-life surveys and in pulmonary function testing.

This technique may offer some advantages over the conventional approaches, which the authors point out in their discussion. There is no need for single lung ventilation with the laparoscopic approach, as well as increased working space and visualization. There may be decreased postoperative pain, especially when compared with thoracotomy. There may be a reduced risk of visceral injury when compared with blind placement of plicating stitches from the chest side of the diaphragm.

This approach may be a valuable tool for the armamentarium of the surgeon asked to plicate an elevated and nonfunctional hemidiaphragm. Careful consideration of thoracoscopic versus laparoscopic approach will need to include consideration of previous abdominal or intrathoracic surgery, as well as other potential concurrent procedures. It may also be prudent when using the abdominal approach in a patient with previous thoracic surgery to routinely incise the diaphragm and inspect the thoracic cavity while inserting the chest tube to avoid inadvertent lung injury.

C. T. Klodell, Jr, MD

The Relationship Between Chest Tube Size and Clinical Outcome in Pleural Infection

Rahman NM, Maskell NA, Davies CWH, et al (Oxford Radcliffe Hosp, Headington, UK; Southmead Hosp, Bristol, UK; Royal Berkshire Hosp, Reading, UK; et al)
Chest 137:536-543, 2010

Background.—The optimal choice of chest tube size for the treatment of pleural infection is unknown, with only small cohort studies reported describing the efficacy and adverse events of different tube sizes.

Methods.—A total of 405 patients with pleural infection were prospectively enrolled into a multicenter study investigating the utility of fibrinolytic therapy. The combined frequency of death and surgery, and secondary outcomes (hospital stay, change in chest radiograph, and lung function at 3 months) were compared in patients receiving chest tubes of differing size (χ^2, t test, and logistic regression analyses as appropriate). Pain was studied in detail in 128 patients.

Results.—There was no significant difference in the frequency with which patients either died or required thoracic surgery in patients receiving chest tubes of varying sizes (< 10F, number dying or needing surgery 21/58 [36%]; size 10-14F, 75/208 [36%]; size 15-20F, 28/70 [40%]; size > 20F, 30/69 [44%]; χ^2trend, 1 degrees of freedom [df] = 1.21, P =.27), nor any difference in any secondary outcome. Pain scores were substantially higher in patients receiving (mainly blunt dissection inserted) larger tubes (< 10F, median pain score 6 [range 4-7]; 10-14F, 5 [4-6]; 15-20F, 6 [5-7]; > 20F, 6 [6-8]; χ^2, 3 df = 10.80, P =.013, Kruskal-Wallis; χ^2trend, 1 df = 6.3, P =.014).

Conclusions.—Smaller, guide-wire-inserted chest tubes cause substantially less pain than blunt-dissection-inserted larger tubes, without any impairment in clinical outcome in the treatment of pleural infection. These results suggest that smaller size tubes may be the initial treatment of choice for pleural infection, and randomized studies are now required.

Trial Registration.—MIST1 trial ISRCTN number: 39138989.

▶ The authors are to be congratulated for undertaking this study drawn from the data of the Multi-center Intrapleural Streptokinase Trial and attempting to dispel the popular thought that only the largest tubes must be used when dealing with complicated pleural space infection. This trial, as originally designed, evaluated the use of fibrinolytic therapy instilled in the chest tube, with hopes of enhancing the efficacy of drainage of the pleural space infection. Many surgeons have been deeply ingrained with the premise that very large tubes (often > 36F) are required to adequately drain complicated pleural space infections. Unfortunately, the majority of patients do not have an interspace large enough to accommodate a tube of that diameter without compression of the intercostal bundles and subsequent intercostal neuralgia. Additionally, it is often concluded that the failure of the initial drainage was due to inadequately sized tube, which subsequently necessitated the surgical drainage of the pleural space.

The authors conclude that the size of the tube has no bearing on outcomes, including death or need for surgery to drain the pleural space. It is also noted that the larger tubes cause much greater patient discomfort. The technique of insertion also plays a role in the comfort of the patient, with the bluntly tunneled tubes causing greater discomfort. Additionally, there was no difference in the frequency of any other adverse events, including the rate at which the tubes were accidentally displaced, between sizes of tubes. We have found that the Thal-Quick (Cook Medical Inc., Bloomington, IN) chest tube is helpful in ensuring proper placement into the fluid collection, reduced patient discomfort, and liberal use of image-guided drainage techniques. Additionally, many would suggest early repeat CT scanning after drainage with further targeted small caliber tube placements to achieve satisfactory drainage of any remaining fluid collections.

This study does support the management of patients with pleural space infections using smaller caliber tubes, which may allow resolution of the process with similar efficacy but with less pain. This is the first prospective study to address this issue and may warrant a follow-up randomized controlled trial.

C. T. Klodell, Jr, MD

Lung Injury Following Thoracoscopic Talc Insufflation: Experience of a Single North American Center

Gonzalez AV, Bezwada V, Beamis JF Jr, et al (McGill Univ Health Centre, Montreal, QC, Canada; Yuma Regional Med Ctr, AZ; Lahey Clinic Med Ctr, Burlington, MA)
Chest 137:1375-1381, 2010

Background.—Thoracoscopic talc insufflation (TTI) has been used to obliterate the pleural space and prevent recurrent pleural effusions or pneumothorax. Reports of acute pneumonitis and ARDS after the use of talc raised concern about its safety. Differences in particle size of various talc preparations may explain the variable occurrence of pneumonitis. We sought to determine the incidence of lung injury after TTI over a 13-year period at our institution.

Methods.—Patients who underwent TTI between January 1994 and July 2007 were identified from a prospectively maintained logbook. The talc used was commercially available sterile talc (Sclerosol). The hospital course was reviewed in detail, and all cases of respiratory insufficiency were examined with regard to onset, suspected cause, and outcome. Talc-related lung injury was defined as the presence of new infiltrates on chest radiograph and increased oxygen requirements, with no other identifiable trigger than talc exposure.

Results.—A total of 138 patients underwent 142 TTIs for recurrent pleural effusions or spontaneous pneumothorax. TTI was performed most frequently for malignant pleural effusions (75.5% of effusions). The median dose of talc was 6 g (range, 2-8 g). Dyspnea with increased oxygen requirements developed within 72 h postprocedure for 12 patients. Four patients (2.8%) had talc-related lung injury, and talc exposure may have contributed to the respiratory deterioration in four additional patients.

Conclusions.—We report the occurrence of lung injury after TTI using the only talc approved by the US Food and Drug Administration. These results reinforce previous concerns regarding the talc used for pleurodesis in North America.

▶ The authors present their single-institution experience over 13 years with thoracoscopic talc insufflation used as a sclerosing agent for pleurodesis. Many agents are used for this purpose, including talc, tetracycline, doxycycline, and bleomycin, but most feel talc is the most economical and efficacious agent. This seems particularly true when the patient has malignant effusions.

There have been scattered reports of pneumonitis and adult respiratory distress syndrome following talc insufflation. Their technique of pleurodesis was both consistent and standardized, with the Food and Drug Administration (FDA)-approved talc, Sclerosol (Byran Corporation, Woburn, MA) being the only agent used. The median talc dose used per procedure was 4 g, with a mean chest tube drainage period of just over 4 days.

They did note an acute lung injury related to talc insufflation of 2.8%, which did not correlate with the total dose of talc received.

Of perhaps greatest interest is the discussion of the different preparations of talc available abroad, when compared with the United States. The talc used abroad tends to be large-particle talc when compared with the talc in the United States. It is thought that the large-particle talc may exceed the size of the pleural stomata and as such not be taken into the circulation. This hypothesis has been corroborated by the autopsy finding of talc crystals in the lung, liver, kidney, heart, and skeletal muscle of a patient who died after insufflation of the smaller particle talc and related acute lung injury published in a different series.

There are currently only 2 small trials comparing the different talc preparations, but these suggested that the smaller talc particles may worsen gas exchange and induce more systemic inflammation. This may warrant further investigation with a larger randomized trial comparing large-particle talc with the current FDA-approved Sclerosol.

C. T. Klodell, Jr, MD

Is Thoracoscopic Decortication Sufficient for the Treatment of Empyema?
Manunga J, Olak J (Kern Med Ctr, Bakersfield, CA)
Am Surg 76:1050-1054, 2010

Before thoracoscopy became popular in the 1990s, thoracotomy and decortication was the treatment of choice for empyema thoracis not responding to tube thoracostomy. An Institutional Review Board-approved, retrospective review of all patients treated for empyema between September 1, 2006, and August 31, 2009, at Kern Medical Center was conducted. A total of 37 patients (male = 33; female = 4) with a mean age of 43.7 years were treated. Empyema developed after community-acquired pneumonia (CAP) in 27, traumatic hemothorax (TH) in nine, and other cause in one. For 34 of 36 patients (91%), a thoracoscopic approach was successful. Two of 36 patients required conversion to thoracotomy, whereas one patient required an initial thoracotomy in each case as a result of tenacious adhesions. Mean duration of the chest tube was 4.1 days in patients with CAP and 4.6 days in patients with TH. Mean length of stay after surgery was 6 days for patients with CAP and 9.1 days for patients with TH. Five of 37 (13.5%) had complications and one patient died (2.7%). Follow-up was complete for 81.1 per cent of patients, none of whom required a subsequent intervention. Compared with the literature, it appears that the conversion rate to thoracotomy, length of chest tube duration, and postoperative length of stay have decreased as experience has increased.

▶ The authors reviewed their experience with thoracic empyema and the use of thoracoscopy as a mechanism to evacuate the loculated effusion. There are many technical tips that make this technique favorable. First, I believe that the insufflation of CO_2 is invaluable. The insufflation pressure should be set to a maximum pressure of 8 to 10 mm Hg so as to not compromise venous return to the heart. This amount of pressure of CO_2 in conjunction with good double-lumen airway control allows the nonadherent lung to be decompressed away from the chest wall and clearly defines the areas of adhesion between the visceral and parietal pleura. The second technical point the authors make is the use of both 0° and 30° thoracoscopes to allow excellent visualization of the entire pleural space. They additionally note copious amounts of irrigation to dilute the degree of contamination of the pleural space. Additionally, they are diligent about checking the re-expansion of the lung while the video camera is still inside the chest. With this technique, they have been successful in removing the chest tubes when drainage is less than a 100 mL per day and has no growth of microorganisms.

Their series is quite respectable with a relatively short duration of chest tube drainage required and a short length of stay. However, it is unclear from the article which patients were converted to chronic empyema tubes and which had their tubes removed.

The advantages of the video-based procedure over traditional thoracotomy include improved visualization of the pleural space, decreased postoperative pain, better cosmesis, and earlier return to work or full function. The only concern I would raise is that their extremely low conversion rate of 5.7% may be related to referral patterns at their institution where they are seeing these patients a little earlier in the disease process. It would certainly seem reasonable to initiate most of these procedures by video thoracoscopic technique and convert to open only when there are dense adhesions related to chronically neglected empyema.

C. T. Klodell, Jr, MD

Should asymptomatic enlarged thymus glands be resected?

Singla S, Litzky LA, Kaiser LR, et al (Univ of Pennsylvania School of Medicine, Philadelphia; The Univ of Texas, Houston; et al)
J Thorac Cardiovasc Surg 140:977-983, 2010

Objective.—Patients frequently have an "enlarged thymus" incidentally identified on imaging. We sought to determine whether thymectomy is appropriate in patients with diffusely enlarged thymus glands.

Methods.—A retrospective review was conducted of patients undergoing thymectomy without myasthenia gravis at 1 institution over 15 years.

Results.—Of 117 patients undergoing thymectomy, 109 patients had complete data. Thirty-six had a gland judged by the surgeon to be diffusely enlarged, and 73 had a discrete mass. Of the 36 diffusely enlarged thymus glands, 18 (50%) occurred in patients with no symptoms referable to the thymus. No patient (0/18; 0%) with an asymptomatic diffusely enlarged thymus gland had a pathologic diagnosis that would have required resection (8 normal; 10 "hyperplasia"). Of the 18 symptomatic patients with diffusely enlarged glands, 4 (22.2%) harbored lymphoma, but none harbored thymoma or other tumor ($P < .05$; symptomatic vs asymptomatic). Of the 73 patients with discrete masses, 45 (61.6%) were symptomatic, and both the symptomatic and asymptomatic patients had a high rate of pathologic diagnoses that represented an indication for resection (53.3% and 42.8%, respectively, harbored thymoma or other tumor). Of the 25 (of 109) patients initially having a diagnosis of thymic hyperplasia, only 3 (12%) had true follicular hyperplasia on re-review of the pathologic condition. Interestingly, an autoimmune disorder developed in 2 (67%) of these 3 patients on long-term follow-up.

Conclusions.—Asymptomatic patients with diffusely enlarged thymus glands can be followed up expectantly because they have a negligible incidence of significant thymic disease; symptomatic patients with diffusely enlarged thymus glands may have lymphoma, so biopsy is appropriate. Half of patients with a discrete mass have tumors requiring resection; imaging advances would be useful to better differentiate among patients within this group.

▶ This article pertains to a clinical difficulty many of us face frequently in the outpatient setting, namely, the incidental discovery of asymptomatic thymic enlargement. The ubiquitous use of CT scanning for a myriad of indications continues to yield relatively high volumes of the enlarged thymic incidentalomas. The onus is then on the surgeon to determine the clinical significance of this finding and coordinate an appropriate follow-up, biopsy, or resection. This study reviews 36 patients with diffusely enlarged thymic glands without discrete lesions. The real basis of this article is the 18 patients with diffusely enlarged thymus glands and no symptoms attributable to thymic pathology. The conclusion of the authors was to demonstrate the appropriateness of serial follow-up rather than biopsy or resection in patients with diffusely enlarged thymus gland but no symptoms. The authors suggest that this subset of patients may be followed with serial CT scanning, and if the mass remained stable for 5 years, follow-up may be terminated. Although the number of patients studied is relatively small, this represents one of the largest experiences to date of this patient subgroup. I believe this article should serve as a springboard to generate interest in a larger scale of evaluation of this patient subset.

One major difficulty with this study is its retrospective nature and that in all patients the glands were resected. The authors draw the conclusion retrospectively that asymptomatic patients with diffuse enlargement of the thymus gland could be managed expectantly. However, the symptoms they report being the most commonly attributable to the thymus, including chest discomfort, shortness of breath, cough, chest fullness, fatigue, and dysphagia, are relatively common when seeing patients in the clinic. I would submit that the proportion of patients deemed asymptomatic is closely related to how diligently one seeks these symptoms. Additionally, considering that the expectant management would require serial radiographic (CT scanning) examination over 5 years, from both a patient convenience and economic standpoint it may be more efficacious to undergo a minimally invasive procedure to remove the gland. I believe this is particularly important, as many find it very difficult to attribute the true symptoms of a patient to the thymus or conversely find patients in their office with no symptoms, as they are frequently nonspecific and unreliable. While I applaud the authors for their contribution to the literature in this area, I believe this study, although important, does not fully elucidate this issue. What would be particularly meaningful would be to better understand how many patients with similar findings were followed without operation during the same time period.

C. T. Klodell, Jr, MD

Video-assisted thoracoscopic bullectomy and talc poudrage for spontaneous pneumothoraces: Effect on short-term lung function

Dubois L, Malthaner RA (The Univ of Western Ontario, London, Ontario, Canada)
J Thorac Cardiovasc Surg 140:1272-1275, 2010

Objective.—We measured lung function before and after video-assisted thoracoscopic apical bullectomy and talc poudrage in patients with spontaneous pneumothoraces.

Methods.—Seventy-two patients were prospectively followed up for 12 months. The indications for surgery were recurrent pneumothoraces (n = 58), bilateral pneumothoraces (n = 8), and persistent air leak (n = 6). There were 46 males and 26 females with mean age of 29 years (range 15−61 years). The results were analyzed using paired *t* tests.

Results.—There were no recurrences. There were 4 complications (5.6%): 1 wound infection, 1 case of pneumonia, and 2 persistent air leaks each lasting 1 week. There were no conversions to open surgery. Preoperative and 6-month pulmonary function test results were available on 41 patients, and 35 patients completed 12-month pulmonary function tests. Twelve-month values (mean percent ± SD) were as follows: Forced expiratory volume in 1 second fell from 95 ± 19 to 89 ± 16 ($P = .02$); forced expiratory volume in 1 second/forced vital capacity ratio was unchanged, 95 ± 12 versus 94 ± 13 ($P = .9$); total lung capacity fell from 106 ± 19 to 98 ± 12 ($P = 0.002$); vital capacity fell from 100 ± 22 to 96 ± 16 ($P = .05$); residual volume fell from 126 ± 32 to 107 ± 29 ($P = .002$); and diffusion capacity for carbon monoxide corrected for alveolar volume was unchanged, 88 ± 15 versus 91 ± 17 ($P = .07$). Flow rates and diffusion capacities were preserved, but lung volumes were slightly reduced at 1 year.

Conclusions.—Video-assisted thoracoscopic apical bullectomy and talc poudrage is an effective treatment for spontaneous pneumothoraces with a low complication rate and recurrence rate and only minor changes in pulmonary function at 1 year.

▶ Primary spontaneous pneumothorax often requires operative treatment including resection of identifiable blebs and obliteration of the pleural space. There are many techniques available for pleural obliteration with various advantages and disadvantages. The most common is probably mechanical pleurodesis with pleural abrasion technique. However, when performed via thoracoscopy, these approaches are associated with a higher recurrence rate than their open counterparts. The authors describe the use of talc using the video-assisted thoracoscopic approach and in such reported a recurrence rate of less than 2%.

Their operative technique includes the use of two 5-mm ports and one 12-mm port through which they inspected for blebs and used the endostapler. Interestingly, even when no bleb or bulla was identified, a minimal apical wedge resection was still performed. They then nebulized 5 g of asbestos-free sterile talc into the pleural space and placed a chest tube. They observed no recurrences at 12 months. The authors admit that critics of the use of talc cite concerns over the potentially negative effect on lung function, its possible carcinogenesis, and the risk of acute respiratory distress syndrome.

While the authors should be commended for their excellent results, I believe that it is critical to notice that their patient cohort had a relatively low mean age of 29 years and a range from 15 to 61 years. I believe that we should be hesitant to perform talc pleurodesis in young patients. While the oncologic risks with the use of asbestos-free talc is essentially zero, there are still many other concerns. It is highly possible that many of these patients will require a second intrapleural procedure for an unrelated issue at some future time point. The added morbidity of reoperative surgery following talc pleurodesis is significant. For those practicing in centers where lung transplants are performed, redoing dissection following talc pleurodesis is dreaded. This dense inflammatory response to talc likely contributes to the high success rate of the described technique but also should give us some pause when considering use of talc in young patients.

C. T. Klodell, Jr, MD

Pre- and Postoperative Management

Impact of Enteral Feeding Protocols on Enteral Nutrition Delivery: Results of a Multicenter Observational Study

Heyland DK, Cahill NE, Dhaliwal R, et al (Queen's Univ, Kingston, Ontario, Canada; Kingston General Hosp, Ontario, Canada; et al)
JPEN J Parenter Enteral Nutr 34:675-684, 2010

Background.—To evaluate the effect of enteral feeding protocols on key indicators of enteral nutrition in the critical care setting.

Methods.—International, prospective, observational, cohort studies conducted in 2007 and 2008 in 269 intensive care units (ICUs) in 28 countries were combined for the purposes of this analysis. The study included 5497 consecutively enrolled, mechanically ventilated, adult patients who stayed in the ICU for at least 3 days. Sites recorded the presence or absence of a feeding protocol operational in their ICU. They provided selected nutritional data on enrolled patients from ICU admission to ICU discharge for a maximum of 12 days. Sites that used a feeding protocol were compared with those that did not.

Results.—On average, protocolized sites used more enteral nutrition (EN) alone (70.4% of patients vs 63.6%, $P = .0036$), started EN earlier (41.2 hours from admission to ICU vs 57.1, $P = .0003$), and used more motility agents in patients with high gastric residual volumes (64.3% of patients vs 49.0%, $P = .0028$) compared with sites that did not use a feeding protocol. Overall nutritional adequacy (61.2% of patients' caloric requirements vs 51.7%, $P = .0003$) and adequacy from EN were higher in protocolized sites compared with nonprotocolized sites (45.4% of requirements vs 34.7%, $P < .0001$). EN adequacy remained significantly higher after adjustment for pertinent patient and ICU level baseline characteristics.

Conclusions.—The presence of an enteral feeding protocol is associated with significant improvements in nutrition practice compared with sites that do not use such a protocol.

▶ It has been firmly established that the presence of a nutritional support team is important to improve the quality and safe use of total parenteral nutrition. A protocol involving the proper use of nutritional support is essential along with the team approach of nurse, pharmacist, and physician. This multi-institutional study evaluated the use of enteral nutrition in intensive care units (ICUs) from institutions with and without nutritional protocols. It is intuitive that better nutritional support would be seen in those institutions with a proper protocol since they would be likely to have some form of a nutritional support team as well. Importantly, nutritional adequacy was achieved to a greater degree in those institutions with a nutritional protocol. It would have been interesting to perform a safety and a cost-benefit analysis regarding the use or nonuse of a nutritional protocol in the care of patients within ICUs.

J. M. Daly, MD

Incidence and Risk Factors of Persistent Air Leak After Major Pulmonary Resection and Use of Chemical Pleurodesis

Liberman M, Muzikansky A, Wright CD, et al (Massachusetts General Hosp, Boston)

Ann Thorac Surg 89:891-898, 2010

Background.—Persistent air leak (PAL; defined as air leak > 5 days) after major pulmonary resection is prevalent and associated with significant morbidity. This study examines an incompletely characterized treatment for the management of PAL, chemical pleurodesis.

Methods.—A retrospective case-control study examining all isolated lobectomies and bilobectomies by thoracotomy was performed. The PALs (1997 to 2006) and controls (2002 to 2006) were identified from a prospective database. Incidence, risk factors, management, and outcome were defined.

Results.—Over 9 years, 78 PALs were identified in 1,393 patients (5.6%). Controls consisted of 700 consecutive patients. Propensity score analysis matching case and controls showed no predictive risk factors for air leak using a logistic regression model. Univariate analysis demonstrated that female gender, smoking history, and forced vital capacity were predictive risk factors. Treatment of PAL consisted of observation (n = 33, 42.3%), pleurodesis (n = 41, 52.6%), Heimlich valve (n = 3, 3.8%), and reoperation (n = 1, 1.3%). Seventy-three patients (93.6%) required no further intervention. One patient required a muscle flap, one readmission for pneumothorax, and one empyema resulting in death. Sclerosis was successful in 40 of 41 patients (97.6%). Mean time to treatment was 8.4 ± 3.6 days, mean duration of air leak was 10.7 ± 4.5, and mean duration of air leak postsclerotherapy was 2.8 ± 2.2 days. Postoperative pneumonia occurred with increased frequency in PAL patients (6 of 45 [13.3%] vs 34 of 700 [4.9%], p = 0.014). PAL was associated with increased length of stay (14.2 vs 7.1 days, p < 0.001) and time with chest tube (11.5 vs 3.4 days, p < 0.001).

Conclusions.—Air leaks remain an important cause of morbidity. Pleurodesis is an effective option in management of PAL after major pulmonary resection.

▶ Persistent air leak following pulmonary resection remains a major problem for surgeons and patients alike. It prolongs the length of stay, occasionally complicates recovery, and serves as a nidus for both surgeon and patient dissatisfaction. The authors present an excellent retrospective review of their large series and detail the use of chemical pleurodesis as therapeutic intervention for air leak. The authors identified an overall low persistent air leak rate of 5.6%, but when leaks were encountered, they were resolved in 97.6% with the use of chemical pleurodesis. When successful, this allows removal of the chest tube and discharge from the hospital, often a more acceptable outcome to the patient when compared with prolonged chest tube drainage with Heimlich valve. The technique used should be closely noted. The sclerosing agent (usually 5 g talc in 50 cc of normal saline) is instilled sterilely via the chest tube, followed by elevation of the Pleurevac flexible tubing for 1 to 2 hours. At no time is the chest tube clamped. Following this time interval, the tube is returned to low suction to allow apposition of the visceral and parietal pleural surfaces, an essential event to allow pleurodesis. The authors present a useful flow diagram that suggests any patient with air leak at 5 days who can safely tolerate a water seal should be considered for chemical pleurodesis. Although not mentioned in the article and only briefly discussed, I find it useful to administer some level of narcotics and anxiolytics to the patients for the initial instillation. Once the initial few minutes have passed, the patients tolerate the procedure well and can actively participate by rolling side to side every 15 minutes to help distribute the sclerosing agent.

C. T. Klodell, Jr, MD

Sutureless pneumostasis using bioabsorbable mesh and glue during major lung resection for cancer: Who are the best candidates?
Ueda K, Tanaka T, Li T-S, et al (Yamaguchi Univ Graduate School of Medicine, Japan)
J Thorac Cardiovasc Surg 139:600-605, 2010

Objective.—Preventing air leaks after major lung resection for cancer is mandatory for successful fast-track surgical intervention. We reported our preliminary results with performance of pneumostasis by combining polyglycolic acid mesh and fibrin glue; however, the advantages of this combination over the conventional method have not been clarified.

Methods.—We controlled air leaks detected during an intraoperative water-seal test by using sutures and fibrin glue before April 2006 and by combining polyglycolic acid mesh and fibrin glue without sutures thereafter. We removed the chest tube the day after the air leaks stopped. For bias reduction in comparison with the 2 historical cohorts, we used the nearest available matching method with the estimated propensity score.

Results.—The durations of chest tube drainage and postoperative hospital stay were significantly shorter in the mesh-and-glue group (n = 61) than in the glue-alone group (n = 61). The incidence of postoperative pulmonary complications was lower in the mesh-and-glue group than in the glue-alone group (0% vs 7%, $P = .042$). According to a stratification analysis, the benefit of combining mesh and glue to reduce the duration of chest tube drainage was limited in patients undergoing upper lobe resection and in patients with severe emphysema undergoing other types of resection.

Conclusion.—Combining bioabsorbable mesh and glue for pneumostasis can reduce the duration of chest tube drainage, postoperative hospital stay, and pulmonary complications after major lung resection for cancer. Patients undergoing upper lobe resection and those with severe emphysema might be the best candidates for this technique.

▶ Air leaks following pulmonary resection remain a difficult and plaguing problem. They mandate the retention of the chest drain with its accompanying discomfort and inconvenience as well as prolong the duration of hospitalization. It is often inconvenient for patient and doctor alike. Many different strategies have been used in an attempt to reduce or eliminate air leaks following resection with variable levels of success. The authors describe a novel technique that uses the combination of polyglycolic acid mesh and fibrin glue and report their results with the technique. Important concepts of their technique include using solution A of the fibrin sealant as a directly applied liquid to the staple line, then applying solution B to create a primary seal. They then soak a piece of the polyglycolic acid mesh in solution A and use it as an onlay patch over the staple line. Finally, solution B is used to adhere the mesh to the staple line. They conclude that the combination of the mesh and the glue were superior to the glue alone. They further conclude that the technique may be particularly useful in patients undergoing upper lobe resection and those with severe emphysema, who in their dataset derived the greatest benefit.

One concern that should be considered is the possible need for reoperative pulmonary resection and the affect of the mesh and glue combination on adhesion formation. The authors make no mention of any patient in whom this technique was used subsequently requiring reoperative resection. This may be a particularly relevant concern when dealing with pulmonary metastatic disease, as this patient subset is particularly prone to need for reentry and reoperative resection.

Overall, this technique seems promising as another viable strategy to help mitigate the deleterious effect of air leaks following pulmonary resection. With the caveat of careful consideration to the potential need for future reoperations, this may be an appropriate technique to consider any time a moderate to large volume of pulmonary parenchyma must be crossed with staplers.

C. T. Klodell, Jr, MD

Pleural Ultrasound Compared With Chest Radiographic Detection of Pneumothorax Resolution After Drainage

Galbois A, Ait-Oufella H, Baudel J-L, et al (Université Pierre et Marie Curie, Paris, France)

Chest 138:648-655, 2010

Background.—Pleural ultrasonography (PU) is more sensitive than chest radiograph (CXR) for diagnosing pneumothorax and could be useful for detecting resolution of pneumothorax after drainage. The aim of this prospective double-blind observational study was to assess PU accuracy during pneumothorax follow-up after drainage.

Methods.—All patients hospitalized with pneumothorax requiring drainage were eligible. After drainage, residual pneumothorax was assessed by CXR and PU (1) 24 h after bubbling in the aspiration device had stopped, (2) 6 h after clamping the pleural catheter, and (3) 6 h after removing the pleural catheter. Pneumothorax indicated by PU but not CXR was confirmed by CT scan or by aspiration of >10 mL of air.

Results.—Forty-four unilateral pneumothoraces were studied (primary spontaneous: 70.5%), and 162 pairs of examinations (CXR and PU) were performed. Twenty residual pneumothoraces were detected by both CXR and PU. Furthermore, PU suspected 14 pneumothoraces that were not identified by CXR; 13 were confirmed. All of these pneumothoraces resulted in therapeutic intervention. Thus, 39% (13/33) of the confirmed residual pneumothoraces were missed by CXR. In patients with primary spontaneous pneumothorax, the positive predictive value of PU for residual pneumothorax diagnosis was 100%; for other pneumothoraces, this value ranged from 90% in the absence of a lung point to 100% when a lung point was observed. PU results were obtained faster than results from CXR (35 ± 34 min vs 71 ± 56 min, $P < .0001$).

Conclusions.—The accuracy of PU is excellent for detecting residual pneumothorax during pneumothorax follow-up after drainage.

▶ The authors present a critical evaluation of a novel approach for the management of pneumothorax following drainage. It represents what may be not only an advance in the way we manage patients after chest tube drainage but also a benefit to patients in reduced radiation exposure, manipulation, and time delay. This technique may offer advantages in that it may detect anterior pneumothorax that are frequently missed by conventional chest radiograph. Bedside ultrasound can be performed in the intensive care unit by relatively briefly trained personnel using routine ultrasound technology. Limitations of this study include use of 8F chest drainage catheters and unknown efficacy of this technique with larger-bore chest tube. The technique relies on 3 signs: the abolition of lung sliding, the A-line sign, and the lung point. It requires the ultrasound probe to be placed perpendicular to the intercostal space and then moved along the anterior axillary line, middle clavicular line, and the outer edge of the scapula. The weaknesses of this technique and study are that it may be a bit oversensitive in that it detected pneumothorax in 39% of patients with a normal chest X-ray. The clinical significance of this otherwise occult pneumothorax is unknown. Additionally, it is unclear if these results are reproducible with a larger chest tubes that are more commonly used. A previous study done on patients with 36F chest tubes demonstrated equivalent results on the first day between chest X-ray and ultrasound.

The pleural ultrasound technique may offer several advantages over conventional chest X-ray in that it is more sensitive for identification of pneumothorax and may allow therapeutic interventions in patients where residual pneumothorax may be particularly deleterious, such as following pleurodesis. This technique may also be beneficial during operations in which we wish to confirm full lung expansion, such as following first rib resection for thoracic outlet syndrome.

C. T. Klodell, Jr, MD

Staging of Non-small Cell Lung Cancer

Decreasing the incidence of prolonged air leak after right upper lobectomy with the anterior fissureless technique
Ng T, Ryder BA, Machan JT, et al (The Warren Alpert Med School of Brown Univ, Providence, RI; Rhode Island Hosp, Providence)
J Thorac Cardiovasc Surg 139:1007-1011, 2010

Objective.—For major pulmonary resections, the incidence of prolonged air leak may be highest after right upper lobectomy. Dissection through an incomplete minor fissure for pulmonary artery exposure may contribute to air leak. We evaluate the efficacy of the anterior fissureless technique in decreasing the incidence of prolonged air leak after right upper lobectomy.

Methods.—Twenty-seven consecutive patients had right upper lobectomy by the classic technique of fissure dissection for pulmonary artery exposure (group A). The next 66 patients had right upper lobectomy by the anterior fissureless technique (group B).

Results.—During the period of group A, we observed a higher incidence of prolonged air leak [22.2% (6/27) vs 6.5% (3/46), $P = .049$] and an increase in hospitalization days (mean 14.8 vs 8.7 days, $P = .021$) after right upper lobectomy as compared with all other lobar resections. Comparing the 2 techniques for right upper lobectomy (group A vs group B), there was no difference in patient characteristics, operative characteristics, morbidity, or mortality. However, there was a difference in the time to air leak cessation (log-rank $P = .002$), incidence of prolonged air leak [22.2% (6/27) vs 7.6% (5/66), $P = .047$], days with chest tube (mean 9.7 vs 6.6 days, $P = .044$), and days in hospital (mean 14.8 vs 8.2 days, $P = .001$) favoring group B. No other factors predicted prolonged air leak after right upper lobectomy.

Conclusions.—The anterior fissureless technique decreases the duration of air leak, incidence of prolonged air leak, days with chest tube, and days in hospital without any noted disadvantages. This technique should be considered when performing right upper lobectomy.

▶ The authors report their findings with a change in practice to an anterior fissureless technique for right upper lobectomy. The anterior fissureless approach has been well described in the past as a method to decrease postoperative air leaks and to facilitate dissection when the fissure is incomplete. This general approach to pulmonary resection that attempts to minimize or entirely avoid any direct dissection through the fissure is essential for all surgeons performing pulmonary resection. This technique is equally applicable to both video-assisted thoracoscopic surgery and open lobectomy. One additional technical pearl to consider is to begin the dissection posteriorly. With careful dissection in the crotch of the bronchus, between the right upper lobe bronchus and the bronchus intermedius, it is possible to cleanly expose the pulmonary artery from behind the fissure. When dissecting in this crotch of the bronchus, there is a constant finding of a lymph node just before the artery. With careful use of cautery, this area can be dissected very cleanly and the lymph node elevated from the artery. The superior segmental artery to the lower lobe is easily seen, and the posterior ascending artery can also often be seen from this view. This additional minute of dissection is time well spent, as the anterior fissureless approach allows for much easier passage of the endostapler. Once the right upper lobe vein is divided (being careful not to injure the right middle lobe vein) and then the anterior pulmonary artery (PA) trunk followed by the posterior ascending artery, the stapler will pass smoothly from anterior to posterior into the space created by the earlier dissection of the bronchial crotch.

The authors also describe their management of the chest tube postoperatively, which includes transition to water seal on postoperative day 1 for all patients with air leak less than or equal to grade 3 and removal of the tube once the air leak has sealed and output is less than 400 mL in a 24-hour period. This evidence-based chest tube management is not yet widespread in all surgeons performing pulmonary resections but is helpful in allowing rapid closure of air leaks and decreasing length of stay.

This general philosophy of avoiding direct dissection through the fissures and parenchyma in attempts to access the PA should be applied in all pulmonary resections, and this technical description to the right upper lobectomy should be seriously considered for all such resections without significant involvement of the fissure with either lymphadenopathy or tumor.

C. T. Klodell, Jr, MD

Limited Resection for the Treatment of Patients With Stage IA Lung Cancer
Wisnivesky JP, Henschke CI, Swanson S, et al (Mount Sinai School of Medicine, NY; New York-Presbyterian Hosp-Weill Cornell Med Ctr; Brigham and Women's Hosp, Boston, MA; et al)
Ann Surg 251:550-554, 2010

Objective.—Lobectomy is the standard of care for stage IA lung cancer. Some small retrospective studies have suggested similar results after limited resection for tumors ≤2 cm in size. The objective of the study was to compare survival after lobectomy and limited resection among Medicare patients with lung cancer.

Methods.—Using the Surveillance, Epidemiology, and End Results registry, linked to Medicare records, we identified 1165 cases of stage I lung cancer ≤2 cm in size that underwent lobectomy or limited resection (segmentectomy or wedge resection). We used logistic regression to determine propensity scores for undergoing limited resection based on the patients' preoperative characteristics. Overall and lung cancer-specific survival of patients treated with lobectomy or limited resection was compared after adjusting for their propensity score.

Results.—Overall, 196 (17%) patients underwent limited resection. For the entire sample, the adjusted hazard ratio for all cause mortality (1.09; 95% confidence interval: 0.85−1.40) or lung cancer-specific death (hazard ratio: 1.39; 95% confidence interval: 0.97−2.01) for patients undergoing limited resection were not significantly different from those having lobectomy. Similarly, we found no significant differences in overall or lung cancer-specific survival for patients treated with limited resection compared with lobectomy when data was analyzed stratifying and matching patients by their propensity scores.

Conclusions.—These results suggest that survival of patients >65 years of age undergoing limited resection or lobectomy for stage IA tumors ≤2 cm appears to be similar. Although these findings should be confirmed in prospective trials, our results suggest that limited resection may be an effective therapeutic alternative for these patients.

▶ In this review, the authors stress that lung cancer is frequently a disease of older adults, with a peak incidence between 65 and 74 years. The current recommendations for anatomic lobectomy in patients with stage IA lung cancer are based on results of a single trial with less than 300 patients. The conclusion of that trial was that the lobectomy group had a lower rate of locoregional recurrence and a trend toward better survival. In this study, a total of 1165 patients were included for analysis; 17% had a limited resection, while 73% had lobectomy. Interestingly, limited resection was more frequently performed among women and in patients with multiple comorbidities and smaller tumors. There were no differences between groups with regard to age, race or ethnicity, marital status, median estimated income, or histologic subtype. Lobectomy was associated with a higher number of lymph nodes sampled. The statistical analysis demonstrated that survival was not significantly different between those with limited resection and lobectomy and that similar results were obtained when lung cancer−specific survival was compared among patients.

Anatomic lobectomy is considered the standard of care for patients with stage IA non−small cell lung cancer. The appropriate role for limited resection for non−small cell lung cancer less than 2 cm in size remains unknown. In this analysis, there were similar survival rates among patients older than 65 years with stage IA lung cancer treated with limited resection or lobectomy. This may certainly warrant a randomized controlled trial, but these data do suggest that more conservative approach may be an acceptable alternative for the surgical treatment of these patients in some circumstances. The study must be interpreted with caution when considering younger individuals, as the risk of death from competing causes is lower; therefore, it's possible that minor increases in probability of lung cancer−related death with limited resection will translate into worst overall survival rates. Additionally, this is a retrospective study, and the allocation of patients for limited resection or lobectomy was not random. A final word of caution is that propensity score methods were used to balance the study groups and control for covariates. However, there are no data about the patient's preoperative lung function involved in that propensity matching this may have allowed selection bias, as patients with limited pulmonary reserve are frequently selected for limited resection. In conclusion, these data suggest that in patients older than 65 years with stage IA lung tumors, limited resection may be an acceptable alternative to lobectomy. However, these findings need to be corroborated by randomized controlled trials. It is essential if one is to apply this limited resection strategy that the lymph node sampling remain consistent with practices during lobectomy to ensure that these patients are being adequately staged and that the data available for future review yield correct conclusions.

C. T. Klodell, Jr, MD

Mediastinoscopy in Patients With Lung Cancer and Negative Endobronchial Ultrasound Guided Needle Aspiration
Defranchi SA, Edell ES, Daniels CE, et al (Mayo Clinic, Rochester, MN)
Ann Thorac Surg 90:1753-1758, 2010

Background.—Endobronchial ultrasound with transbronchial needle aspiration (EBUS-TBNA) has been proposed as a safe, less-invasive alternative to mediastinoscopy to stage mediastinal lymph nodes in patients with lung cancer. We evaluated the negative predictive value of EBUS-TBNA in lung cancer patients suspected of having N2 nodal metastases.

Methods.—This study is a single-institution retrospective review of cases with suspected or confirmed lung cancer undergoing mediastinoscopy after a negative EBUS-TBNA between June 2006 and February 2008.

Results.—A total of 494 patients underwent EBUS-TBNA during the study period. Twenty-nine patients with suspected or confirmed lung cancer had a negative EBUS-TBNA and underwent subsequent mediastinoscopy. Mediastinoscopy was performed for findings suspicious of N2 disease based on noninvasive imaging. Mediastinoscopy found metastatic nodes in eight of 29 patients (28%) for a patient-specific negative predictive value of EBUS-TBNA of 72% (95% CI, 56% to 89%). Mediastinal lymph node dissection found four further patients with positive N2 nodes (19%). The EBUS-TBNA and mediastinoscopy sampled the same lymph node station on 36 occasions in the 29 patients. The average lymph node size was 10 mm. Mediastinoscopy was positive in 5 of 36 stations, for a nodal-specific negative predictive value of EBUS-TBNA of 86% (95% CI, 75% to 97%).

Conclusions.—Endobronchial ultrasound with transbronchial needle aspiration can effectively sample mediastinal lymph node stations in patients with lung cancer. However, in this early experience, 28% of patients with high clinical suspicion of nodal disease had N2 mediastinal nodal metastases confirmed by mediastinoscopy despite negative EBUS-TBNA.

▶ The authors sought to evaluate the negative predictive value of endobronchial ultrasound (EBUS)—guided transbronchial needle biopsy in patients suspected of having N2 nodal metastasis. They selected patients with a high level of suspicion of N2 nodal involvement and subjected them to EBUS-guided needle biopsy and then followed with surgical mediastinoscopy. The authors report on 29 patients who had suspected or confirmed lung cancer and a negative EBUS-guided biopsy but still high clinical suspicion based on CT or positron emission tomography (PET) scan positivity. They defined radiographic suspicion as a lymph node of more than 1 cm in its minor axis on CT scan or PET positive. Their technique of mediastinoscopy was fairly routine, although the article does not specify whether this was the newer video mediastinoscopy technique. Interestingly, even in patients who had both negative EBUS biopsy and mediastinoscopy, there were still 4 of 21 patients at the time of lobectomy and mediastinal lymph node dissection who were found to have positive N2 nodal disease.

Many have steadily moved from the use of mediastinoscopy and toward the increased use of EBUS-guided transbronchial needle biopsy for staging the N2 nodal stations in patients with enlarged mediastinal lymph nodes. This practice is often based on a perception that mediastinoscopy is an invasive procedure, requires general anesthesia, and carries a small but measurable risk of potentially significant complications. It is important for us to remember that mediastinoscopy does offer the ability to sample tissue from all pretracheal lymph nodes and the subcarinal space under direct vision. Furthermore, this study serves to reinforce the fact that patients with radiographic evidence of N2 nodal metastasis and a negative EBUS should probably still be offered surgical video mediastinoscopy for definitive staging of mediastinum and consideration of subsequent neoadjuvant chemoradiotherapy if they are found to have N2 nodal disease preoperatively.

C. T. Klodell, Jr, MD

Video-Assisted Mediastinoscopy Compared With Conventional Mediastinoscopy: Are We Doing Better?

Anraku M, Miyata R, Compeau C, et al (Univ of Toronto, Ontario, Canada)
Ann Thorac Surg 89:1577-1581, 2010

Background.—Conventional mediastinoscopy (CM) is recently being replaced by video-assisted mediastinoscopy (VAM), with potentially better yield and better safety profile for VAM.

Methods.—All 645 mediastinoscopies (505 CM, 140 VAM) performed between May 2004 and May 2008 were reviewed. Numbers of stations biopsied, total number of lymph nodes dissected, pathology results, and complications were recorded. Patients were divided into two groups: staging for lung cancer group (n = 500) and diagnostic group (n = 145). The staging group was further analyzed, using 304 patients who eventually underwent thoracotomy to evaluate accuracy and negative predictive value of mediastinoscopy, comparing between the two methods (233 CM, 71 VAM).

Results.—Average age was 65 years (range, 26 to 91), and 382 were male. There was no mortality. Eight complications (1.2%) occurred, more in the VAM group (3.8%) than in the CM group (0.8%; $p = 0.04$). The total number of dissected nodes was higher in the VAM group than in the CM group (7.0 ± 3.2 versus 5.0 ± 2.8, $p < 0.001$), and so was the number of stations sampled (3.6 versus 2.6, $p < 0.01$). Sensitivity was higher for VAM (95% versus 92.2%, $p =$ not significant), and so was the negative predictive value (98.6% versus 95.7%, $p =$ not significant). Most false negative biopsies (8 of 11, 73 %) occurred in station 7.

Conclusions.—Both methods are safe. More lymph nodes and stations were evaluated by VAM, with trend toward higher negative predictive value. The higher rate of minor complications seen with VAM might be related to a more aggressive and thorough dissection.

▶ This article compares the video-assisted versus conventional mediastinoscopy approaches. The authors present a well-done study in which they review 505 patients who underwent conventional mediastinoscopy and compare with 140 patients who underwent video-assisted mediastinoscopy approaches. Using the numbers of lymph nodes biopsied, the total numbers that were dissected, and pathology results compared, they ultimately conclude that more lymph nodes were able to be evaluated more safely with video-assisted approach. This is a critical time for an article such as this to be published in that we are currently in a state of flux between the use of endobronchial ultrasound and more traditional mediastinoscopy for staging of the N2 nodal basins. I believe this article is of particular interest and importance to those practicing in teaching institutions. Although conventional mediastinoscopy is quite safe in experienced hands, the use of the video-assisted mediastinoscopy yields not only better visualization and illumination but also magnification. This allows much more detailed and possibly safer dissection. With the video-assisted technique, the anatomic structures are viewed on a magnified video screen as opposed to down the shaft of the mediastinum scope, which makes structures easier to identify. Additionally, for those practicing in teaching institutions, the comfort provided to the attending physician from the complete visualization of all the trainee is doing is immeasurable. Additionally, during times of difficult dissection when the attending physician is operating, all that is being done is on the video screen, again enhancing the learning opportunities for all. The use of video-assisted mediastinoscopy should and will replace conventional mediastinoscopy for essentially all indications.

C. T. Klodell, Jr, MD

Article Index

Chapter 1: General Considerations

Chapter 2: Trauma

Chapter 3: Burns

Chapter 4: Critical Care

Chapter 5: Transplantation

Chapter 6: Surgical Infection

Chapter 7: Endocrine

Chapter 8: Nutrition

Chapter 9: Wound Healing

Chapter 10: Gastrointestinal

Chapter 11: Oncology

Chapter 12: Vascular Surgery

Chapter 13: General Thoracic Surgery

Author Index

417

Pr
CPI Group (UK) Ltd, Croydon, CR0 4YY
08/05/2025
1864678-0011